Osteoporosis in Orthopedics

Yoichi Shimada • Naohisa Miyakoshi
Editors

Osteoporosis in Orthopedics

Assessment and Therapeutic Options

Springer

Editors
Yoichi Shimada
Department of Orthopedic Surgery
Akita University Graduate School of Medicine
Akita, Japan

Naohisa Miyakoshi
Department of Orthopedic Surgery
Akita University Graduate School of Medicine
Akita, Japan

ISBN 978-4-431-55777-7 ISBN 978-4-431-55778-4 (eBook)
DOI 10.1007/978-4-431-55778-4

Library of Congress Control Number: 2015951965

Springer Tokyo Heidelberg New York Dordrecht London

Printed on acid-free paper

Springer Japan KK is part of Springer Science+Business Media (www.springer.com)

Preface

Osteoporosis, a skeletal disorder characterized by low bone mass and compromised bone strength resulting in increased bone fragility and susceptibility to fracture, is a major public health concern in aged societies around the world. Pharmacotherapy with antiosteoporotic agents is an essential treatment for osteoporosis as a "metabolic" bone disease. However, because its pathophysiology is multifactorial and the clinical features are varied, we have to reconsider this disease from many aspects. In this book, we have focused on recent interest regarding assessments and therapeutic options of osteoporosis from the point of view of orthopedics.

The contributors of this book's chapters are today's frontrunners in the research fields of osteoporosis who are publishing high-quality articles. They are all Japanese orthopedic surgeons who have been conducting studies from basic research to specific orthopedic surgeries. In Japan, orthopedic surgeons usually treat osteoporotic patients via a variety of strategies including pharmacotherapy, surgery, and exercise. The authors' comprehensive expertise in both mineral metabolism and orthopedics has contributed to excellent progress in the research fields of osteoporosis worldwide.

The first part of this book mainly discusses basic research and assessment tools. This part includes in vivo and in vitro studies showing the importance of mechanical stimulation on bone, mechanisms of osteoporosis-related bone pain, collagen cross-links as a determinant of bone quality, and hip structure analysis and finite element analysis as new assessment tools for osteoporosis. The second part of the book then discusses clinical factors affecting the conditions of osteoporosis and osteoporosis-related fractures. The importance of the changes in the geometry of the lower extremities for atypical femoral fractures and the relationship of osteoporosis to other age-related conditions including spondylosis and sarcopenia are explained in monographs.

The third part of this book focuses on new clinical applications of antiosteoporotic agents. Although numerous lines of evidence have shown the effectiveness of the antiosteoporotic agents particularly on bone mineral density, some agents have a possibility of being used for other specific effects. This part thus focuses on the extraskeletal effects of vitamin D and the bone-healing ability of teriparatide after fractures and osteosynthetic surgeries. The last part of the book discusses exercise and osteoporosis. In addition to pharmacotherapy, management of physical conditions by exercise is also very important for preventing fractures and maintaining the quality of life in patients with osteoporosis.

This book aims to provide a comprehensive understanding of osteoporosis, which has multifactorial pathophysiology and requires multifaceted countermeasures. Clinicians, researchers, medical students, and staff who are curious about osteoporosis will learn of new trends in assessments and treatment options. The book will also be attractive to orthopedic and spine surgeons who need extensive knowledge of osteoporosis and mineral metabolism for their patients' care. We hope that this book will serve as an important source of information for readers in many specialties treating osteoporosis.

We thank the outstanding authors who contributed to this book for their time and effort. We are also grateful to Springer Japan for the opportunity to share this knowledge with others.

Akita, Japan

Naohisa Miyakoshi
Yoichi Shimada

Contents

Part I
Basic Research and Assessments

Chapter 1
Skeletal Adaptation to Mechanical Strain: A Key Role in Osteoporosis

Toshihiro Sugiyama, Yoon Taek Kim, and Hiromi Oda

Abstract Wolff's law indicates that mechanical loading plays a central role in controlling skeletal strength, as evidenced by marked bone gain in the dominant arms of professional tennis players or rapid bone loss in the weight-bearing sites of astronauts during space flight. Among various experimental methods of mechanical stimulation, the noninvasive axial loading model of the mouse tibia/fibula is useful to assess both cortical and trabecular compartments in vivo. The bone normally responds to local mechanical environment at each skeletal site to maintain resultant "elastic" deformation (strain), and this mechanical strain-related feedback control, known as the mechanostat, acts continuously throughout the physiologic range as recently shown in humans as well as animals. The response of the bone to mechanical loads would be impaired with aging but can be enhanced by intermittent treatment with parathyroid hormone. Increased bone strength by an osteoporosis drug results in decreased bone strain, suggesting that the effect of osteoporosis therapy is limited by skeletal adaptation to mechanical strain, which confirms the attractive efficacy of alternative drugs of mechanical strain-related stimulus such as anti-sclerostin antibodies. In contrast, although lower bone quality is linked to weaker bone strength, the mechanostat could compensate mineral-related, but not collagen-related, impairment of bone quality. Bone mechanobiology is important toward a cure for osteoporosis.

Keywords Wolff's law • Mechanical loading • Mechanostat • Mechanical strain • Bone quality

1.1 Introduction

German orthopedic surgeon, Julius Wolff, essentially established the concept of skeletal adaptation to mechanical environment, known as Wolff's law, in the nineteenth century [1–3]. Harold Frost developed this law in the 1960s and

---

T. Sugiyama (✉) • Y.T. Kim • H. Oda
Department of Orthopaedic Surgery, Saitama Medical University, 38 Morohongo, Moroyama, Saitama 350-0495, Japan
e-mail: tsugiym@saitama-med.ac.jp

Y. Shimada, N. Miyakoshi (eds.), *Osteoporosis in Orthopedics*,
DOI 10.1007/978-4-431-55778-4_1

suggested that the skeleton adapts to mechanical stimulation through control of bone strength by resultant "elastic" deformation (strain) of the tissue, and the mechanical strain-related feedback control has been called the mechanostat [4]. Quantifying mechanical strain on bone surfaces during locomotion by gauges was introduced by Lance Lanyon, also in the 1960s; their experiments in various living animals, including humans, demonstrated the uniformity in peak strain magnitudes and maximum strain rates experienced [5]. Consequently, mechanical strain plays a central role in controlling skeletal strength; for example, increased bone strain in the dominant arms of professional tennis players can induce marked bone gain, while decreased bone strain at the weight-bearing sites of astronauts during space flight would cause rapid bone loss.

Lanyon and colleagues mostly established the fundamental rules about how mechanical strain stimulates the bone [5]. For example, (1) bone formation induced by mechanical loading positively correlates with the peak strain magnitude [6, 7]; (2) the rate of change of strain magnitude is another critical determinant [8, 9] and the bone responds to dynamic, but not static, mechanical loading [10, 11]; (3) the number of cycles of mechanical loading required to maximally stimulate bone formation is surprisingly small [12, 13]; (4) novel, unusual direction of mechanical loading results in higher mechanical strain-related stimulus [7, 12]; and (5) mechanical loading stimulates bone formation independently of bone resorption [14, 15]. In addition, rest interruption between mechanical loading cycles restores the mechanosensitivity of the bone [16, 17].

Osteoporosis is associated with fragility fractures, especially in older women, which could result in significant morbidity and mortality, and its major causes include menopause and aging. It has been generally reported that aging would impair skeletal response to mechanical strain [18–20]. In addition, although the mechanosensitivity of the bone might not be diminished early after ovariectomy-induced estrogen deficiency [21–23], accumulating evidence has consistently shown the involvement of the receptors of estrogen [23–25]. Here we introduce the noninvasive axial loading model of the mouse tibia/fibula to assess both cortical and trabecular compartments in vivo and discuss the mechanostat from a clinical point of view.

1.2 The Axial Loading Model of the Mouse Tibia/Fibula

There are a number of experimental models to study the adaptation of the bone to mechanical loading in vivo [5]. Early experiments in animals such as rabbits [10], sheep [8], turkeys [11], and rats [7, 26, 27] have been followed by those in mice [28–36]. Among these, the noninvasive axial loading model of the mouse tibia/fibula that enables to assess both cortical and trabecular compartments [32, 33, 36] is especially useful. Skeletally mature female C57BL/6 mice can be generally selected for experiments relating to osteoporosis [20, 22, 36–44], because this mouse strain has been extensively used as the background of genetically modified animals in the field of bone research and also shows a good response to mechanical loading [45]. It is important to note that there were several modifications of the original loading regimen [32, 37, 38, 41]; for example, a lower strain rate and a higher static preload could be associated with a loss of trabecular bone in the proximal tibia. Although one possible disadvantage to use rodents such as the rat and mouse in osteoporosis research is that intracortical bone remodeling only occurs at very low levels, this point would have less influence because mechanical loading stimulates bone modeling independently of bone resorption [14, 15].

In vitro experimental approaches are also essential to elucidate the mechanisms by which the bone responds to mechanical stimuli; fluid flow are generally used in osteocytic cells as this would be a natural stimulus within a canalicular network, while mechanical strain can be directly applied in osteoblastic cells because these cells are located on bone surfaces [46–48]. Regardless of the methods, however, it is not easy to replicate the situation of skeletal loading, and findings in vitro should be always investigated in vivo; for example, the inconsistency has been reported in association with cyclooxygenase-2 [43, 49], focal adhesion kinase [50], and connexin 43 [51].

1.2.1 Examples of Experimental Findings

1.2.1.1 Continuous Response

It has been generally believed that the mechanostat includes an adapted state called lazy zone where the strength of the bone remains constant over a wide range of peak strain magnitudes [4]. An experiment was performed to test this hypothesis [41]. In brief, skeletally mature female C57BL/6 mice were right sciatic neurectomized to minimize natural loading in their right tibiae, and these tibiae were subjected to external axial loading (40 10-s rest-interrupted cycles) on alternate days for 2 weeks from the fifth day, with a peak dynamic load magnitude ranging from 0 to 14 N (peak strain magnitude: 0–5000 με) and a constant loading rate of 500 N/s (maximum strain rate: 75,000 με/s) (Fig. 1.1). High-resolution micro-computed tomography (μCT) was used to quantify variables of three-dimensional cortical and trabecular bone structure at precisely comparable sites of the loaded and contralateral control limbs. As a result, multilevel regression analysis showed the continuously positive relationship between mechanical loading/strain and bone mass/strength without the lazy zone (Fig. 1.2).

Notably, the above continuous response in the mechanostat is consistent with the results in humans [52] as well as other experimental models [6, 53, 54]. This is entirely compatible with studies in which bones under normal physical activity are additionally subjected to mechanical loading [20, 55, 56] showing osteogenic responses only above certain levels of peak strain magnitude, because artificial (external) loading would stimulate the bone only when this stimulus exceeds that already derived from natural (internal) loading.

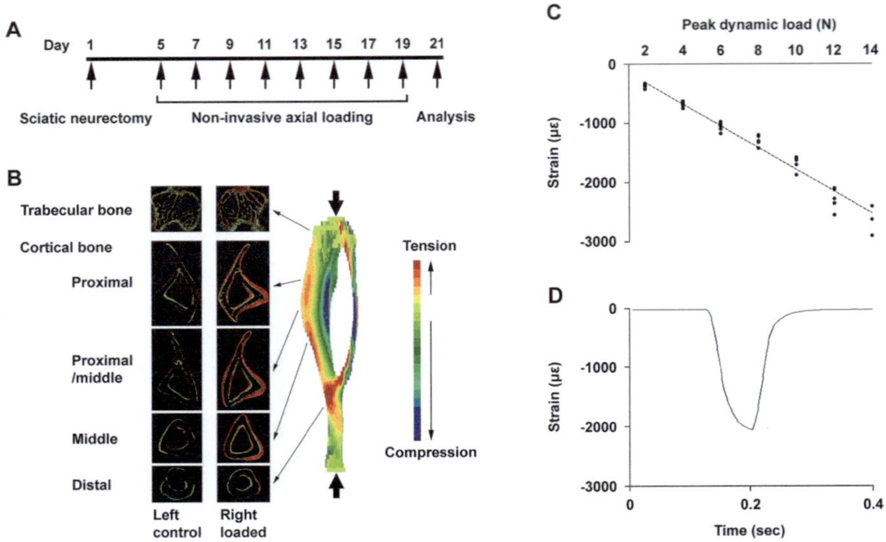

Fig. 1.1 The mouse noninvasive tibia axial loading model. (**a**) Overview of the experimental design. (**b**) Loading-related osteogenesis labeled by calcein green on the first day of loading and alizarin red on the last day of loading and loading-induced strain distribution by finite element analysis. (**c**) Relationship between peak dynamic load and strain on the center of the lateral surface in the right proximal/middle tibiae, where predominant osteogenesis can be induced, in 17-week-old mice with right sciatic neurectomy. (**d**) Representative strain recording, induced by a peak dynamic load of 12 N, on the center of the lateral surface in the right proximal/middle tibiae of 17-week-old mice with right sciatic neurectomy (Adapted from Sugiyama et al. [41])

1.2.1.2 Local Control

Most in vivo experiments of external mechanical loading use animals in which artificial loads are applied to the bones on one side, and the osteogenic responses in the loaded bones have been generally compared with those in the non-loaded contralateral pair. For this approach to be valid, it is essential that the adaptive response of the loaded bones is confined to those bones and does not influence their contralateral controls. However, this assumption has been challenged by recent reports showing the systemic effects of mechanical loading [57–59].

This possibility was investigated [38]. In brief, skeletally mature female C57BL/6 mice were randomly assigned to one of the following three groups; all groups were treated with isoflurane anesthesia three times a week for 2 weeks (approximately 7 min/day). During each anesthetic period, the right tibiae/fibulae in the DYNAMIC + STATIC group were subjected to dynamic loading superimposed upon a static preload to hold the bones. The right tibiae/fibulae in the STATIC group received the static preload alone, while the NOLOAD group received no artificial loading. Bilateral tibiae, fibulae, femora, ulnae, and radii were analyzed by high-resolution μCT and histomorphometry. As a result, the adaptive response in both cortical and trabecular regions of the bones subjected to dynamic loading, even

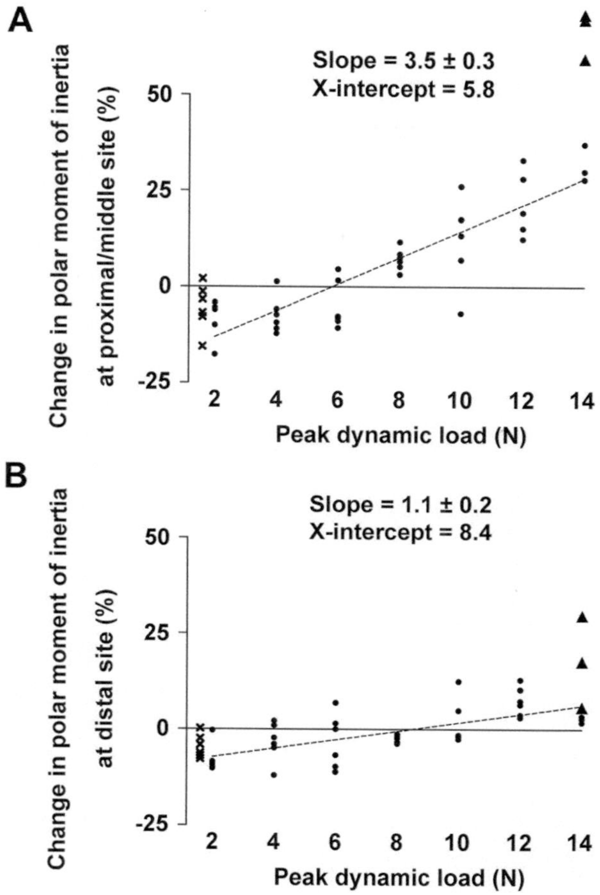

Fig. 1.2 Relationship between peak dynamic load and the change ([*right–left*]/*left*) in polar moment of inertia (J), a parameter of structural bone strength, in the tibiae of 20-week-old mice that received right sciatic neurectomy and axial loading in the right tibia. (**a**) Proximal/middle site. (**b**) Distal site. Best-fit and SE values of slope and best-fit values of x-intercept are shown. ● = mice with no apparent woven bone formation, **X** = mice without external dynamic loading, ▲ = mice with apparent woven bone formation. Note that **X** ($n = 6$) and ▲ ($n = 3$) were excluded for the multilevel regression analyses (Adapted from Sugiyama et al. [41])

when this response was sufficiently vigorous to stimulate woven bone formation, was confined to the loaded bones and did not involve changes in other bones that are adjacent, contralateral, or remote to them (Figs. 1.3 and 1.4).

The above local control in the mechanostat has been confirmed by recent studies [60, 61]. In contrast, the systemic effects of mechanical loading [57–59] might be associated with the loading regimen [38]. Nevertheless, the protocol of mechanical loading should be designed to produce a realistic physiological stimulus capable of stimulating a measurable osteogenic response while avoiding collateral stimulation associated with trauma and interference with blood supply both within the bone and around the loading cups. It is therefore important to note that any loading protocol using the contralateral non-loaded bone as a control can be accepted only after validation of the local control.

1.2.1.3 Osteoporosis Drugs

Parathyroid Hormone

Several in vivo experiments of external loading in rats have shown that intermittent treatment with parathyroid hormone (iPTH) and high-magnitude loading synergistically increase bone formation [62–65]. Although high-impact exercise to increase bone strength would be difficult for older patients with skeletal fragility, iPTH could reduce the loading level necessary to stimulate a loading-related anabolic effect.

An experiment was performed to investigate this concept [37]. In brief, female C57BL/6 mice from 13 to 19 weeks of age were given daily injections of vehicle or iPTH (1–34) at low (20 μg/kg/day), medium (40 μg/kg/day), or high (80 μg/kg/day) dose. For three alternate days per week during the last 2 weeks of this treatment, the tibiae and ulnae on one side were subjected to dynamic axial loading. Two levels of peak load magnitude, one sufficient to engender an osteogenic response and the other insufficient to do so, were applied. The whole tibiae and ulnae were analyzed by high-resolution μCT and histomorphometry. As a result, in the tibia, loading at a level sufficient by itself to stimulate osteogenesis produced an osteogenic response in the low-dose iPTH (1–34)-treated trabecular bone and in the proximal and middle cortical bone treated with all doses of iPTH (1–34). In the ulna, loading at a level that did not by itself stimulate osteogenesis was osteogenic at the distal site when combined with high-dose iPTH (1–34). At both levels of loading, there were synergistic effects in cortical bone volume of the proximal tibia and distal ulna between loading and high-dose iPTH (1–34) (Fig. 1.5). Images of fluorescently labeled bones confirmed that such synergism resulted from increases in both endosteal and periosteal bone formation. No woven bone was induced by iPTH (1–34) or either level of loading alone, whereas the combination of iPTH (1–34) and the sufficient level of loading stimulated woven bone formation on endosteal and periosteal surfaces of the proximal cortex in the tibiae. Consistent with these experimental data, daily treatment with teriparatide could synergistically produce bone gain with physiological levels of mechanical loading in humans [66].

Bisphosphonate

The combination effects of bisphosphonates and mechanical loading were studied in a variety of external loading models in rodents. As mentioned earlier, mechanical loading can stimulate bone formation independently of bone resorption [14], and pamidronate did not change osteogenesis caused by loading in the rat tail [15]. Similarly, alendronate, risedronate, and zoledronic acid at clinical doses did not influence periosteal expansion induced by loading in the rat ulna [67]. In contrast, the response of the cortical bone to loading was impaired by zoledronic acid in the

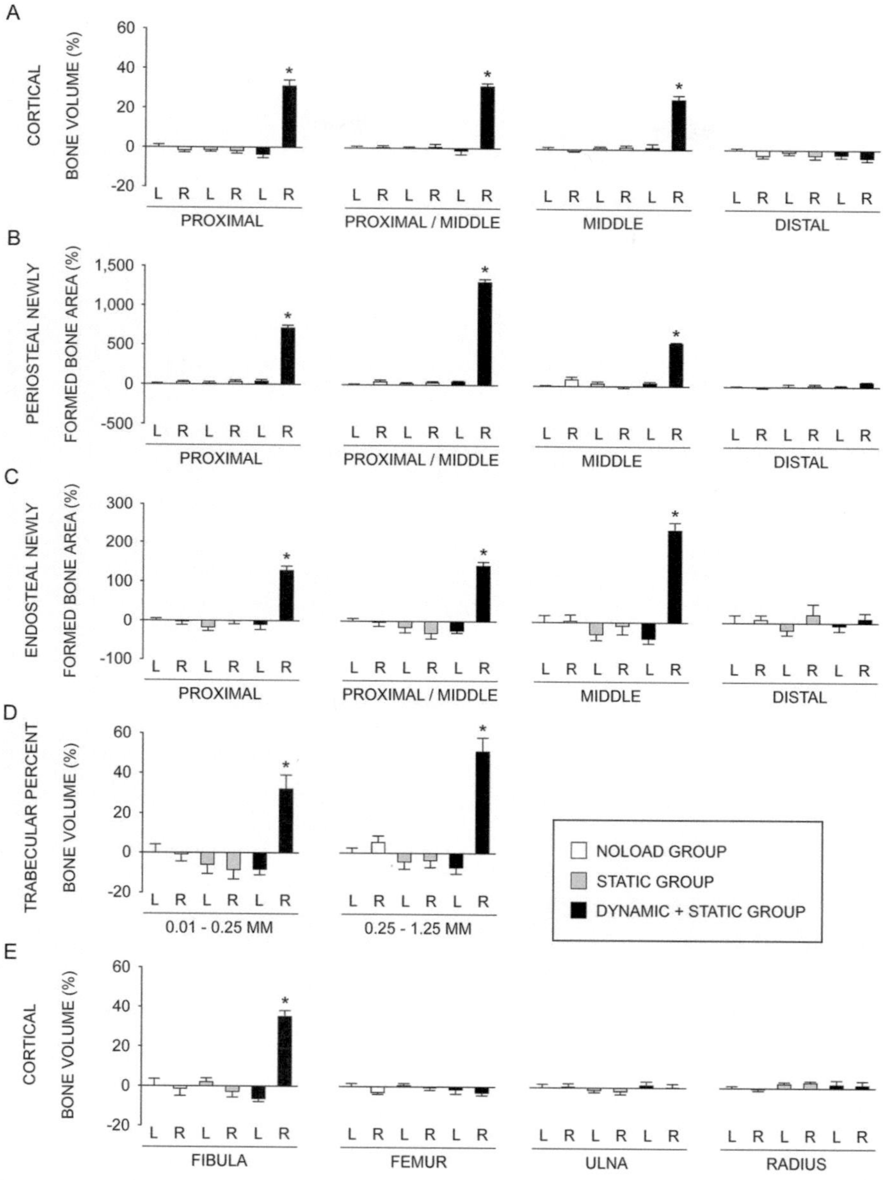

Fig. 1.3 Relative values, analyzed by μCT and histomorphometry, of the *left* and *right* bones in the NOLOAD, STATIC, and DYNAMIC + STATIC groups compared to the left bones in the NOLOAD group. *L* left, *R* right. (**a**) Cortical bone volume analyzed by μCT at the proximal (25 % of the bone's length from its proximal end), proximal/middle (37 %), middle (50 %), and distal (75 %) sites of the tibia. (**b**) Periosteal labels and inter-label bone area, analyzed by histomorphometry, normalized by total cortical bone area at the proximal, proximal/middle, middle, and distal sites of the tibia. (**c**) Endosteal labels and inter-label bone area, analyzed by histomorphometry, normalized by total cortical bone area at the proximal, proximal/middle, middle, and distal sites of the tibia. (**d**) Trabecular percent bone volume analyzed by μCT at two sites 0.01–

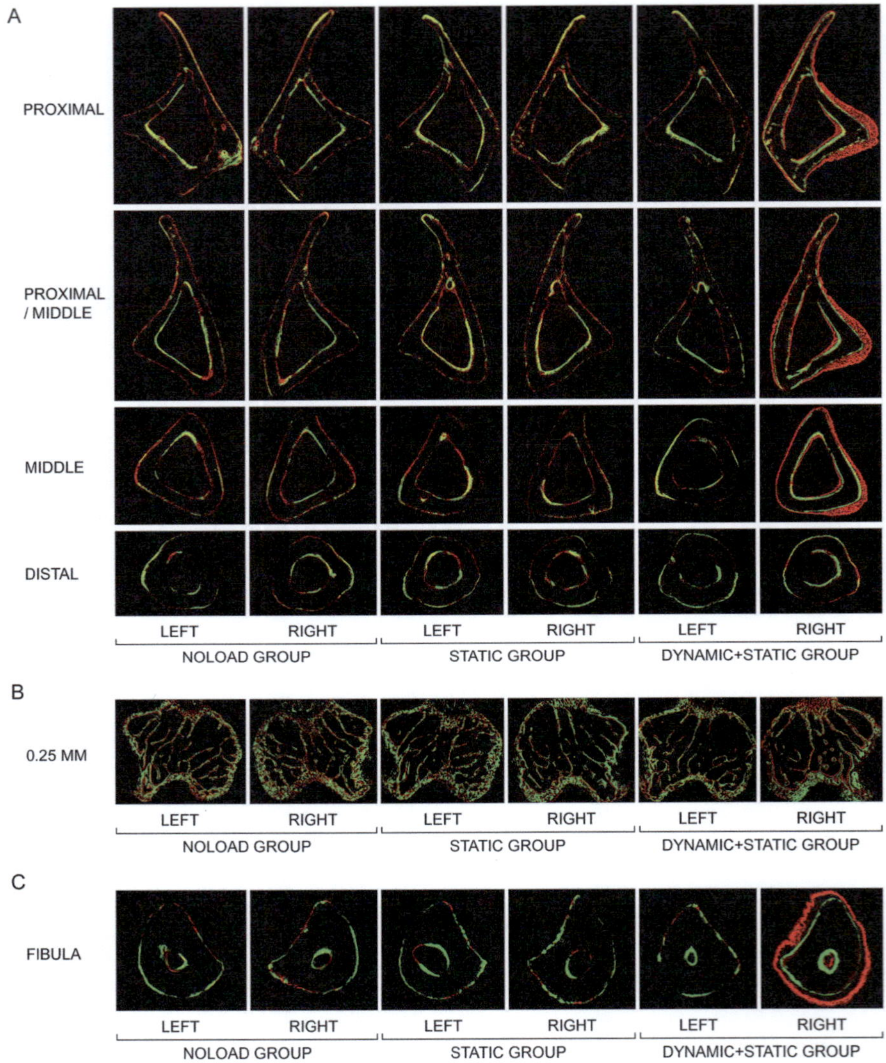

Fig. 1.4 Representative transverse fluorochrome-labeled images. (**a**) Cortical bone at the proximal (25 % of the bone's length from its proximal end), proximal/middle (37 %), middle (50 %), and distal (75 %) sites of the tibia. (**b**) Trabecular bone at the site 0.25 mm distal to the growth plate in the proximal tibia. (**c**) Cortical bone at the middle (50 %) site of the fibula. *Green*: calcein label injected on the first day of loading (day 1). *Red*: alizarin label injected on the last day of loading (day 12) (Adapted from Sugiyama et al. [38])

Fig. 1.3 (continued) 0.25 mm (containing primary spongiosa) and 0.25–1.25 mm (secondary spongiosa) distal to the growth plate in the proximal tibia. (**e**) Cortical bone volume analyzed by μCT at the middle (50 %) site of the fibula, femur, ulna, and radius. Data are the mean ± SE ($n = 6$–7). *$P < 0.05$ versus all other five values by one-way ANOVA followed by a post hoc Bonferroni or Dunnett's T3 test (Adapted from Sugiyama et al. [38])

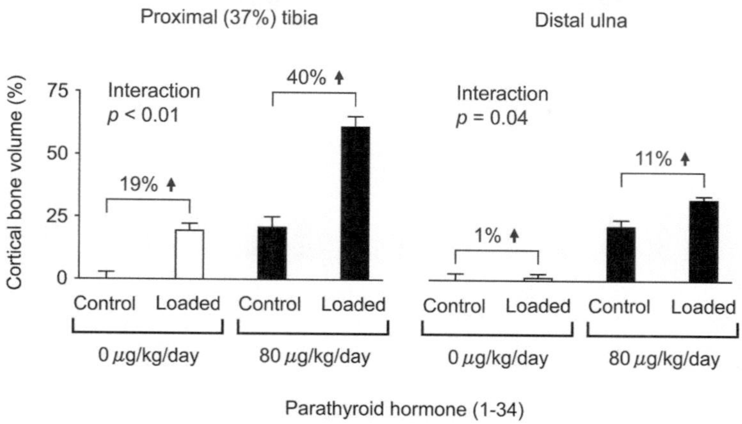

Fig. 1.5 Relative effect of 6 weeks of high-dose iPTH (1–34) and 2 weeks of mechanical loading alone or in combination on cortical bone volume at the proximal (37 %) tibia and distal ulna in 19-week-old female C57BL/6 mice. Levels of peak load: sufficient to engender an osteogenic response in the tibia and insufficient to do so in the ulna. Mean ± SE ($n = 5$–8). Interaction between high-dose iPTH (1–34) and mechanical loading by two-way ANOVA (Adapted from Sugiyama et al. [37])

mouse tibia [68] and minodronate at higher doses but not the optimal dose for osteoporosis treatment in the rat tibia [69].

An experiment was performed to assess the separate and combined effects of risedronate and mechanical loading on the trabecular and cortical bone [39]. In brief, 17-week-old female C57BL/6 mice were given daily subcutaneous injections of vehicle or risedronate at a dose of 0.15, 1.5, 15, or 150 μg/kg/day for 17 days. From the fourth day of treatment, the right tibiae were subjected to mechanical loading for three alternate days per week for 2 weeks. Trabecular and cortical sites in the tibiae were analyzed by high-resolution μCT and histomorphometry. As a result, in the non-loaded tibiae, treatment with the higher doses of risedronate at 15 or 150 μg/kg/day resulted in higher trabecular bone volume and trabecular number than in vehicle-treated controls, whereas such treatment was associated with no differences in cortical bone volume at any dose. In the loaded tibiae, loading induced increases in trabecular and cortical bone volume compared with contralateral controls primarily through increased trabecular thickness and periosteal expansion, respectively, independently of risedronate treatment. In conclusion, the response to mechanical loading in both trabecular and cortical bone in mice was not impaired by risedronate, even over a 1000-fold dose range (Fig. 1.6). This is consistent with mechanical loading-related bone modeling [14]; formation and resorption occur on different surfaces during bone modeling, and thus, modeling-based bone formation and resorption are not coupled. In considering the optimization of clinical treatments for osteoporosis, it is reassuring that antiresorptive therapy and mechanical loading can exert independent beneficial effects.

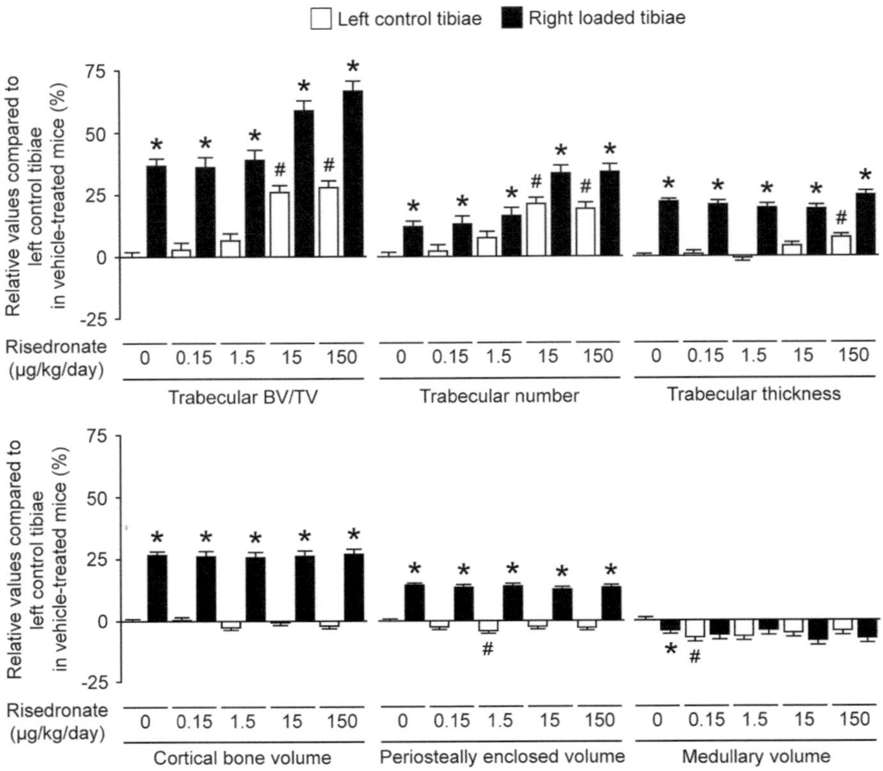

Fig. 1.6 Relative values of trabecular and cortical μCT parameters of the left control and right loaded tibiae in mice treated with vehicle or risedronate at a dose of 0.15, 1.5, 15, or 150 μg/kg/day compared to the left control tibiae in vehicle-treated mice. Values were obtained from mixed model analysis including body weight and are presented as mean ± SE ($n = 20$ in vehicle treatment and $n = 10$ in risedronate treatments). $^{\#}P < 0.05$ versus left control tibiae in vehicle-treated mice and $^{*}p < 0.05$ versus left control tibiae in each treatment with vehicle or risedronate by mixed model analysis followed by Bonferroni adjustment (Adapted from Sugiyama et al. [39])

1.3 The Mechanostat-Based Clinical Perspectives

In addition to other chronic diseases such as hypertension, hypercholesterolemia, and diabetes, a treat-to-target strategy was recently applied in rheumatoid arthritis and has now been discussed in osteoporosis. An important goal of osteoporosis therapy is to achieve normal risk of hip fracture associated with significant morbidity and mortality, but the anti-fracture efficacies of currently approved osteoporosis drugs are limited [70–72]. Here, it is important to note that the human skeleton normally adapts to mechanical environment [52, 73–76].

1.3.1 Limitation of Osteoporosis Therapy

The adult skeleton in humans would continuously respond to change in mechanical environment to maintain resultant strain of the bone [52, 76], while increased bone strength by an osteoporosis drug results in decreased bone strain regardless of suppressing bone resorption or promoting bone formation. This suggests that the effect of osteoporosis therapy is limited by skeletal adaptation to mechanical strain, i.e., the natural homeostatic system in the skeleton (Fig. 1.7) [77, 78], which is consistent with the fact that there exists a powerful effect that returns bone mass to its pretreatment level after the withdrawal of treatment with osteoporosis agents. In addition, this theory can provide a new significant insight into the mechanisms by which vitamin D or warfarin affects the skeleton [79–81].

A strategy to reduce the limitation of osteoporosis therapy is pharmacologically enhancing skeletal response to mechanical stimulation. Advantages of this strategy include increasing bone strength safely in a structural appropriate manner, depending on local mechanical environment at each skeletal site. Among drugs currently approved for the treatment of osteoporosis, only intermittent treatment with parathyroid hormone would have such a possibility; although high-impact exercise to increase bone strength is not easy for older patients with skeletal fragility, teriparatide has been suggested to have a synergistic effect with even low, physiological levels of mechanical loading in animals [37] and humans [66].

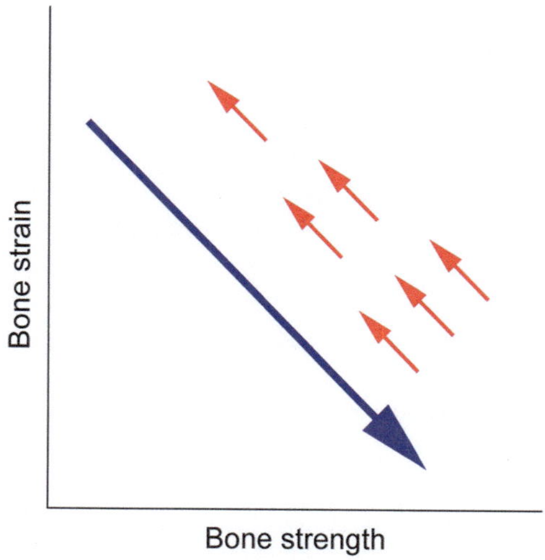

Fig. 1.7 Mechanical strain-related feedback control of bone strength: natural homeostatic system in the skeleton. A *long arrow* indicates the effect of osteoporosis therapy that increases bone strength and thus decreases bone strain from physical activity, regardless of suppressing bone resorption or promoting bone formation or increasing bone quantity or quality. *Short arrows* indicate the negative feedback control of bone strength that returns bone strain to its pretreatment level (Adapted from Sugiyama et al. [77])

There is, however, a disadvantage of the strategy to enhance skeletal response to mechanical stimulation. The skeleton is adapted to the mechanical environment resulting from habitual physical activity, but not to the unusual direction of mechanical force by falls. As a result, the enhancement of bone response to daily physical activity might not efficiently reduce the risk of fall-related hip or non-vertebral fractures. One approach to overcome this disadvantage is to find an agent that has the effect of mechanical strain. For example, it has been shown in animals that the production of sclerostin secreted by osteocytes is increased by skeletal disuse and decreased by skeletal loading [36, 42, 82–84].

1.3.2 Alternative Drugs of Mechanical Strain-Related Stimulus

Consequently, anti-sclerostin antibodies such as romosozumab and blosozumab can be considered as the alternative drugs of mechanical strain-related stimulus [85]. The latest findings include marked modeling-based bone formation by romosozumab in monkeys [86] and rapidly increased bone formation as well as decreased bone resorption by romosozumab [87, 88] and blosozumab [89, 90] in postmenopausal women. In contrast to bone remodeling, modeling-based bone formation and resorption are not coupled, and mechanical stimulation is a natural uncoupling factor that stimulates bone formation and inhibits bone resorption.

In phase 2 studies of postmenopausal women with low areal bone mineral density (BMD), romosozumab and blosozumab markedly increased areal BMD at the lumbar spine and hip dose-dependently, but areal BMD at the one-third radius was not changed even by the highest dose of romosozumab [88] or blosozumab [90]. Experimental evidence that the production of sclerostin secreted by osteocytes is increased by skeletal disuse and decreased by skeletal loading [36, 42, 82–84] implies that even the highest doses of romosozumab and blosozumab were not enough for the radius because the levels of sclerostin expression in non-weight-bearing bones such as the radius could be higher than those in weight-bearing bones such as the lumbar spine and hip. Several lines of evidence to support this hypothesis include (1) patients with sclerosteosis due to deficiency of sclerostin have higher areal BMD at the radius as well as the lumbar spine and hip [91] and (2) appropriate doses of anti-sclerostin antibodies effectively increase bone mass in animals with skeletal disuse or unloading [92, 93]. If correct, the highest doses of romosozumab and blosozumab are unlikely to cause unwanted bony overgrowth at non-weight-bearing sites such as the face and skull in postmenopausal women with osteoporosis, while further higher doses of these drugs would be required to improve skeletal fragility in patients with reduced physical activity.

The existence of other mechanotransduction pathways independent of sclerostin [94], however, indicates that treatment with an anti-sclerostin antibody cannot escape from the mechanostat-related limitation of osteoporosis therapy (Fig. 1.7)

[77]. In fact, both romosozumab and blosozumab treatments in postmenopausal women with low areal BMD showed that marked changes in circulating bone formation and resorption markers returned to the pretreatment levels within a year despite the continued treatments [88, 90]. This theory is also compatible with the relation between circulating sclerostin and bone mass; sclerostin-related high bone mass in patients with sclerosteosis or van Buchem disease and heterozygous carriers of these diseases is linked to lower levels of circulating sclerostin [95, 96], while circulating sclerostin and bone mass in normal women and men have a positive correlation [97, 98]. The discrepancy suggests that higher bone mass associated with other mechanotransduction pathways independent of sclerostin would cause lower mechanical strain in the skeleton and thus could result in compensatory higher sclerostin production according to the mechanostat.

1.3.3 Bone Quality Associated with Mineral Versus Collagen

Fall-related fracture occurs if the energy from the fall is higher than that the bone can absorb. Force-displacement curve obtained from a biomechanical test shows that energy absorption, the area under the curve, represents bone fragility and an ideal strategy for the improvement of bone fragility is to increase both of the force and displacement at failure [99] (Fig. 1.8a).

From a material point of view, stiffness and toughness of bone tissue generally depend on mineral and collagen, respectively [100]. There is a yield force at which a bone begins to deform plastically, and mechanical strain from normal physical activity would be linked to the pre-yield "elastic" deformation associated with mineral, but not to the post-yield "plastic" deformation associated with collagen (Fig. 1.8b). Consequently, mechanical strain-related feedback control could compensate mineral-related, but not collagen-related, impairment of bone quality to maintain "elastic" deformation [78]. Indeed, this theory is compatible with clinical data relating to bone quality. Examples of the mechanostat-based compensation for mineral-related impairment of bone quality would include rickets/osteomalacia and use of warfarin [77, 79–81], while the impairment of bone quality associated with collagen cross-links significantly contributes to skeletal fragility in diabetes [101–103].

Finally, it is possible to speculate that daily treatment with teriparatide improves bone fragility at the hip through the mechanostat-based "modeling-related direct" and "remodeling-related compensatory" mechanisms (Fig. 1.8c). The enhancement of skeletal response to mechanical loading [37, 62–66] would result in the former effect. In contrast, a decrease in the degree of mineralization after the treatment [104] might act to improve bone fragility if compensated efficiently, because compensatory bone gain by the mechanostat to maintain the pre-yield "elastic" deformation could increase the yield force at which a bone begins to deform plastically and thus the energy that the bone can absorb. This possibility is supported by histomorphometric data showing that 1 or 2 years of the treatment

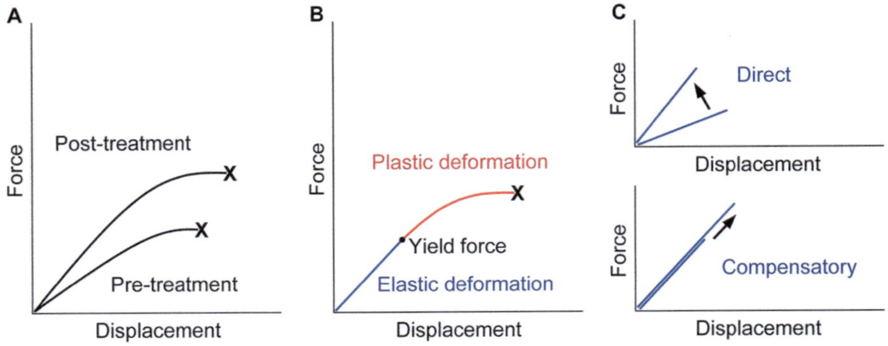

Fig. 1.8 Force-displacement curve of a bone. (**a**) Treatment with an ideal osteoporosis drug improves bone fragility by increasing both the force and displacement at failure. **X** denotes fracture. (**b**) The curve would consist of the pre-yield "elastic" deformation associated with mineral and the post-yield "plastic" deformation associated with collagen. Consequently, mechanical strain-related feedback control, the mechanostat, could work against mineral-related, but not collagen-related, impairment of bone quality. **X** denotes fracture. (**c**) The pre-yield "elastic" deformation can be modified by osteoporosis therapy that directly enhances the response to mechanical loading and increases the slope of the curve (*upper*) or lowers mineral-related bone quality and results in compensatory bone gain by the mechanostat to maintain the slope of the curve (*lower*). Note that, in the latter case, the yield force can be increased if compensated efficiently (Adapted from Sugiyama et al. [78])

results in increases in modeling- and remodeling-based bone formation [105], because the mechanostat suggests that the former "modeling-related direct" effect does not continue for a long time [77].

References

1. Wolff J (1892) Das Gesetz der Transformation der Knochen. Verlag von August Hirschwald, Berlin
2. Wolff J (1986) The law of bone remodelling. Springer, Berlin
3. Brand RA (2010) Biographical sketch: Julius Wolff, 1836–1902. Clin Orthop Relat Res 468:1047–1049
4. Frost HM (2003) Bone's mechanostat: a 2003 update. Anat Rec A: Discov Mol Cell Evol Biol 275:1081–1101
5. Meakin LB, Price JS, Lanyon LE (2014) The contribution of experimental in vivo models to understanding the mechanisms of adaptation to mechanical loading in bone. Front Endocrinol 5:154
6. Rubin CT, Lanyon LE (1985) Regulation of bone mass by mechanical strain magnitude. Calcif Tissue Int 37:411–417
7. Turner CH, Akhter MP, Raab DM, Kimmel DB, Recker RR (1991) A noninvasive, in vivo model for studying strain adaptive bone modeling. Bone 12:73–79
8. O'Connor JA, Lanyon LE, MacFie H (1982) The influence of strain rate on adaptive bone remodelling. J Biomech 15:767–781

9. Turner CH, Owan I, Takano Y (1995) Mechanotransduction in bone: role of strain rate. Am J Physiol 269:E438–E442
10. Hert J, Liskova M, Landa J (1971) Reaction of bone to mechanical stimuli. 1. Continuous and intermittent loading of tibia in rabbit. Folia Morphol 19:290–300
11. Lanyon LE, Rubin CT (1984) Static vs dynamic loads as an influence on bone remodelling. J Biomech 17:897–905
12. Rubin CT, Lanyon LE (1984) Regulation of bone formation by applied dynamic loads. J Bone Joint Surg Am 66:397–402
13. Umemura Y, Ishiko T, Yamauchi T, Kurono M, Mashiko S (1997) Five jumps per day increase bone mass and breaking force in rats. J Bone Miner Res 12:1480–1485
14. Pead MJ, Skerry TM, Lanyon LE (1988) Direct transformation from quiescence to bone formation in the adult periosteum following a single brief period of bone loading. J Bone Miner Res 3:647–656
15. Jagger CJ, Chambers TJ, Chow JW (1995) Stimulation of bone formation by dynamic mechanical loading of rat caudal vertebrae is not suppressed by 3-amino-1-hydroxypropylidene-1-bisphosphonate (AHPrBP). Bone 16:309–313
16. Robling AG, Burr DB, Turner CH (2001) Recovery periods restore mechanosensitivity to dynamically loaded bone. J Exp Biol 204:3389–3399
17. Srinivasan S, Weimer DA, Agans SC, Bain SD, Gross TS (2002) Low-magnitude mechanical loading becomes osteogenic when rest is inserted between each load cycle. J Bone Miner Res 17:1613–1620
18. Rubin CT, Bain SD, McLeod KJ (1992) Suppression of the osteogenic response in the aging skeleton. Calcif Tissue Int 50:306–313
19. Srinivasan S, Gross TS, Bain SD (2012) Bone mechanotransduction may require augmentation in order to strengthen the senescent skeleton. Ageing Res Rev 11:353–360
20. Meakin LB, Galea GL, Sugiyama T, Lanyon LE, Price JS (2014) Age-related impairment of bones' adaptive response to loading in mice is associated with sex-related deficiencies in osteoblasts but no change in osteocytes. J Bone Miner Res 29:1859–1871
21. Hagino H, Raab DM, Kimmel DB, Akhter MP, Recker RR (1993) Effect of ovariectomy on bone response to in vivo external loading. J Bone Miner Res 8:347–357
22. Sugiyama T, Galea GL, Lanyon LE, Price JS (2010) Mechanical loading-related bone gain is enhanced by tamoxifen but unaffected by fulvestrant in female mice. Endocrinology 151:5582–5590
23. Windahl S, Saxon L, Borjesson A, Lagerquist M, Frenkel B, Henning P, Lerner UH, Galea GL, Meakin LB, Engdahl C, Sjogren K, Antal MC, Krust A, Chambon P, Lanyon LE, Price JS, Ohlsson C (2013) Estrogen receptor-α is required for the osteogenic response to mechanical loading in a ligand-independent manner involving its activation function 1 but not 2. J Bone Miner Res 28:291–301
24. Lee K, Jessop H, Suswillo R, Zaman G, Lanyon L (2003) Bone adaptation requires oestrogen receptor α. Nature 424:389
25. Galea GL, Price JS, Lanyon LE (2013) Estrogen receptors' roles in the control of mechanically adaptive bone (re)modeling. Bonekey Rep 2:413
26. Chambers TJ, Evans M, Gardner TN, Turner-Smith A, Chow JW (1993) Induction of bone formation in rat tail vertebrae by mechanical loading. Bone Miner 20:167–178
27. Torrance AG, Mosley JR, Suswillo RF, Lanyon LE (1994) Noninvasive loading of the rat ulna in vivo induces a strain-related modeling response uncomplicated by trauma or periostal pressure. Calcif Tissue Int 54:241–247
28. Akhter MP, Cullen DM, Pedersen EA, Kimmel DB, Recker RR (1998) Bone response to in vivo mechanical loading in two breeds of mice. Calcif Tissue Int 63:442–449
29. Lee KC, Maxwell A, Lanyon LE (2002) Validation of a technique for studying functional adaptation of the mouse ulna in response to mechanical loading. Bone 31:407–412

30. Gross TS, Srinivasan S, Liu CC, Clemens TL, Bain SD (2002) Noninvasive loading of the murine tibia: an in vivo model for the study of mechanotransduction. J Bone Miner Res 17:493–501
31. Judex S, Donahue LR, Rubin C (2002) Genetic predisposition to low bone mass is paralleled by an enhanced sensitivity to signals anabolic to the skeleton. FASEB J 16:1280–1282
32. de Souza RL, Matsuura M, Eckstein F, Rawlinson SC, Lanyon LE, Pitsillides AA (2005) Non-invasive axial loading of mouse tibiae increases cortical bone formation and modifies trabecular organization: a new model to study cortical and cancellous compartments in a single loaded element. Bone 37:810–818
33. Fritton JC, Myers ER, Wright TM, van der Meulen MC (2005) Loading induces site-specific increases in mineral content assessed by microcomputed tomography of the mouse tibia. Bone 36:1030–1038
34. Zhang P, Tanaka SM, Jiang H, Su M, Yokota H (2006) Diaphyseal bone formation in murine tibiae in response to knee loading. J Appl Physiol 100:1452–1459
35. Webster DJ, Morley PL, van Lenthe GH, Muller R (2008) A novel in vivo mouse model for mechanically stimulated bone adaptation – a combined experimental and computational validation study. Comput Methods Biomech Biomed Eng 11:435–441
36. Moustafa A, Sugiyama T, Saxon LK, Zaman G, Sunters A, Armstrong VJ, Javaheri B, Lanyon LE, Price JS (2009) The mouse fibula as a suitable bone for the study of functional adaptation to mechanical loading. Bone 44:930–935
37. Sugiyama T, Saxon LK, Zaman G, Moustafa A, Sunters A, Price JS, Lanyon LE (2008) Mechanical loading enhances the anabolic effects of intermittent parathyroid hormone (1–34) on trabecular and cortical bone in mice. Bone 43:238–248
38. Sugiyama T, Price JS, Lanyon LE (2010) Functional adaptation to mechanical loading in both cortical and cancellous bone is controlled locally and is confined to the loaded bones. Bone 46:314–321
39. Sugiyama T, Meakin LB, Galea GL, Jackson BF, Lanyon LE, Ebetino FH, Russell RG, Price JS (2011) Risedronate does not reduce mechanical loading-related increases in cortical and trabecular bone mass in mice. Bone 49:133–139
40. Saxon LK, Jackson BF, Sugiyama T, Lanyon LE, Price JS (2011) Analysis of multiple bone responses to graded strains above functional levels, and to disuse, in mice in vivo show that the human Lrp5 G171V High Bone Mass mutation increases the osteogenic response to loading but that lack of Lrp5 activity reduces it. Bone 49:184–193
41. Sugiyama T, Meakin LB, Browne WJ, Galea GL, Price JS, Lanyon LE (2012) Bones' adaptive response to mechanical loading is essentially linear between the low strains associated with disuse and the high strains associated with the lamellar/woven bone transition. J Bone Miner Res 27:1784–1793
42. Moustafa A, Sugiyama T, Prasad J, Zaman G, Gross TS, Lanyon LE, Price JS (2012) Mechanical loading-related changes in osteocyte sclerostin expression in mice are more closely associated with the subsequent osteogenic response than the peak strains engendered. Osteoporos Int 23:1225–1234
43. Sugiyama T, Meakin LB, Galea GL, Lanyon LE, Price JS (2013) The cyclooxygenase-2 selective inhibitor NS-398 does not influence trabecular or cortical bone gain resulting from repeated mechanical loading in female mice. Osteoporos Int 24:383–388
44. Meakin LB, Sugiyama T, Galea GL, Browne WJ, Lanyon LE, Price JS (2013) Male mice housed in groups engage in frequent fighting and show a lower response to additional bone loading than females or individually housed males that do not fight. Bone 54:113–117
45. Kodama Y, Umemura Y, Nagasawa S, Beamer WG, Donahue LR, Rosen CR, Baylink DJ, Farley JR (2000) Exercise and mechanical loading increase periosteal bone formation and whole bone strength in C57BL/6J mice but not in C3H/Hej mice. Calcif Tissue Int 66:298–306

46. Klein-Nulend J, Bacabac RG, Bakker AD (2012) Mechanical loading and how it affects bone cells: the role of the osteocyte cytoskeleton in maintaining our skeleton. Eur Cell Mater 24:278–291
47. Thompson WR, Rubin CT, Rubin J (2012) Mechanical regulation of signaling pathways in bone. Gene 503:179–193
48. Galea GL, Price JS (2015) Four-point bending protocols to study the effects of dynamic strain in osteoblastic cells in vitro. Methods Mol Biol 1226:117–130
49. Alam I, Warden SJ, Robling AG, Turner CH (2005) Mechanotransduction in bone does not require a functional cyclooxygenase-2 (COX-2) gene. J Bone Miner Res 20:438–446
50. Castillo AB, Blundo JT, Chen JC, Lee KL, Yereddi NR, Jang E, Kumar S, Tang WJ, Zarrin S, Kim JB, Jacobs CR (2012) Focal adhesion kinase plays a role in osteoblast mechanotransduction in vitro but does not affect load-induced bone formation in vivo. PLoS One 7, e43291
51. Lloyd SA, Loiselle AE, Zhang Y, Donahue HJ (2014) Shifting paradigms on the role of connexin43 in the skeletal response to mechanical load. J Bone Miner Res 29:275–286
52. Christen P, Ito K, Ellouz R, Boutroy S, Sornay-Rendu E, Chapurlat RD, van Rietbergen B (2014) Bone remodelling in humans is load-driven but not lazy. Nat Commun 5:4855
53. Schulte FA, Ruffoni D, Lambers FM, Christen D, Webster DJ, Kuhn G, Muller R (2013) Local mechanical stimuli regulate bone formation and resorption in mice at the tissue level. PLoS One 8, e62172
54. Ellman R, Spatz J, Cloutier A, Palme R, Christiansen BA, Bouxsein ML (2013) Partial reductions in mechanical loading yield proportional changes in bone density, bone architecture, and muscle mass. J Bone Miner Res 28:875–885
55. Turner CH, Forwood MR, Rho JY, Yoshikawa T (1994) Mechanical loading thresholds for lamellar and woven bone formation. J Bone Miner Res 9:87–97
56. Sawakami K, Robling AG, Ai M, Pitner ND, Liu D, Warden SJ, Li J, Maye P, Rowe DW, Duncan RL, Warman ML, Turner CH (2006) The Wnt co-receptor LRP5 is essential for skeletal mechanotransduction but not for the anabolic bone response to parathyroid hormone treatment. J Biol Chem 281:23698–23711
57. Sample SJ, Behan M, Smith L, Oldenhoff WE, Markel MD, Kalscheur VL, Hao Z, Miletic V, Muir P (2008) Functional adaptation to loading of a single bone is neuronally regulated and involves multiple bones. J Bone Miner Res 23:1372–1381
58. Wu Q, Sample SJ, Baker TA, Thomas CF, Behan M, Muir P (2009) Mechanical loading of a long bone induces plasticity in sensory input to the central nervous system. Neurosci Lett 463:254–257
59. Sample SJ, Collins RJ, Wilson AP, Racette MA, Behan M, Markel MD, Kalscheur VL, Hao Z, Muir P (2010) Systemic effects of ulna loading in male rats during functional adaptation. J Bone Miner Res 25:2016–2028
60. McKenzie JA, Silva MJ (2011) Comparing histological, vascular and molecular responses associated with woven and lamellar bone formation induced by mechanical loading in the rat ulna. Bone 48:250–258
61. Willie BM, Birkhold AI, Razi H, Thiele T, Aido M, Kruck B, Schill A, Checa S, Main RP, Duda GN (2013) Diminished response to in vivo mechanical loading in trabecular and not cortical bone in adulthood of female C57Bl/6 mice coincides with a reduction in deformation to load. Bone 55:335–346
62. Chow JW, Fox S, Jagger CJ, Chambers TJ (1998) Role for parathyroid hormone in mechanical responsiveness of rat bone. Am J Physiol 274:E146–E154
63. Hagino H, Okano T, Akhter MP, Enokida M, Teshima R (2001) Effect of parathyroid hormone on cortical bone response to in vivo external loading of the rat tibia. J Bone Miner Metab 19:244–250
64. Li J, Duncan RL, Burr DB, Gattone VH, Turner CH (2003) Parathyroid hormone enhances mechanically induced bone formation, possibly involving L-type voltage-sensitive calcium channels. Endocrinology 144:1226–1233

65. Kim CH, Takai E, Zhou H, von Stechow D, Muller R, Dempster DW, Guo XE (2003) Trabecular bone response to mechanical and parathyroid hormone stimulation: the role of mechanical microenvironment. J Bone Miner Res 18:2116–2125
66. Poole KE, Treece GM, Ridgway GR, Mayhew PM, Borggrefe J, Gee AH (2011) Targeted regeneration of bone in the osteoporotic human femur. PLoS One 6, e16190
67. Feher A, Koivunemi A, Koivunemi M, Fuchs RK, Burr DB, Phipps RJ, Reinwald S, Allen MR (2010) Bisphosphonates do not inhibit periosteal bone formation in estrogen deficient animals and allow enhanced bone modeling in response to mechanical loading. Bone 46:203–207
68. Stadelmann VA, Bonnet N, Pioletti DP (2011) Combined effects of zoledronate and mechanical stimulation on bone adaptation in an axially loaded mouse tibia. Clin Biomech 26:101–105
69. Nagira K, Hagino H, Kameyama Y, Teshima R (2013) Effects of minodronate on cortical bone response to mechanical loading in rats. Bone 53:277–283
70. Kawai M, Modder UI, Khosla S, Rosen CJ (2011) Emerging therapeutic opportunities for skeletal restoration. Nat Rev Drug Discov 10:141–156
71. Crandall CJ, Newberry SJ, Diamant A, Lim YW, Gellad WF, Booth MJ, Motala A, Shekelle PG (2014) Comparative effectiveness of pharmacologic treatments to prevent fractures: an updated systematic review. Ann Intern Med 161:711–723
72. Kanis JA, McCloskey E, Branco J, Brandi ML, Dennison E, Devogelaer JP, Ferrari S, Kaufman JM, Papapoulos S, Reginster JY, Rizzoli R (2014) Goal-directed treatment of osteoporosis in Europe. Osteoporos Int 25:2533–2543
73. Sugiyama T, Taguchi T, Kawai S (2002) Adaptation of bone to mechanical loads. Lancet 359:1160
74. Sugiyama T, Kawai S (2004) Quantitative ultrasound, skeletal quality, and fracture risk. Lancet 363:1076–1077
75. Sugiyama T, Taguchi T (2005) Cortical stability of the femoral neck and hip fracture risk. Lancet 366:1525–1526
76. Bhatia VA, Edwards WB, Johnson JE, Troy KL (2015) Short-term bone formation is greatest within high strain regions of the human distal radius: a prospective pilot study. J Biomech Eng 137:011001
77. Sugiyama T, Kim YT, Oda H (2015) Osteoporosis therapy: a novel insight from natural homeostatic system in the skeleton. Osteoporos Int 26:443–447
78. Sugiyama T, Torio T, Sato T, Matsumoto M, Kim YT, Oda H (2015) Improvement of skeletal fragility by teriparatide in adult osteoporosis patients: a novel mechanostat-based hypothesis for bone quality. Front Endocrinol 6:6
79. Sugiyama T, Tanaka S, Miyajima T, Kim YT, Oda H (2014) Vitamin D supplementation and fracture risk in adults: a new insight. Osteoporos Int 25:2497–2498
80. Sugiyama T, Yoshioka H, Sakaguchi K, Kim YT, Oda H (2015) An evidence-based perspective on vitamin D and the growing skeleton. Osteoporos Int 26:1447–1448
81. Sugiyama T, Kugimiya F, Kono S, Kim YT, Oda H (2015) Warfarin use and fracture risk: an evidence-based mechanistic insight. Osteoporos Int 26:1231–1232
82. Robling AG, Niziolek PJ, Baldridge LA, Condon KW, Allen MR, Alam I, Mantila SM, Gluhak-Heinrich J, Bellido TM, Harris SE, Turner CH (2008) Mechanical stimulation of bone in vivo reduces osteocyte expression of Sost/sclerostin. J Biol Chem 283:5866–5875
83. Tu X, Rhee Y, Condon KW, Bivi N, Allen MR, Dwyer D, Stolina M, Turner CH, Robling AG, Plotkin LI, Bellido T (2012) Sost downregulation and local Wnt signaling are required for the osteogenic response to mechanical loading. Bone 50:209–217
84. Ke HZ, Richards WG, Li X, Ominsky MS (2012) Sclerostin and dickkopf-1 as therapeutic targets in bone diseases. Endocr Rev 33:747–783
85. Sugiyama T, Torio T, Miyajima T, Kim YT, Oda H (2015) Romosozumab and blosozumab: alternative drugs of mechanical strain-related stimulus toward a cure for osteoporosis. Front Endocrinol 6:54

86. Ominsky MS, Niu QT, Li C, Li X, Ke HZ (2014) Tissue-level mechanisms responsible for the increase in bone formation and bone volume by sclerostin antibody. J Bone Miner Res 29:1424–1430
87. Padhi D, Jang G, Stouch B, Fang L, Posvar E (2011) Single-dose, placebo-controlled, randomized study of AMG 785, a sclerostin monoclonal antibody. J Bone Miner Res 26:19–26
88. McClung MR, Grauer A, Boonen S, Bolognese MA, Brown JP, Diez-Perez A, Langdahl BL, Reginster JY, Zanchetta JR, Wasserman SM, Katz L, Maddox J, Yang YC, Libanati C, Bone HG (2014) Romosozumab in postmenopausal women with low bone mineral density. N Engl J Med 370:412–420
89. McColm J, Hu L, Womack T, Tang CC, Chiang AY (2014) Single- and multiple-dose randomized studies of blosozumab, a monoclonal antibody against sclerostin, in healthy postmenopausal women. J Bone Miner Res 29:935–943
90. Recker R, Benson C, Matsumoto T, Bolognese M, Robins D, Alam J, Chiang AY, Hu L, Krege JH, Sowa H, Mitlak B, Myers S (2015) A randomized, double-blind phase 2 clinical trial of blosozumab, a sclerostin antibody, in postmenopausal women with low bone mineral density. J Bone Miner Res 30:216–224
91. Gardner JC, van Bezooijen RL, Mervis B, Hamdy NA, Lowik CW, Hamersma H, Beighton P, Papapoulos SE (2005) Bone mineral density in sclerosteosis; affected individuals and gene carriers. J Clin Endocrinol Metab 90:6392–6395
92. Tian XY, Jee WS, Li X, Paszty C, Ke HZ (2011) Sclerostin antibody increases bone mass by stimulating bone formation and inhibiting bone resorption in a hindlimb-immobilization rat model. Bone 48:197–201
93. Spatz JM, Ellman R, Cloutier AM, Louis L, van Vliet M, Suva LJ, Dwyer D, Stolina M, Ke HZ, Bouxsein ML (2013) Sclerostin antibody inhibits skeletal deterioration due to reduced mechanical loading. J Bone Miner Res 28:865–874
94. Morse A, McDonald M, Kelly N, Melville K, Schindeler A, Kramer I, Kneissel M, van der Meulen MC, Little DG (2014) Mechanical load increases in bone formation via a sclerostin-independent pathway. J Bone Miner Res 29:2456–2467
95. van Lierop AH, Hamdy NA, Hamersma H, van Bezooijen RL, Power J, Loveridge N, Papapoulos SE (2011) Patients with sclerosteosis and disease carriers: human models of the effect of sclerostin on bone turnover. J Bone Miner Res 26:2804–2811
96. van Lierop AH, Hamdy NA, van Egmond ME, Bakker E, Dikkers FG, Papapoulos SE (2013) Van Buchem disease: clinical, biochemical, and densitometric features of patients and disease carriers. J Bone Miner Res 28:848–854
97. Modder UI, Hoey KA, Amin S, McCready LK, Achenbach SJ, Riggs BL, Melton LJ III, Khosla S (2011) Relation of age, gender, and bone mass to circulating sclerostin levels in women and men. J Bone Miner Res 26:373–379
98. Szulc P, Bertholon C, Borel O, Marchand F, Chapurlat R (2013) Lower fracture risk in older men with higher sclerostin concentration: a prospective analysis from the MINOS study. J Bone Miner Res 28:855–864
99. Turner CH (2002) Biomechanics of bone: determinants of skeletal fragility and bone quality. Osteoporos Int 13:97–104
100. Fratzl P, Gupta HS, Paschalis EP, Roschger P (2004) Structure and mechanical quality of the collagen-mineral nano-composite in bone. J Mater Chem 14:2115–2123
101. Saito M, Marumo K (2010) Collagen cross-links as a determinant of bone quality: a possible explanation for bone fragility in aging, osteoporosis, and diabetes mellitus. Osteoporos Int 21:195–214
102. Garnero P (2012) The contribution of collagen crosslinks to bone strength. Bonekey Rep 1:182
103. Leslie WD, Rubin MR, Schwartz AV, Kanis JA (2012) Type 2 diabetes and bone. J Bone Miner Res 27:2231–2237

104. Borggrefe J, Graeff C, Nickelsen TN, Marin F, Gluer CC (2010) Quantitative computed tomographic assessment of the effects of 24 months of teriparatide treatment on 3D femoral neck bone distribution, geometry, and bone strength: results from the EUROFORS study. J Bone Miner Res 25:472–481
105. Ma YL, Zeng Q, Donley DW, Ste-Marie LG, Gallagher JC, Dalsky GP, Marcus R, Eriksen EF (2006) Teriparatide increases bone formation in modeling and remodeling osteons and enhances IGF-II immunoreactivity in postmenopausal women with osteoporosis. J Bone Miner Res 21:855–864

Chapter 2
Osteoclast-Mediated Pain in Osteoporosis

Kousuke Iba and Toshihiko Yamashita

Abstract Recent studies have indicated that osteoporosis patients experience idiopathic skeletal pain independent of those fractures or deformity; additionally, bisphosphonate, an effective drug for postmenopausal osteoporosis treatment, improves that skeletal pain. However, the etiology of this pain is still unknown. In this chapter, we demonstrate several data in the basis with our experiments using ovariectomized mouse model and speculate the mechanism of osteoclast-mediated pain in osteoporosis.

We have shown that pathological changes leading to increased bone resorption by osteoclast activation were related to the induction of pain-like behavior in OVX mice. This pain-like behavior was improved by the treatment with bisphosphonate. In addition, the antagonists of transient receptor potential vanilloid type 1 (TRPV1) and antagonist of acid-sensing ion channel (ASIC) 3 which are acid-sensing nociceptors and an inhibitor of vacuolar H^+-ATPase known as an proton pump improved the threshold value of pain-like behaviors accompanying an improvement in the acidic environment in the bone tissue based through osteoclast inactivation. Moreover, the antagonist to P2X2/3 receptor as an ATP ligand nociceptor improved the pain-like behavior in OVX mice. These results indicated that the skeletal pain accompanying osteoporosis is possibly associated with the acidic microenvironment caused by osteoclast activation, and P2X2/3 might have a role in osteoporosis patients under a high bone turnover state.

Keywords Transient receptor potential vanilloid type 1 • Acid-sensing ion channel • P2X • Skeletal pain • Osteoporosis

2.1 Skeletal Pain in Osteoporosis Patients

Osteoporosis is a major health-care concern and risk factor for fractures in the current aging society [1]. The most common problems due to osteoporosis are impairments in activities of daily living (ADL) and skeletal pain resulting from and

K. Iba (✉) • T. Yamashita
Department of Orthopaedic Surgery, Sapporo Medical University School of Medicine, South 1, West 16, Chuo-ku, Sapporo, Hokkaido 060-8543, Japan
e-mail: iba@sapmed.ac.jp

Y. Shimada, N. Miyakoshi (eds.), *Osteoporosis in Orthopedics*,
DOI 10.1007/978-4-431-55778-4_2

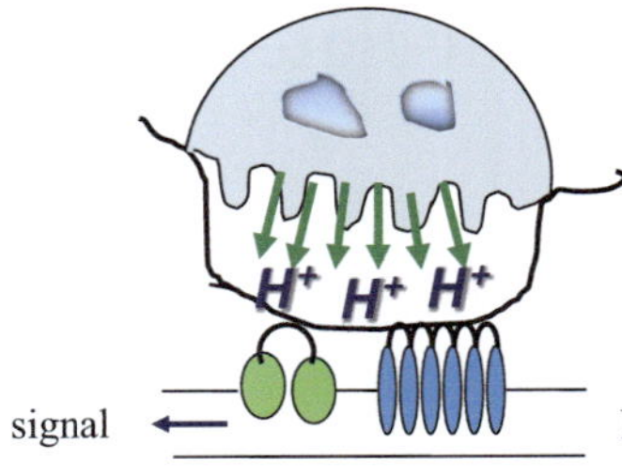

Fig. 2.1 The mechanism of induction for cancer-induced bone pain. The acidic microenvironment created by activated osteoclast-stimulated nocicepotors, which results in skeletal pain as the mechanism observed for cancer-induced bone pain

associated with osteoporotic fractures and skeletal deformities [2]. In contrast, osteoporosis patients may also show idiopathic skeletal pain in the absence of fractures or skeletal deformities [3, 4]. Several studies have indicated that osteoporosis patients also experience idiopathic skeletal pain independent of those fractures or deformity [3–5]. Moreover, recent studies also demonstrated that bisphosphonate (BP), which is an effective drug for postmenopausal osteoporosis treatment [6, 7], improves skeletal pain [3, 4, 8]. Although the etiology of this pain is still unknown [3–5], one of the mechanisms underlying the induction of idiopathic skeletal pain in osteoporosis patient is indicated to be the acidic microenvironment created by activated osteoclasts, which results in pain through the same mechanism as that observed for cancer-induced bone pain [9, 10] (Fig. 2.1). Then, the improvement effect of BP on idiopathic skeletal pain in osteoporosis patients could be worked via the inhibition of osteoclast activity as an anti-bone resorption drug [3, 4, 8]. In addition, the previous studies showed that bone pain associated with bone disorders, such as metastatic bone diseases [11], Paget's disease of bone [12], and osteogenesis imperfecta [13], may also be related to increased osteoclastic bone resorption, suggesting that osteoporosis-related bone pain is caused by increased osteoclastic bone resorption. In this chapter, we demonstrate several data in the basis with our experiments using ovariectomized mouse model and speculate the mechanism osteoclast-mediated pain in osteoporosis.

2.2 Assessment of Pain-Like Behavior in Ovariectomized (OVX) Mice as a Model of Postmenopausal Osteoporosis

Skeletal pain in OVX mice as a model of postmenopausal osteoporosis and that in OVX mice treated with BP were evaluated to elucidate mechanisms causing osteoporosis-related bone pain. OVX mice reveal osteoporotic changes 6 weeks after the surgery, of which total femoral bone mineral density (BMD) was significantly lower in the OVX group than in the sham group. Serum tartrate-resistant acid phosphatase 5b (TRAP5b), a bone resorption marker, was significantly higher in the OVX mice compared with the sham mice 4 weeks after surgery.

2.2.1 Evaluation of Pain-Like Behavior and Bone Metabolism in OVX Mice

2.2.1.1 Assessment of Pain-Like Behavior

Behavioral tests were conducted just after OVX and every 2 weeks thereafter. Thermal nociceptive testing (paw-flick test) was conducted using an analgesimeter (Plantar test 7370, Ugo Basile, Italy). The mice were unrestrained, and radiant heat was applied to the plantar surface of the left hind paw until it was actively withdrawn by the animal. Paw withdrawal latency (PWL) was considered to be an index of the thermal nociceptive threshold, and a decrease in this measurement indicated thermal hyperalgesia [14]. Mechanical allodynia (von Frey test) was measured using von Frey monofilaments on the left hind paw. The von Frey withdrawal threshold was determined by adjusting the stimulus intensity between 0.2 and 10 g equivalents of force and was estimated using the Dixon nonparametric test [15]. Motor functions were measured using the rotarod test, a test associated with pain-like behavior. The mice were placed on a cylinder, and the speed of rotation was set to 32 rotations/min. Latency to the fall from the rotarod was recorded. Lower values on these behavioral tests indicated greater skeletal pain [16].

2.2.1.2 Assessment of Skeletal Pain by Immunohistochemistry of Spinal Cord

We assessed skeletal pain by measuring c-Fos expression in the spinal cord, a functional marker of nociception [17]. The c-fos proto-oncogene is an immediate early gene and is expressed in response to both noxious and non-noxious stimuli [18, 19]. The L4–L5 segment of the spinal cord was immune-stained with c-Fos, and the number of c-Fos-labeled neurons in laminae I–II of that was counted.

In addition, a 0.02 mg/kg of body weight dose of alendronate (Merck & Co., Inc., NJ, USA), a BP, was administered to OVX mice subcutaneously once per day for 2 and 4 weeks after surgery (OVX + BP) [20, 22]. Behavioral tests, serum TRAP5b measurements, and immunohistochemical tests were performed in the sham and OVX mice.

2.2.2 Pain-Like Behavior After OVX and the Influence of BP

OVX mice had lower pain threshold on the paw-flick test and von Frey test, 4, 6, 8, and 10 weeks after surgery, compared with the sham mice (Fig. 2.2a, b), and the rotarod test showed a lower threshold 6 and 8 weeks after surgery (Fig. 2.2c). OVX mice were treated with BP (OVX + BP) for 2 weeks. The pain thresholds of the

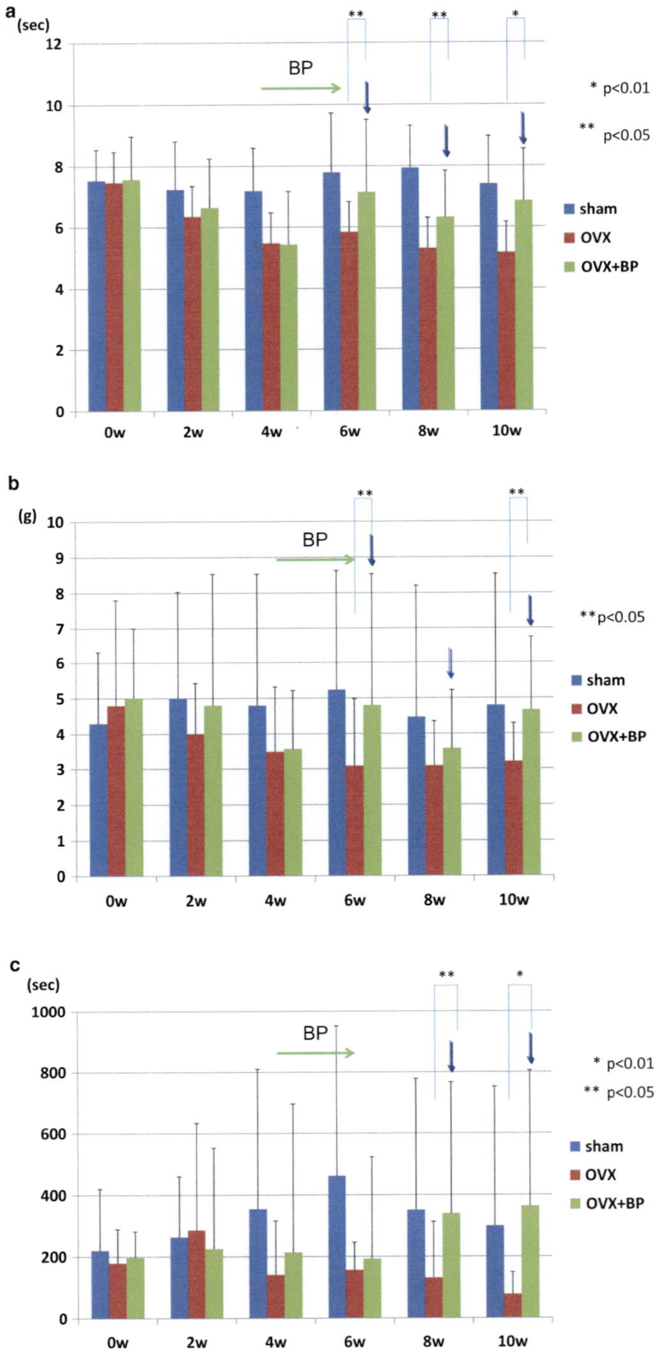

Fig. 2.2 The measurement of pain-like behavior. OVX mice showed a significant decrease in pain threshold value on the paw-flick test (**a**) and von Frey test (**b**) at 4, 6, 8, and 10 weeks after OVX and on the rotarod test (**c**) at 6 and 10 weeks, compared with the sham mice ($*p < 0.05$). The OVX-induced decrease was significantly improved at 2, 4, and 6 weeks after BP administration

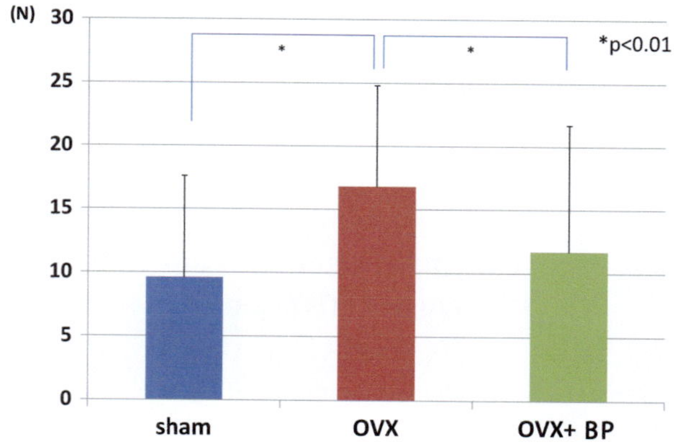

Fig. 2.3 Immunostaining for c-Fos in transverse sections of the L4–L5 level of the lumbar spinal cord. The number of c-Fos immunoreactive neurons in OVX mice (OVX) was significantly greater than that in both sham mice (sham) and OVX mice after BP administration (OVX + BP) (Figures were modified from Ref. [22])

OVX mice improved significantly in all tests after administrating BP, and these effects remained 4 weeks after discontinuing BP treatment (Fig. 2.2a-c). The decreased pain threshold value due to OVX was improved significantly 2 weeks after administering BP (OVX + BP). These effects maintained until 10 weeks after discontinuing BP treatment [22].

The serum TRAP5b was significantly related to the pain threshold value, with correlation on the paw-flick test, on the von Frey test, and on the rotarod test. Furthermore, BP's reduction in pain-like behavior was associated with decreased serum TPAP5b levels.

The number of c-Fos immunoreactive neurons, a marker of nociception, in laminae I–II of the dorsal horn of the spinal cord was significantly greater in the OVX mice than in the sham mice (Fig. 2.3). Those neurons were significantly lower in the OVX + BP mice than in the OVX mice (Fig. 2.3). These results, therefore, suggest that OVX mice with osteoporosis have greater skeletal pain than normal mice. In addition, the higher serum TRAP5b levels associated with OVX decreased significantly following BP treatment and were significantly correlated with pain threshold values [22], further suggesting that the skeletal pain accompanying osteoporosis is possibly associated with osteoclastic activity.

Several studies show that estrogen decrease associated with OVX increases skeletal pain by augmenting nociceptive pathway excitability in the peripheral and central neuronal systems [23–25]. BP may also directly suppress the release of neurotransmitters or inflammatory mediators in the nervous system [26–29]. Estrogen decrease due to OVX may have caused skeletal pain by directly influencing the nervous system in our study. However, more than 80 % of intravenously administered BP is taken up by bone tissue within 24 h and remains in the tissue for a long duration [30]. Furthermore, our results suggest that the BP

Fig. 2.2 (continued) (OVX + BP). These effects were maintained until 4 weeks after the discontinuation of BP treatment. *post-op* (weeks), weeks after the surgery; *BP* (*arrow*), 2-week treatment with BP from 4 to 6 weeks after the ovariectomy (Figures were modified from Ref. [22])

improvement of pain-like behavior was maintained even after discontinuing treatment for more than 4 weeks (Fig. 2.2). Therefore, the pain-like behavior associated with OVX and the inhibitory effects of BP are likely reflected by bone metabolic changes.

2.3 Mechanism of Skeletal Pain Induction Related to Osteoclast Activation

Osteoclasts degrade bone minerals by secreting protons through vacuolar H^+-ATPases (V-ATPase), creating an acidic microenvironment [31, 32]. Acid causes pain through acid-sensing nociceptors [33, 34]. Two main classes of these nociceptors, TRPV1 and acid-sensing ion channels (ASICs), are expressed in sensory neurons innervating the bone [34] and elicit pain signals when activated by acid stimuli [34, 35]. Previous studies of bone pain in a metastatic cancer model show that the acidic microenvironment created by bone-resorbing osteoclasts activates TRPV1 [9, 36, 37].

2.3.1 Acidic Environment in Bone by Activated Osteoclast and the Influence of BP

Histochemical findings in bone tissue demonstrated that the number of TRAP-positive osteoclasts in OVX mice was increased in comparison with that in sham mice (Fig. 2.4). In contrast, the number of TRAP-positive osteoclasts in OVX + BP was lower than that in OVX mice (Fig. 2.4). The V-ATPase expression was greater in OVX mice than that in sham or OVX + BP mice, respectively (Fig. 2.5). These findings, which osteoclast activity and V-ATPase expression were increased in OVX mice, indicated that the skeletal pain accompanying osteoporosis is possibly associated with the acidic microenvironment resulting from osteoclast activation [22].

2.3.2 Involvement of Acid-Sensing Nociceptors in Skeletal Pain Induction Related to Osteoclast Activation

With regard to the induction of pain through acid-sensing nociceptors, two main classes of these nociceptors, transient receptor potential channel vanilloid subfamily member 1 (TRPV1) and acid-sensing ion channels (ASICs), are expressed in the sensory neurons innervating the bone [34, 35] and elicit pain signals when activated by acid stimuli [33, 34]. TRPV1 is a member of a family of polymodal and

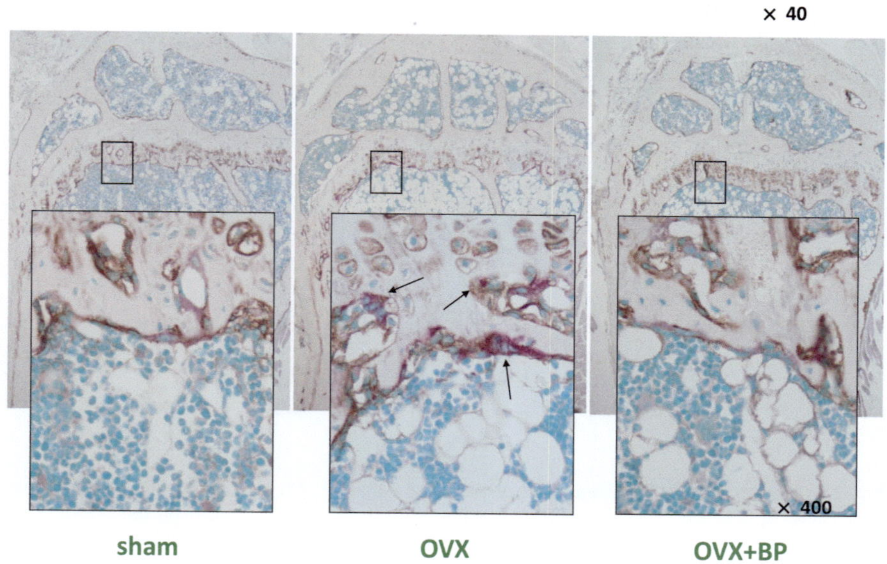

Fig. 2.4 Staining for TRAP in femora. Figures show double staining for localized ALP-positive osteoblasts (*brown color*) and TRAP-reactive osteoclasts (*red*) in the femoral trabeculae of sham, OVX, and OVX + BP mice. OVX mice demonstrate several TRAP-reactive osteoclasts (*black arrow*), while the other groups had a few flattened TRAP-positive osteoclasts (Figures were modified from Ref. [22])

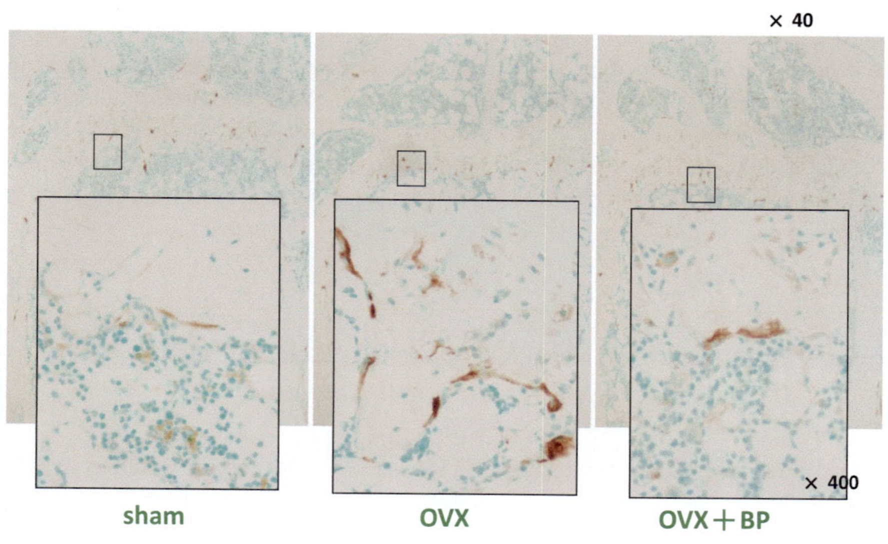

Fig. 2.5 The histochemical detection of V-ATPase in femora. The immunoreactivity against V-ATPase (*brown color*). There are many V-ATPase-immunopositive osteoclasts on the bone surfaces in the OVX group, while only a few flattened immunoreactive osteoclasts can be seen in the sham and OVX + BP groups (Figures were modified from Ref. [22])

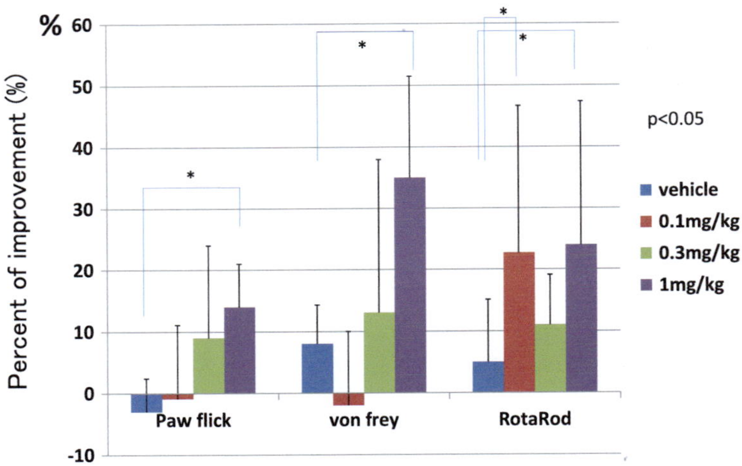

Fig. 2.6 Effects of a TRPV1 antagonist on pain-like behavior. All tests were conducted 6 weeks after OVX. A TRPV1 antagonist (SB366791), at a dose of 1 mg/kg, improved the threshold of pain-like behavior compared with the baseline value at 30 min after administration

nonselective cation channels that are predominantly expressed by sensory nerve fibers and sensitized by protons [21] and improved the threshold [22]. ASICs are a major group of acid-sensing nociceptors and are expressed in sensory neurons innervating the bone and known to be related to the acid-induced pain [34, 35] in a similar manner as another important nociceptor TRPV1 [21, 22]. According to our study, the antagonists of TRPV1 or ASIC significantly improved the threshold value for pain-like behavior in OVX mice (Fig. 2.6) [22 and unpublished data]. In general, the secretion of protons by osteoclasts through V-ATPase is known as an acidification pathway during bone resorption [32]. We also demonstrated that a V-ATPase inhibitor significantly improved pain-like behavior in OVX mice (unpublished data). These results support our hypothesis that the acidic microenvironment produced by osteoclasts activates acid-sensing nociceptors and contributes to bone pain.

2.3.3 Involvement of P2X Receptors in Skeletal Pain Induction Related to Osteoclast Activation

Extracellular adenosine triphosphate (ATP) and P2X receptors, which is a P2X receptor ligand, are implicated in nociceptive signaling under both normal and pathologic pain states. P2X receptors, which include seven subunits (P2X1–P2X7) belonging to the ligand-gated ion channel family, are activated by extracellular ATP [38, 39]. In the periphery, ATP can be released as a result of tissue injury, visceral distension, or sympathetic activation and can excite nociceptive primary afferents by acting as homomeric P2X3 or heteromeric P2X2/3 receptors

[38]. Recent studies have demonstrated that the level of ATP is increased by osteoclast activation under a high bone turnover state in osteoporosis and that several P2X receptor subunits exist in bone tissue [40–42]. Particularly, many studies have demonstrated that P2X7 receptor expressed in osteoclasts or osteoblasts and had significant roles in bone homeostasis or in association with pathogenesis of osteoporosis [43–46]. However, there are relatively few studies concerning expression and function of P2X2 [45] or P2X3 receptors in the bone. A recent study has indicated that a P2X3 receptor could contribute to bone cancer pain through the upregulation of increased local ATP levels in bone tissue [42]. P2X3 receptor, a specific ATP-sensitive ligand-gated ion channel, is selectively localized on peripheral and central processes of sensory afferent neurons and participates in the role of nociceptive signaling [47, 48]. The P2X3 receptor is natively expressed as a functional homomer and as a heteromultimeric combination with the P2X2 receptor [47–49]. Based on the results of those studies, we also hypothesize that increased local ATP underlying a high bone turnover state in osteoporosis activates the P2X receptor in bone tissue, and those activated P2X2/3 might has a role in the induction of skeletal pain.

We, therefore, examined effects of P2X2/3 and P2X3 antagonists on pain-like behaviors in OVX mice and demonstrated that those selective antagonists improved the threshold value of pain-like behavior in OVX mice compared with that in control mice treated with the vehicle alone. Significant improvement was observed in the pain threshold value of the paw flick test and the von Frey test after the administration (Fig. 2.6, unpublished data).

2.3.4 Involvement of Cytokines in Skeletal Pain Induction Related to Osteoclast Activation

We examined the expression of several inflammatory cytokines, IL-1β, IL-6, and TNF-α, in bone tissue as the expression of these cytokines is involved in chronic pain and is related to P2X receptor activation [39]. The expression of IL-1β, IL-6, and TNF-α in bone tissue was confirmed by reverse transcription-polymerase chain reaction RT-PCR. The expression level of Il-1β was significantly increased in OVX mice in comparison with that in sham mice, whereas no significant differences in expression of IL-6 and TNF-α were observed between the OVX and sham mice (unpublished data). Previous reports have indicated that P2X7 receptors regulate IL-1β secretion from bone marrow-derived macrophages [50] and the ATP-dependent activation of P2X7 receptors contributes to the release of cytokines of the IL-1 superfamily [51]. Thus, we speculate that P2X2/3 antagonists might directly inhibit IL-1β expression which in turn could be related to the observed improvements in pain-like behavior in OVX mice. We believe additional studies are needed to further elucidate the mechanisms.

2.4 Osteoclast-Mediated Pain in Osteoporosis

Our study demonstrated that OVX mice with osteoporosis have greater skeletal pain than normal mice and the higher serum TRAP5b levels associated with OVX decreased significantly following BP treatment and were significantly correlated with pain threshold values, further suggesting that the skeletal pain accompanying osteoporosis is possibly associated with osteoclastic activity. In addition, the antagonists of three types of nociceptors, TRPV1, ASIC3, and P2X2/3, improved the threshold values of pain-like behavior in OVX mice. Currently, our clinical study also showed that the low back pain in osteoporosis patients was significantly related to the level of bone resorption markers, but not to the value of BMD, the level of degenerative change, and the past history of old vertebral fractures [52].

We, therefore, speculate that inhibition of acid environment formation or improvement in the high bone turnover state resulting from osteoclast inactivation is one of mechanisms by which BP treatment improves skeletal pain in osteoporosis patients. Thus, antagonists to ASIC3 and P2X2/3 might be potential drug targets for the improvement of skeletal pain related to pathological conditions such as high bone turnover in osteoporosis, Paget's disease of the bone, or bone metastatic cancer.

References

1. Gass M, Dawson HB (2006) Preventing osteoporosis-related fractures: an overview. Am J Med 119:S3–S11
2. National Osteoporosis Foundation (2010) Clinician's guide to prevention and treatment of osteoporosis. National Osteoporosis Foundation, Washington, DC
3. Kann P, Schulz G, Schehler B, Beyer J (1993) Backache and osteoporosis in perimenopausal women. Med Klin 88:9–15
4. Iwamoto J, Takeda T, Sato Y, Uzawa M (2004) Effect of alendronate on metacarpal and lumbar bone mineral density, bone resorption and chronic back pain in postmenopausal women with osteoporosis. Clin Rheumatol 23:383–389
5. Cummings SR, Melton LJ (2002) Osteoporosis I: epidemiology and outcomes of osteoporotic fractures. Lancet 359:1761–1767
6. Ghinoi V, Brandi ML (2002) Clodronate: mechanisms of action on bone remodeling and clinical use in osteometabolic disorders. Expert Opin Pharmacother 3:1643–1656
7. Benford HL, McGowan NW, Helfrich MH, Nuttall ME, Rogers MJ (2001) Visualization of bisphosphonate-induced caspase-3 activity in apoptotic osteoclasts in vitro. Bone 28:465–473
8. Ohtori S, Akazawa T, Murata Y, Kinoshita T, Yamashita M, Nakagawa K, Inoue G, Nakamura J, Orita S, Ochiai N, Kishida S, Takasa M, Eguchi Y, Yamauchi K, Suzuki M, Aoki Y, Takahashi K (2010) Risedronate decreases bone resorption and improves low back pain in postmenopausal osteoporosis patients without vertebral fractures. J Clin Neurosci 17:209–213
9. Nagae M, Hiraga T, Wakabayashi H et al (2006) Osteoclasts play a part in due to the inflammation adjacent to bone. Bone 39:1107–1115
10. Lozano-Ondoua AN, Symons-Liguori AM, Vanderah TW (2013) Cancer induced bone pain: mechanisms and models. Neurosci Lett 537:52–59

11. Fulfaro F, Casuccio A, Ticozzi C, Ripamonti C (1998) The role of bisphosphonates in the treatment of painful metastatic bone disease. Pain 78:157–169
12. Iba K, Takada J, Wada T, Yamashita T (2010) Five-year follow-up of Japanese patients with Paget's disease of the bone after treatment with low-dose oral alendronate: a case series. J Med Case Rep 4:166
13. Astrom E, Soderhall S (2002) Beneficial effect of long term intravenous bisphosphonate treatment of osteogenesis imperfect. Arch Dis Child 86:356–364
14. Kawamata T, Ji W, Yamamoto J, Niiyama Y, Furuse S, Namiki A (2008) Contribution of transient receptor vanilloid subfamily 1 to endothelin-1-induced thermal hyperalgesia. Neuroscience 15:1067–1076
15. Luger NM, Sabino MA, Schwei MJ, Mach DB, Pomonis JD, Keyser CP, Rathbun M, Clohisy DR, Honore P, Yaksh TL, Mantyh PW (2002) Efficacy of systemic morphine suggests a fundamental difference in the mechanisms that generate bone cancer vs. inflammatory pain. Pain 99:397–406
16. Crawley JN (1999) Behavioral phenotyping of transgenic and knockout mice: experimental design and evaluation of general health, sensory functions, motor abilities, and specific behavioral tests. Brain Res 835:18–26
17. Hamba M, Muro M, Hiraide T, Ozawa H (1994) Expression of c-fos like protein of in the rat brain after injection of interleukin-1-beta into the gingiva. Brain Res Bull 34:61–68
18. Takayama B, Kikuchi S, Konno S, Sekiguchi M (2008) An immunohistochemical study of the antinociceptive effects of calcitonin in ovariectomized rats. BMC Muscloskelet Disord 9:164
19. Hunt SP, Pini A, Evan G (1987) Induction of c-fos like protein in spinal cord neurons following sensory stimulation. Nature 328:632–634
20. Shoji S, Tabuchi M, Miyazawa K, Yabumoto T, Tanaka M, Kadota M, Maeda H, Goto S (2010) Bisphosphonate inhibits bone turnover in OPG−/−mice via a depressive effect on both osteoclasts and osteoblasts. Calcif Tissue Int 87:181–192
21. Caterina MJ, Leffler A, Malmberg AB et al (2000) Impaired nociception and pain sensation in mice lacking the capsaicin receptor. Science 288:306–313
22. Abe Y, Iba K, Sasaki K et al (2015) Inhibitory effect of bisphosphonate on osteoclast function contributes to improved skeletal pain in ovariectomized mice. J Bone Miner Metab 33:125–134
23. Akesson K (2003) New approaches to pharmacological treatment of osteoporosis. Bull World Health Organ 81:657–664
24. Sanoja R, Cervero F (2010) Estrogen-dependent changes in visceral afferent sensitivity. Auton Neurosci 153:84–89
25. Sanoja R, Cervero F (2005) Estrogen-dependent abdominal hyperalgesia induced by ovariectomy in adult mice: a model of functional abdominal pain. Pain 118:243–253
26. Bonabello A, Galmozzia MR, Bruzzesea T, Zara GP (2001) Analgesic effect of bisphosphonates in mice. Pain 91:269–275
27. Orita S, Ohtori S, Koshi T, Yamashita M, Yamauchi K, Inoue G, Suzuki M, Eguchi Y, Kamoda H, Arai G, Ishikawa T, Miyagi M, Ochiai N, Kishida S, Takaso M, Aoki Y, Toyone T, Takahashi K (2010) The effects of risedronate and exercise on osteoporotic lumbar rat vertebrae and their sensory innervations. Spine 35:1974–1982
28. Van Offel JF, Schuerwegh AJ, Bridts CH, Bracke PG, Stevens WJ, De Clerck LS (2001) Influence of cyclic intravenous pamidronate on proinflammatory monocytic cytokine profiles and bone density in rheumatoid arthritis treated with low dose prednisolone and methotrexate. Clin Exp Rheumatol 19:13–20
29. Le Goff B, Heymann D (2011) Pharmacodynamics of bisphosphonates in arthritis. Expert Rev Clin Pharmacol 4:633–641
30. Roelofs AJ, Coxon FP, Ebetino FH, Lundy MW, Henneman ZJ, Nancollas GH, Sun S, Blazewska KM, Bala JL, Kashemirov BA, Khalid AB, Mckenna CE, Rogers MJ (2010) Fluorescent risedronate analogues reveal bisphosphonate uptake by bone marrow monocytes and localization around osteocytes in vivo. J Bone Miner Res 25:606–616

31. Teitelbaum SL (2000) Bone resorption by osteoclasts. Science 289:1504–1508
32. Rousselle AV, Heymann D (2002) Osteoclastic acidification pathways during bone resorption. Bone 30:533–540
33. Julius D, Basbaum AI (2001) Molecular mechanisms of nociception. Nature 413:203–210
34. Mantyh PW, Clohisy DR, Koltzenburg M, Hunt SP et al (2002) Molecular mechanisms of cancer pain. Nat Rev Cancer 2:201–209
35. Mach DB, Rogers SD, Sabino MC, Luger NM, Schwei MJ, Keyser CP, Pomonis JD, Clohisy DR, Adams DJ, O'Leary P, Mantyh PW (2002) Origins of skeletal pain: sensory and sympathetic innervation of the mouse femur. Neuroscience 113:155–166
36. Caterina MJ, Schumacher MA, Tominaga M, Rosen TA, Levine JD (1997) The capsaicin receptor: a heat-activated ion channel in the pain pathway. Nature 389:816–824
37. Nagae M, Hiraga T, Yoneda T (2007) Acidic microenvironment created by osteoclasts causes bone pain associated with tumor colonization. J Bone Miner Metab 25:99–104
38. Chizh BA, Illes P (2000) P2X receptors and nociception. Pharmacol Rev 53:553–568
39. Inoue K (2007) P2 receptors and chronic pain. Purinergic Signal 3:135–144
40. Rumney RMH, Wang N, Agrawal A, Gartland A (2012) Purinergic signaling in bone. Front Endocrinol (Lausanne) 3:116
41. Wang N, Gartland A (2014) Targeting P2 receptors-current progress in treating musculoskeletal disease. Curr Opin Pharmacol 16:122–126
42. Wu JX, Xu MY, Miao XR et al (2012) Functional up-regulation of P2X3 receptors in dorsal root ganglion in a rat model of bone cancer pain. Eur J Pain 16:1378–1388
43. Gallagher JA, Buckley KA (2002) Expression and function of P2 receptors in bone. J Musculoskelet Neuronal Interact 2(5):432–439
44. Pellegatti P, Falzoni S, Donvito G, Lemaire I, Di Virgilio F (2011) P2X receptor drives osteoclast fusion by increasing the extracellular adenosine concentration. FASEB J 25 (4):1264–1274
45. Hoebertz A, Townsend-Nicholson A, Glass R, Burnstock G, Arnett TR (2000) Expression of P2 receptors in bone and cultured bone cells. Bone 27:502–510
46. Grol MW, Panupinthu N, Korcok J, Sims SM, Dixon SJ (2009) Expression, signaling, and function of P2X7 receptors in bone. Purinergic Signal 5:205–221
47. Chen CC, Akopian AN, Sivilotti L, Colquhoun D, Brunstock G, Wood JN (1995) A P2X purinoceptor expressed by a subset of sensory neuron. Nature 377(6548):428–431
48. Lewis C, Neidhart S, Holy C, North RA, buell G, Surprenant A (1995) Coexpression of P2X2 and P2X3 receptor subunits can account for ATP-gated currents in sensory neurons. Nature 377(6548):432–435
49. Lynch KJ, Touma E, Niforatos W, Kage KL, Burgard EC, van Biesen T, Kowaluk EA, Jarvis MF (1999) Molecular and functional characterization of human P2X(2) receptors. Mol Pharmacol 56(6):1171–1181
50. Verhoef PA, Kertesy SB, Lundberg K et al (2005) Inhibitory effects of chloride on the activation of caspase-1, IL-1β secretion, and cytolysis by the P2X7 receptor. J Immunol 175:7623–7634
51. Martin U, Scholler J, Gurgel J et al (2009) Externalization of the leaderless cytokine IL-1F6 occurs in response to lipopolysaccharide/ATP activation of transduced bone marrow macrophages. J Immunol 183:4021–4030
52. Abe Y, Iba K, Sasaki K, Kanaya K, Takada J, Yamashita T (2013) Effect of bisphosphonate on the low back pain in osteoporosis patients. Orthop Surg Traumatol 3:283–287 (Japanese)

Chapter 3
Collagen Cross-Links as a Determinant of Bone Quality

Mitsuru Saito and Keishi Marumo

Abstract A reduction in sex hormones from middle age and increasing age and an increase in oxidative stress related to lifestyle-related diseases can also reduce bone material properties in terms of collagen posttranslational modification and cross-link formation. These changes lead to both qualitative and quantitative abnormalities in collagen, which is the major bone matrix protein. The intermolecular cross-link formation of collagen, which regulates bone material attributes, is a mechanism independent of bone remodeling. In other words, cross-link formation is controlled by the environment surrounding the bone matrix, comprising cellular functions, oxidative stress, and glycation level. Because oxidative stress is also a risk factor of arteriosclerosis and cardiovascular event, there is link between low bone quality and lifestyle-related disease. High levels of pentosidine in urine or blood, or mild hyperhomocysteinemia which suggests bone collagen abnormalities, might be used as surrogate markers for evaluating bone quality, assessing the risk of bone fracture. Patients with osteoporosis can be divided into three types on the basis of bone density and with bone quality. We are entering an age in which the treatment of osteoporosis will be personalized, with drugs administered depending on these types.

Keywords Bone quality • Collagen cross-link • Advanced glycation end products • Oxidative stress

3.1 Introduction

Bone mineral density (BMD) decreases after menopause, resulting in increased risk of bone fracture. In the 2010 Consensus Development Conference, the National Institute of Health (NIH) proposed the concept of bone quality as a factor that affects bone strength as well as BMD. At the conference, osteoporosis was defined as a disorder that decreases bone strength and bone strength is determined by BMD

M. Saito (✉) • K. Marumo
Department of Orthopaedic Surgery, The Jikei University School of Medicine, 3-25-8, Nishi-Shimbashi, Minato-ku, Tokyo 105-8461, Japan
e-mail: xlink67@gol.com

Y. Shimada, N. Miyakoshi (eds.), *Osteoporosis in Orthopedics*,
DOI 10.1007/978-4-431-55778-4_3

and bone quality [1]. Bone quality is determined by bone material properties and structural properties (microstructure: porosity of the cortical bone and trabecular structure of the cancellous bone) [2].

BMD and microstructure are mainly regulated by bone remodeling. Approximately 40 % of the cancellous bone and 4–7 % of the cortical bone are continually replaced annually due to bone remodeling, enabling bone structure and BMD to be maintained. In the remodeling process, there is minimal reduction in bone mass because the level of bone resorption due to osteoclasts is similar to the level of bone formation due to osteoblasts. However, the level of resorption can exceed the level of formation due to aging, reduced estrogen levels associated with menopause, or reduced androgen levels in men. Bone microstructure deteriorates and BMD decreases in such individuals.

Bone material properties are affected by various factors. Aging bone tissue is repaired in the process of bone remodeling. However, deterioration of bone material properties markedly advances due to increases in oxidative stress, glycation stress, reactive oxygen species, and carbonyl stress associated with aging and reduced sex hormone levels. Bone material properties are determined by the quality of the structural components. The structural components of the bone consist of mineral components made of hydroxyapatite and organic components made of collagen proteins. Collagen accounts for approximately 20 % of bone by weight but 50 % of bone by volume [2]. Bone is like a reinforced concrete building where collagen is the reinforcing bars and minerals are concrete. When reinforced concrete building deteriorates, repair work is done to prevent a collapse. In coastal-reinforced concrete structures, reinforcing bars rust severely due to salt air damage, and earthquake resistance decreases even if repair work is periodically performed. A similar process has been shown to occur in bones [2]. That is, collagen deteriorates with age due to increases in reactive oxygen species, oxidative stress, glycation stress, and carbonyl stress which correspond to salt air damage in reinforced concrete buildings. As a result, bone strength decreases. Approximately 30 % of bone strength is determined by bone quality in primary osteoporosis. When lifestyle disease-related osteoporosis, secondary osteoporosis, was examined, poor bone quality was found to markedly decrease bone strength [3, 4]. These lifestyle diseases included diabetes, arteriosclerosis, and renal impairment.

In osteoporosis, bone strength is decreased due to excessive collagen deterioration with age. This decreased bone strength cannot be explained by increased bone remodeling. In other words, deterioration of bone collagen cannot be assessed using markers (bone formation and bone resorption markers) that reflect bone remodeling or using calcium-based analysis. Deterioration of collagen is affected by reduction in osteoblast function and by glycation and oxidative stress involving matrix proteins [2]. Therefore, the assessment of fracture risk needs to evaluate material properties of collagen as well as structures and calcium-based parameters that are dependent on bone remodeling. Such assessment is necessary to evaluate fracture risk with good accuracy. In recent basic and clinical studies, the authors of the present article found that osteoporosis is not of a single disease type but can be classified into multiple types depending on BMD and bone collagen and proposed tailor-made treatment according to this classification [5].

3.2 Bone Collagen

Collagen maturity and deterioration with age are determined by the formation of intermolecular cross-links in posttranslational modification [2]. Collagen is made by strong bonds created from bridges between collagen molecules or "cross-links" (corresponding to beams connecting reinforcing bars in the building structure analogy). Collagen cross-links are classified into two types. One type is a genetically regulating enzymatic cross-linking. It involves an orderly bonding of molecules due to the actions of enzymes whose secretion is regulated by osteoblasts. This type of cross-link enables appropriate elasticity as mineralization is induced, and the resulting bone has flexibility and strength [6–8]. Thus, this type of cross-link is "beneficial and good bonding" (Figs. 3.1 and 3.2). The other type is an advanced glycation end product (AGE) cross-link, a "detrimental" senescent cross-link. It involves disorderly bonding of molecules, and the resulting bone is excessively rigid and becomes brittle like porcelain [2] (Figs. 3.1 and 3.2). Fragility of bone exhibits decreased enzymatic cross-linking and increased disadvantageous AGEs [2–4], and such detrimental intermolecular cross-linking of collagen occurs through a mechanism that is independent of bone remodeling. This mechanism is regulated by cellular function and systemic factors, such as oxidative stress and glycation (Figs. 3.1 and 3.3). Based on the aforementioned findings, one can increase the accuracy in the assessment of bone fracture risk by simultaneously measuring BMD and assessing bone quality from the perspective of collagen [2, 4, 9–11]. The amount of AGEs in bone is positively correlated with serum and urinary pentosidine levels. High levels of serum and urinary pentosidine are factors of fracture risk [9–11]. Pentosidine is one of the AGEs and has been used as a surrogate marker that reflects the total amount of AGEs. Methods are being developed to measure pentosidine levels in body tissues and fluids [2]. In 2012, the Japan Osteoporosis Society published the Japanese Guidelines for the Use of Biomarkers of Bone Turnover in Osteoporosis (Life Science Publishing). This publication described the following as bone matrix markers: serum and urinary pentosidine and homocysteine, which induces abnormal collagen cross-linking. The Japan Osteoporosis Society also published the Japanese 2013 Guidelines for Prevention and Treatment of Osteoporosis and the Clinical Practice Guide on Fracture Risk Associated with Lifestyle-Related Diseases. These two publications included the concept involving the mechanism of bone fragility caused by deterioration of bone collagen. Our laboratory was the first in the world to develop this concept. In these publications, our laboratory members were contributing authors in charge of the content related to the aforementioned, and the concept of osteoporosis was greatly changed in Japan.

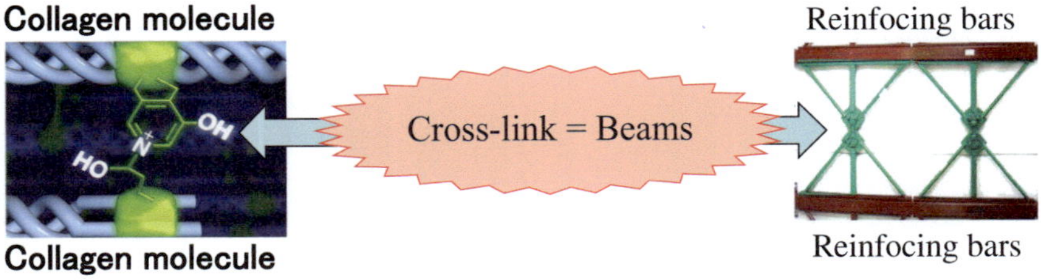

	Enzymatic crosslinks	Advanced glycation end products (AGEs)
Triggers	Enzymatic reaction Lysyl oxidase	Oxidative stress, glycation, Carbonyl stress
	Essential for calcification	Inhibiting calcification
Bone strength	⬆ Flexible, Stout	⬇ Fragile
	Immature and mature crosslinks	Senescent crosslinks

Fig. 3.1 Roles of collagen enzymatic and nonenzymatic AGEs cross-links. The strength of collagen fibers, aggregation of collagen molecules, is determined by collagen cross-links, which bond adjacent molecules. In an analogy with building structures, collagen cross-links correspond to beams that connect reinforcing bars. Collagen cross-links can be classified into two types: enzymatic cross-links that increase bone strength and detrimental, nonphysiological AGEs cross-links that weaken the bone

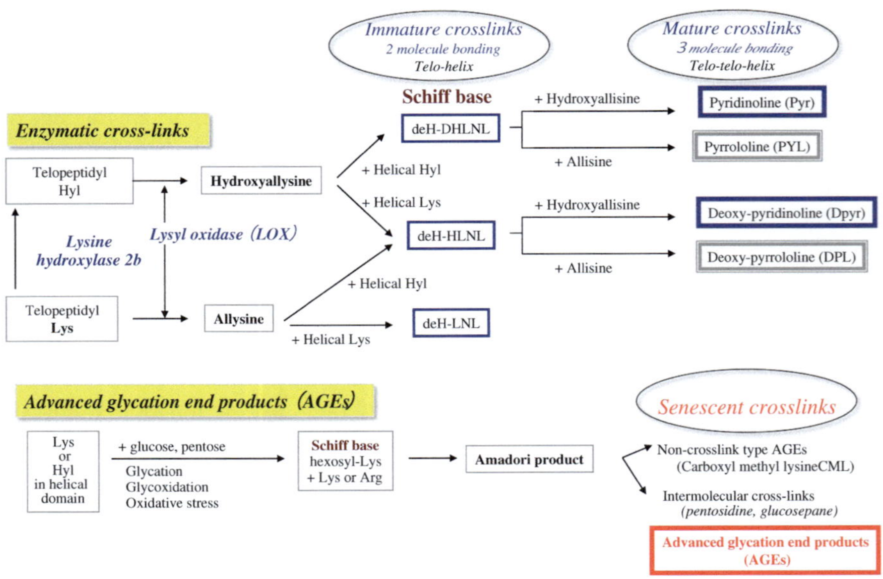

Fig. 3.2 Biochemistry of collagen cross-links

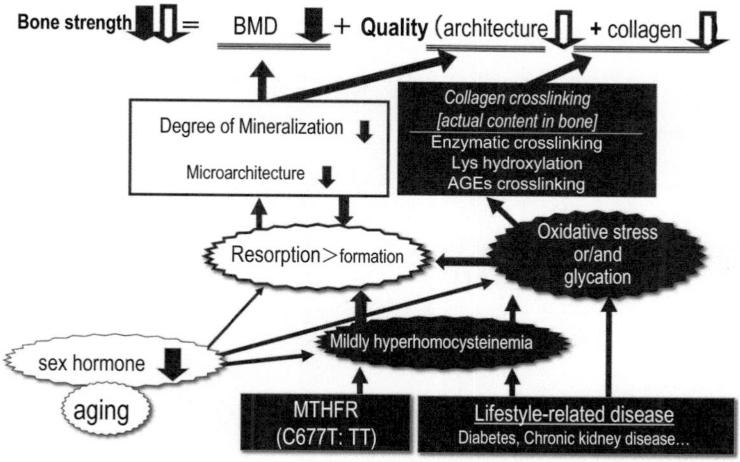

Fig. 3.3 Mechanism of reduction in bone strength. Bone quality is determined by bone material qualities and structural properties (microstructure). Sex hormone deficiency, aging, and lifestyle-related diseases induce not only reduction in bone mineral density (*BMD*) but also reduction in bone quality, particularly involving an AGE increase in collagen. Thus, bone strength is negatively affected. BMD and bone microstructure are parameters of bone strength that are dependent on bone remodeling. Material properties among bone quality factors are inhibited by the level of cellular function and the environment of the matrix surroundings (oxidative stress and glycation level)

3.3 Bone Quality Estimation

Oxidation and glycation increase when there is primary osteoporosis [12–14] (Fig. 3.4a), diabetes [15] (Fig. 3.4b), or renal failure [16] (Fig. 3.4c). In these diseases, we have shown that reduced formation of enzymatic cross-links and excessive AGE formation are induced in bone collagen, resulting in reduced bone strength. It has also been reported that AGEs increase in bone collagen with aging and bone strength decreases [2–4, 17]. Bone remodeling is increased due to aging and reduced sex hormones in both men and women. When bone remodeling is increased, collagen metabolism greatly increases. Therefore, it was unexpected that AGEs increase in bone collagen because AGEs are formed in proteins with long life-spans. However, there are factors related to AGE formation other than the life-span of matrix. If there is an environment that increases oxidation, glycation, or carbonyl stress (such as aging and lifestyle-related diseases), AGE formation is easily induced even with increased remodeling and shortened collagen life-span [2]. Not surprisingly, if bone remodeling is decreased and oxidation and glycation are increased, AGE formation is markedly increased in bone collagen. Diabetes corresponds to this type of pathological condition [15]. The aforementioned findings indicate that the assessment of bone fragility needs not only to measure calcium-based parameters and bone metabolism markers reflecting bone remodeling but also to simultaneously evaluate the deterioration of bone quality.

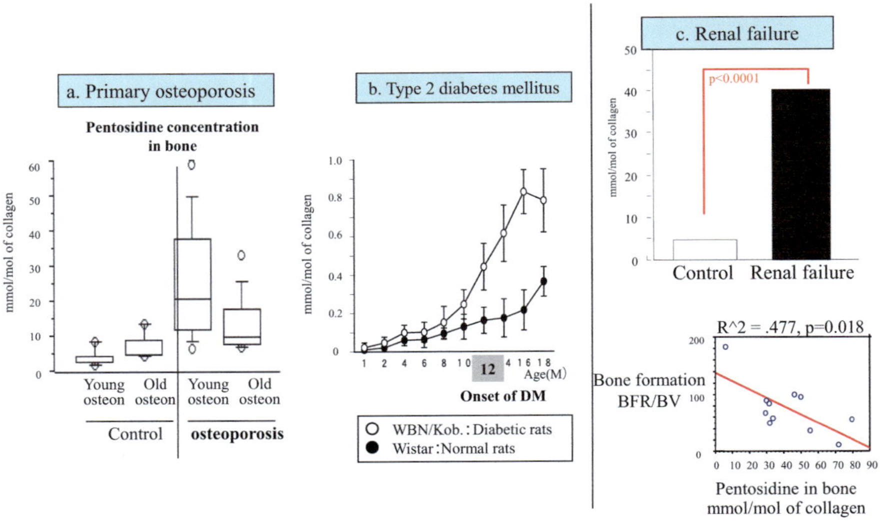

Fig. 3.4 AGE cross-linking pentosidine in bone collagen. (**a**) Excessive pentosidine formation in bone collagen in patients with primary osteoporosis. Bones were analyzed by dividing them into those with young osteons and those with old osteons. In a patient group with bone fractures, pentosidine was also increased even in young osteons, and AGE formation was seen from early stages of bone formation (References [12, 13]). (**b**) Collagen cross-links and bone strength in spontaneously diabetic rats. Pentosidine increased with progression of diabetes (–○-: WBN/Kob rats, –●-: Wistar rats). $*p < 0.05$: Comparison of age-matched controls and Wistar rats [15]. (**c**) AGE pentosidine concentrations in bone collagen and bone morphometry in hemodialysis patients. In hemodialysis patients, pentosidine levels increased markedly in bone, and the rate of bone formation decreased with such increase [16]

From such a perspective, one needs to understand the mechanism of detrimental AGE cross-linking and beneficial enzymatic cross-linking in collagen [2–4].

3.4 Roles of Enzymatic Cross-Links in Bone (Figs. 3.1 and 3.2)

The formation of enzymatic cross-links is strictly regulated by the expression of enzyme lysyl oxidase during collagen maturation and promote mineralization. The total number of such cross-links is dependent on the activity of lysyl oxidase, an enzyme secreted by osteoblasts themselves [6–8]. This cross-link formation plateaus before osteoid mineralizes [8]. If the enzyme activity is not sufficiently increased before osteoid mineralization, formation of enzymatic cross-links is decreased, and collagen fibers with sufficient strength cannot be formed [15]. We have shown that enzymatic cross-links were decreased 25 % when there was deficiency of vitamin B6, which is an essential cofactor for lysyl oxidase activity, and that bone strength was reduced without a decrease in BMD in healthy rats [18] and diabetic rats [15]. In another study, we examined a rat model of glucocorticoid-induced osteoporosis in which bone fracture risk increases before BMD decreases. Enzymatic cross-link formation decreased due to the inhibitory effect of glucocorticoid on lysyl oxidase, and bone strength decreased despite high BMD [19]. These results indicate that enzymatic cross-links are beneficial cross-links that positively affect bone strength. In a physiological environment, the total number of enzymatic cross-links peaks in human bone from childhood to 30 years of age, and there is no excessive induction of such cross-linking [20, 21].

3.5 Roles of AGEs in Bone (Figs. 3.1 and 3.2)

AGE formation is induced by increased oxidative stress and carbonyl stress and persistent hyperglycemia. Pentosidine and glucosepane are common AGE cross-links [2]. Bone tissue analysis has shown that the amount of pentosidine formed is positively correlated with the total amount of AGEs and that pentosidine can be used as a surrogate marker of overall AGEs [2]. They form in proteins with long life-spans because AGEs form in a time-dependent manner in a physiological environment [2, 12, 13, 20]. Pentosidine increases in bone collagen with aging, and bone strength decreases [2]. If patients have diseases that increase glycation or oxidation, excessive AGE formation occurs, which greatly exceeds time-dependent AGE formation [2–4, 14–16]. AGEs decrease bone strength in two ways. One way is by directly affecting cross-link formation [2–4]. The other way is by decreasing osteoblast function via cell surface receptors for AGE (RAGE) and by decreasing biological function through induction of apoptosis [22, 23]. When excised bone block was incubated by sugar solution to induce AGE cross-linking, the strength of these bone blocks was reduced, which is independent of BMD. Thus, bone strength is decreased not only with decreased cell function but also with excessive cross-linking alone due to AGEs. This result is important in better understanding deterioration of bone quality [24].

3.6 Age-Related Changes in Pentosidine Concentration in Bone, Serum, and Urine

Urinary [10] and serum [25] pentosidine levels increase with age just as pentosidine levels in bone collagen increase with age. The age-related AGE increase in bone is a phenomenon observed in both men and women [12, 13, 17, 20, 26].

Currently, the established methods of pentosidine measurement are precision instrumental analysis using high-performance liquid chromatography (HPLC) and enzyme-linked immunosorbent assay (ELISA) using antibodies against pentosidine. Measurements using ELISA are covered by the Japanese national health insurance as a routine test for patients with renal impairment (measured at SRL, Shinjuku-ku, Tokyo, Japan). In one study, our laboratory examined the correlation between pentosidine levels in bone collagen and serum and urinary pentosidine levels. In this study, samples from orthopedic surgery patients ($n = 100$) were used, and correlation was examined between measurements by HPLC and measurements by ELISA [27]. The results showed that pentosidine levels measured by HPLC were positively correlated among samples of bone collagen, blood, and urine. However, plasma pentosidine levels measured by ELISA were not significantly correlated with urinary or bone pentosidine levels measured by HPLC. One reason is that current ELISA method uses heat treatment as pretreatment for pentosidine measurement [28]. It has been indicated that AGEs such as pentosidine and carboxymethyllysine are increased as artifacts when heat treatment is used. Artifacts do not occur in acidic conditions even when heat treatment is used, and improvement in the pretreatment method should be considered based on such a finding [28]. Improved ELISA methods are currently being developed that enable measurement without heat treatment, and there is a potential in this method.

3.7 Bone Quality Markers: Pentosidine and Homocysteine

It is known that decreased enzymatic cross-linking and increased pentosidine formation in bone occur in primary osteoporotic patients (15–25 patients) with femoral neck fractures [2–4] (Fig. 3.4a). This result was consistent with the finding in our collaborative study with Shiraki et al. in which a high urinary pentosidine concentration was a fracture risk factor independent of BMD [10]. In the study of Shiraki et al., 432 postmenopausal women untreated for osteoporosis were examined longitudinally with the end point of incident vertebral fracture. The results showed that the highest quartile group of urinary pentosidine (creatinine correction: 47.5 pM/mg Cr) was a fracture risk factor (odds ratio: 1.3) independent of BMD, age, bone metabolism markers, prevalent fracture, and renal function (creatinine clearance) (Fig. 3.5). This risk was higher than that for BMD, a traditional fracture risk factor. In another report, we showed that serum homocysteine levels were high in patients with high pentosidine levels in bone collagen [13]. Homocysteine inhibits lysyl oxidase activity and causes decreased formation of beneficial cross-links. Simultaneously, homocysteine increases oxidative stress, which promotes AGE formation in collagen [14]. Mild hyperhomocysteinemia has been shown to be a fracture risk factor independent of BMD in studies such as the Rotterdam study [29], Framingham study [30], and Women's Health Initiative (WHI) cohort study [31]. Thus, hyperhomocysteinemia began to be considered a factor that reduces bone quality [2, 4, 32]. In a recent study, meta-analysis showed that hyperhomocysteinemia is a fracture risk factor independent of BMD in both men and women [33].

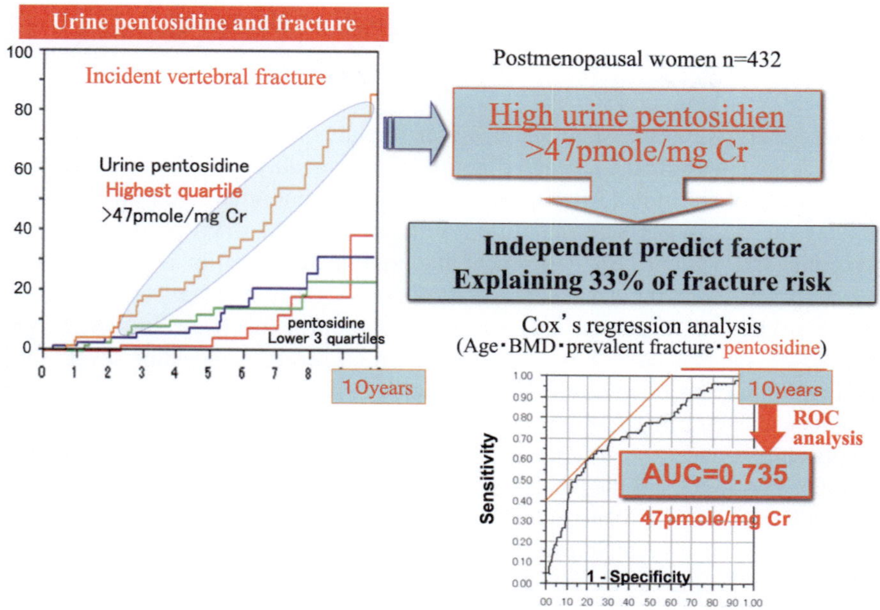

Fig. 3.5 Urinary pentosidine levels and fracture risk. A prospective study was conducted on 432 postmenopausal women using incident fracture as an end point. The results showed that the highest quartile group of urinary pentosidine (creatinine correction: 47.5 pM/mg Cr) was a fracture risk factor independent of BMD, age, bone metabolism markers, prevalent fracture, and renal function (creatinine clearance). In addition, 93 % of incident vertebral fractures could be explained by BMD, prevalent fracture, age, and urinary pentosidine concentration, and a high urinary pentosidine level was shown to be a predictor of fracture, which was attributed 33 % of the fracture risk (AUC = 0.735) [10]

In one study, we used ovariectomized rabbits to examine whether hyperhomocysteinemia induces AGE formation in bone collagen [14]. The results showed that when hyperhomocysteinemia was induced using a 1 % methionine diet, decreased enzymatic cross-linking in bone collagen and increased pentosidine formation were induced, and bone strength decreased without a decrease in BMD. Even in a general population, high serum homocysteine levels induce cross-link abnormalities in bone collagen and are thought to increase the fracture risk by reducing bone quality [2]. Recently, the OFELY study indicated that many fracture events occurred in patients with high urinary pentosidine levels, and a replication study was performed to investigate the importance of bone quality assessment [34].

3.8 Other Factors for Poor Bone Quality: Diabetes and Chronic Kidney Disease

In meta-analysis, Vestergaard showed that fractures occur in patients with type 2 diabetes and high BMD, and deterioration of bone quality began to be considered as the cause of fractures [35]. The authors of the present article examined spontaneously diabetic WBN/Kob rats. The results showed that when persistent hyperglycemia and vitamin B6 deficiency due to impaired insulin action develop, enzymatic cross-linking decreases and AGE cross-linking increases in bone collagen, resulting in decreased bone strength without a decrease in BMD [15] (Fig. 3.4b). Other studies have reported that high serum pentosidine levels [36] and high urinary pentosidine levels [37] become independent fracture risk factors in patients with type 2 diabetes. These results were consistent with the aforementioned relationship between pentosidine increase in bone collagen and decrease in bone strength. The authors of the present article found that pentosidine levels increase in bone collagen when oxidative stress increases with increased AGE formation in collagen and when renal impairment occurs, which increases oxidative and carbonyl stress [16] (Fig. 3.4c). In addition, the authors showed that osteoblast function decreased as AGE formation increased in bone collagen [16]. Clinical application of bone quality markers can also be expected in patients with diabetes and renal impairment [2–4].

3.9 Classification of Osteoporosis by BMD and Bone Quality Markers (Fig. 3.6)

The increased fracture risk associated with aging cannot be explained by decreased BMD alone or by decreased bone quality alone. The degrees to which BMD and bone quality decrease vary by individual. In one study, our laboratory examined 502 postmenopausal women (Nagano cohort study) and assessed the fracture risk by type of bone fragility. Bone fragility of each woman was classified into one of the following three types based on BMD and bone quality [6] (Fig. 3.6): osteoporosis with low BMD, osteoporosis with low bone quality, and osteoporosis with a combination of both types (osteoporosis with low BMD + low bone quality). Patients with low BMD osteoporosis have BMD of <70 % of young adult mean (YAM). Patients with low bone quality osteoporosis have high serum levels of homocysteine or urinary pentosidine. When the fracture risk was compared with patients who had BMD of >80 % of YAM, the fracture risk was increased 3.6-fold in patients with low BMD osteoporosis and was increased 1.5-fold in patients with low bone quality osteoporosis. It was increased markedly at 7.2-fold in patients with low BMD + low bone quality osteoporosis due to their synergistic effect. The ratio of patients by type was 5:3:2 for low BMD type, low bone quality type, and

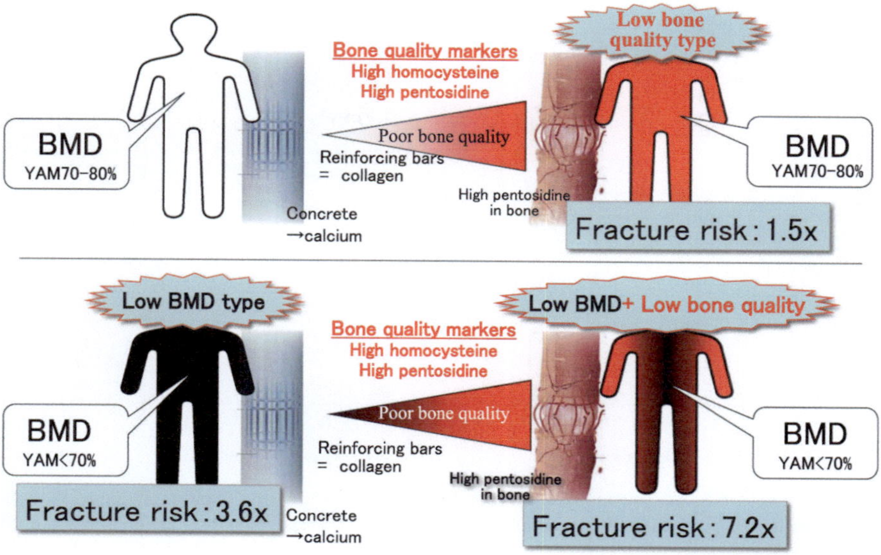

Fig. 3.6 Classification of osteoporosis by BMD and bone quality markers (homocysteine and pentosidine). Increases in fracture risk in osteoporosis were divided into three patterns using the finding that hyperhomocysteinemia causes AGE (pentosidine) accumulation in bone. "Low bone quality osteoporosis" is a condition in which fracture risk increases with the presence of abnormal homocysteine metabolism alone, even if the BMD is ≥ 70 % of young adult mean (*YAM*). "Low BMD osteoporosis" is a condition in which fracture risk increases due to low BMD even if homocysteine metabolism is satisfactory. "Low BMD + low bone quality osteoporosis" is a condition in which both BMD and homocysteine metabolism decrease. The fracture risk was increased 1.5-fold in patients with low bone quality osteoporosis, 3.6-fold in patients with low BMD osteoporosis, and 7.2-fold in patients with low BMD + low bone quality osteoporosis. *YAM* young adult mean BMD (Modified from Shiraki et al. [9])

low BMD + low bone quality type, respectively, showing that the low bone quality type was not rare.

3.10 Potential of Therapeutic Drug Use Based on BMD and Bone Quality Markers

In a recent study, the authors of the present article have shown that drugs for osteoporosis can be used based on osteoporosis type classified by BMD and bone quality [38]. Bisphosphonate, anti-resorption, was administered to 251 postmenopausal patients with osteoporosis, and factors were analyzed which affected incident bone fractures after drug administration began. The study examined BMD, bone resorption and formation markers, presence or absence of prevalent fracture, age, and bone quality markers (plasma homocysteine and urinary pentosidine) at baseline. The results showed that independent risk factors for incident fracture were

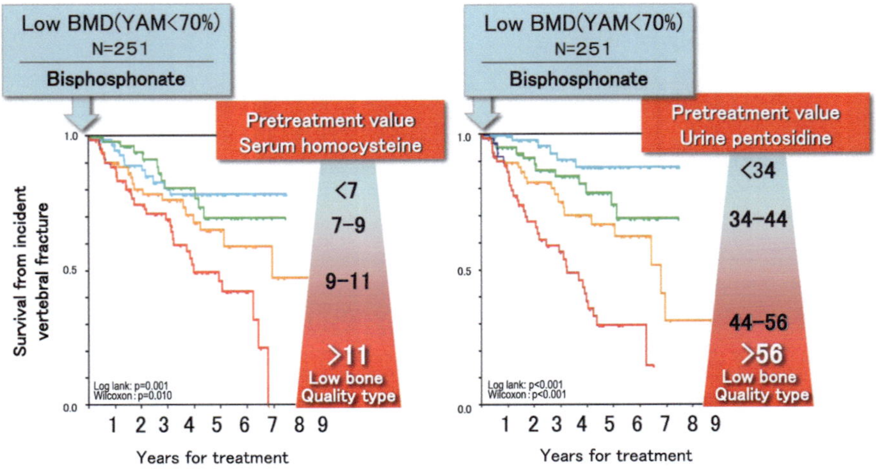

Fig. 3.7 Usefulness of preliminary measurements of bone quality markers in patients with resistance to bisphosphonates. Bisphosphonates were administered to 251 postmenopausal patients with osteoporosis (low BMD). A longitudinal study was performed on incident fractures in these patients after bisphosphonate administration was begun. Even when bone metabolism markers improved and BMD increased, there was a lower preventive effect on fracture in patients with higher bone quality marker levels (serum homocysteine and urinary pentosidine levels) at the beginning of treatment [38]

a high plasma homocysteine level and a high urinary pentosidine level at the commencement of treatment. Even when BMD was increased, the risk for incident fracture was increased 1.6-fold in patients with low BMD + low bone quality osteoporosis (Fig. 3.7). Bisphosphonates inhibit bone resorption and increase BMD but do not affect the formation of enzymatic cross-links in bone collagen [38]. In addition, bone collagen renewal is inhibited when metabolism is excessively inhibited long term by bisphosphonates. Then AGE cross-links increase in a time-dependent manner and microcracks develop in bone. Thus, it is important to monitor the level of bone metabolism over time using bone resorption and formation markers in clinical practice. The aforementioned findings indicate the need to improve the quality of bone collagen in addition to the importance of increased BMD in patients with low BMD + low bone quality osteoporosis [5].

3.11 Usefulness of Bone Quality Marker Level as a Risk Factor for Severe Vertebral Collapse

In the Nagano cohort study, the authors of the present article examined 1475 postmenopausal women and found that bone quality markers can be an independent risk factor for severe vertebral collapse (collapse of vertebral height of ≥40 %) [39] (Fig. 3.8). Low BMD was also extracted as a risk factor for severe vertebral

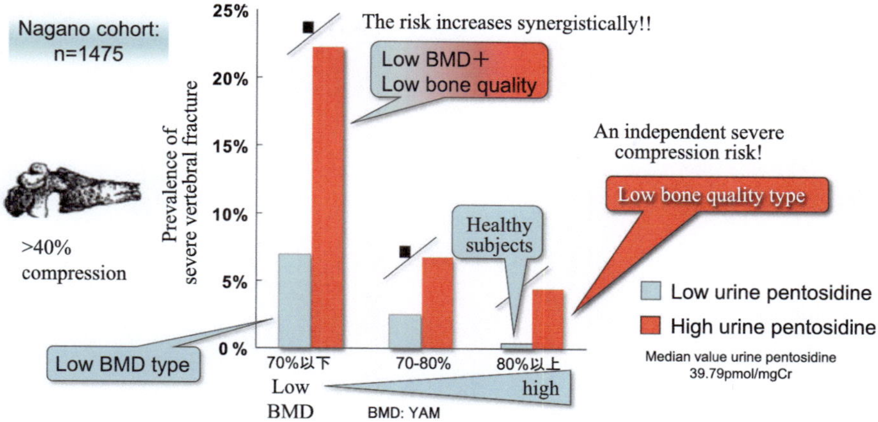

Fig. 3.8 High levels of bone quality markers as a risk factor for severe vertebral collapse. Since severe vertebral collapse is an independent risk factor for subsequent incident fracture, it can be considered a "severe type" of osteoporosis. BMD and bone quality are each an independent risk factor for severe vertebral collapse. The Nagano cohort study showed that the risk for severe collapse is greatly increased in patients with "low BMD + low bone quality osteoporosis" in which there is abnormality in both BMD and bone quality. In the building structure analogy, concrete corresponds to BMD and reinforcing bars correspond to collagen. When concrete and reinforcing bars deteriorate, the likelihood of building collapse becomes higher. Once the building begins to collapse, it can completely collapse easily [39]

collapse, but the frequency of severe vertebral collapse markedly increased when there was a high level of urinary pentosidine, a bone quality marker. Thus, one must be mindful that when patients have both low BMD and high urinary pentosidine levels, the risk for incident fracture increases and simultaneously the risk for severe vertebral collapse increases. Such patients with severe collapse are in a high risk group for incident fracture (vertebral or proximal femoral fracture). Therefore, it is necessary to assess both BMD and bone quality and to provide proper therapeutic intervention.

3.12 Drugs and Vitamins that Improve Bone Quality from the Perspective of Bone Collagen (Table 3.1) Vitamins B6 and K2

Vitamin B6 is an essential coenzyme for lysyl oxidase, an enzyme involved in the formation of enzymatic cross-links. It is also a vitamin with an anti-AGE effect. The authors of the present article used diabetic WBN/Kob rats that develop increased AGE cross-links associated with increased oxidative stress and hyperglycemia and that develop decreased enzymatic cross-links due to B6 deficiency. The rats received pyridoxal 5′-phosphate as vitamin B6, and its effects on

Table 3.1 Effects of drugs on BMD and bone quality

		Anti-resorption	Antioxidant, homocysteine reduction	Osteoblastic function improvement, minimodeling		Osteoblastic function improvement	Osteoblastic function improvement, new bone formation
		Bisphosphonate	SERM	Active vitamin D3		Vit. K2 Vit. B6	PTH (teriparatide)
BMD	Mineralization	↑	↗	Alfacalcidol	Eldecalcitol	→	↑
				→	↗		
Bone quality	**Enzymatic cross-links**	→	↑	↑	↑	↑	↑
	AGEs	→ or ↗	↓	→	↓	↓	↓
	Reference	[21]	[14]	[19, 42]		[40]	[45]

bone strength, BMD, and bone quality were examined [40]. The same rats received menatetrenone as vitamin K2, menatetrenone (MK4), which can improve bone quality by acting on osteoblasts. Its effects on the aforementioned items were examined [40]. The results showed that no significant improvement in bone collagen or bone strength was observed with 2-month administration of vitamin B6 and vitamin K2. However, enzymatic cross-links significantly increased and AGE cross-links significantly decreased with 4-month administration. Bone strength was found to significantly increase even without an increase in BMD. It can be said that vitamin B6 has the potential as a drug that improves bone quality. In Japan, menatetrenone can be used as a drug for osteoporosis and can be expected to show effectiveness in low bone quality osteoporosis.

3.13 Active Form of Vitamin D3

The active form of vitamin D3 acts as the nutrient vitamin D, which promotes calcium absorption from the intestine. It also has a pharmacological effect by binding to intranuclear receptors in osteoblasts, the vitamin D receptors (VDRs). The active form of vitamin D3 has been shown to improve bone collagen cross-link formation by acting on osteoblasts. To an osteoblastic cell culture system, Nagaoka et al. added native vitamin D or alfacalcidol as an active form of vitamin D3, and the effect on collagen cross-links was examined. They showed that only alfacalcidol increased lysyl oxidase activity and promoted the formation of enzymatic cross-links [41]. The authors of the present article administered alfacalcidol to ovariectomized rats of an osteoporosis model and found that bone strength increased due to increased enzymatic cross-links in bone collagen [42]. In other words, the active form of vitamin D3 can be thought to be a drug that improves bone quality. More recently, we reported that eldecalcitol (ELD), an active form of vitamin D analog, approved for the treatment of osteoporosis in Japan, increases lumbar spine bone mineral density (BMD), suppresses bone turnover markers, and improves bone quality in terms of both enzymatic and AGEs cross-link formation in ovariectomized monkey model [43]. Bone antiresorptive agents such as bisphosphonates slow down bone remodeling so that bone mineralization, bone microdamage, and nonenzymatic collagen cross-links all increase. Bone anabolic agents such as parathyroid hormone decrease bone mineralization and bone microdamage by stimulating bone remodeling. ELD did not fit into either category. Histological analysis indicated that the ELD treatment strongly suppressed bone resorption by reducing the number of osteoclasts while also stimulating focal bone formation without prior bone resorption (bone minimodeling). These bidirectional activities of ELD may account for its unique effects on bone quality.

3.14 Selective Estrogen Receptor Modulators (SERMs)

Oxidative stress and serum homocysteine concentration cause deterioration in bone quality, and they are decreased by SERMs [44, 45]. The authors of the present article induced hyperhomocysteinemia in ovariectomized rabbits and administered raloxifene to them. The bone mineralization levels and collagen cross-links were analyzed, and the increase in bone strength was examined [14]. In this rabbit model, cross-link abnormalities were observed that were similar to those observed in human osteoporosis with low bone quality, which the authors reported in another report. In other words, there was induction of decreased enzymatic cross-link formation and increased AGE cross-link pentosidine formation, and bone strength was decreased without a decrease in BMD. When raloxifene was used as a SERM in the same model, BMD and bone metabolism markers did not show clear changes after 4-month administration. However, the serum homocysteine concentration was reduced approximately 40 %. When collagen cross-links were analyzed, enzymatic cross-links were significantly increased, and AGE cross-links were decreased (65 % decrease) due to raloxifene administration. Based on the aforementioned results, raloxifene was thought to be suitable for patients without markedly decreased BMD and with high urinary and serum pentosidine levels or high serum homocysteine levels, markers for bone quality.

3.15 Teriparatide (Parathyroid Hormone)

Parathyroid hormone regulates calcium and promotes both bone formation and resorption. Hyperparathyroidism occurs when there is continuous and excessive action of parathyroid hormone. It is a condition in which bone remodeling is markedly increased (bone resorption > bone formation), resulting in osteoporosis. When continuous administration or intermittent administration of once a week is used, bone mass is increased where an increase in bone formation exceeds an increase in bone resorption and bone quality improves. Consequently, fracture risk decreases. Teriparatide is an agent that promotes bone formation and contains a sequence of 34 N-terminal amino acids identical to the biologically active region of parathyroid hormone. The authors of the present article used ovariectomized monkeys with a bone quality abnormality similar to human osteoporosis. Teriparatide was administered to said monkeys for 18 months, and analysis was performed on the following parameters which determine bone strength: bone mass, bone mineralization level, bone microstructure, bone collagen content, and collagen cross-links [46]. The results showed that teriparatide administration not only increased BMD but also significantly increased collagen content and enzymatic cross-links and decreased AGE cross-link pentosidine. This improvement in bone collagen cross-links was shown to be an independent factor that increases bone strength. These results indicate that teriparatide is suitable for patients who have osteoporosis with low BMD + low bone quality. There are patients who develop incident fractures despite receiving oral drugs for osteoporosis (including bisphosphonates) for at least one year. In such patients, clinicians should consider changing the drug to teriparatide because some patients could also have low bone quality.

3.16 Conclusion

The concept of bone quality was included in three Japanese guidelines: the Japanese 2013 Guidelines for Prevention and Treatment of Osteoporosis, the Clinical Practice Guide on Fracture Risk Associated with Lifestyle-related Diseases, and the Japanese Guidelines for the Use of Biomarkers of Bone Turnover in Osteoporosis. Our laboratory was responsible for writing chapters in these three guidelines.

In summary, when physiological, enzymatic-dependent cross-links decrease between bone collagen molecules and AGEs (aged cross-links) increase, bone strength decreases and fracture risk increases. Pentosidine is a surrogate marker whose level reflects the total amount of AGEs. A pentosidine increase in bone collagen occurs by a mechanism independent of an increase in bone resorption. The pentosidine increase is caused by (1) hyperhomocysteinemia, (2) increased oxidative stress, (3) increased carbonyl stress, or (4) increased glycation. Thus, existing bone resorption markers cannot be used to assess excessive collagen deterioration associated with aging. Serum homocysteine and urinary and serum pentosidine can potentially be bone quality (matrix) markers for predicting fracture risk caused by decreased bone quality, which cannot be assessed by BMD alone. Pentosidine and homocysteine measurements are presently not covered by the Japanese national insurance for the evaluation of osteoporosis. However, the 2012 Japanese Guidelines for the Use of Biomarkers of Bone Turnover in Osteoporosis mentioned that pentosidine and homocysteine might be used in future clinical practice as bone matrix markers to evaluate fracture risks, if further evidence is accumulated. It should be noted that there are some issues related to measurement. When an ELISA method is used to measure serum pentosidine (analysis that can be currently outsourced), heat treatment is used as a pretreatment. Heat treatment has been shown to cause AGE artifact formation and greatly lowers the accuracy at low pentosidine concentrations. Thus, it is necessary to improve the ELISA method and to confirm its correlation with HPLC method. In addition, blood and urinary pentosidine concentrations are affected by renal function, and pentosidine levels increase with age not only in bone but also in the blood vessels, cartilage, and skin. In the Nagano cohort study, the authors of the present article found that a high urinary pentosidine level was an independent fracture risk factor even after correction for renal function (creatinine clearance). Therefore, pentosidine is not a marker that merely reflects decreased bone quality due to renal impairment. In addition, formation of AGE increases in collagen in a “population with excessive aging” having increased systemic oxidative stress. Therefore, arteriosclerosis can develop, and simultaneously bone fractures can occur due to deterioration in bone quality. In other words, serum pentosidine and urinary pentosidine can be considered "markers for excessive aging" that predict cardiovascular events and bone fractures due to bone quality deterioration. Osteoporosis has various manifestations depending on the combinations of different levels of BMD and bone quality. Thus, it is necessary to simultaneously assess both BMD and bone quality and to select a more effective drug or a combination of drugs.

Conflicts of Interest The authors declare no conflict of interest regarding this review article.

References

1. NIH consensus Development Panel on Osteoporosis Prevention, Diagnosis, and Therapy (2001) Osteoporosis prevention, diagnosis and therapy. JAMA 285:785–795
2. Saito M, Marumo K (2010) Collagen cross-links as a determinant of bone quality: a possible explanation for bone fragility in aging, osteoporosis, and diabetes mellitus. Osteoporos Int 21: 195–214
3. Saito M, Marumo K (2013) Bone quality and diabetes. Front Endocrinol. doi:10.3389/fendo.2013.00072
4. Saito M, Kida Y, Kato S et al (2014) Diabetes, collagen, and bone quality. Curr Osteoporos Rep 12:181–188
5. Saito M, Marumo K (2011) Tailor-made treatment and drug choice in osteoporosis: importance of bone density and quality associated in the variety of bone strength determinants. Bone 25:25–32 (in Japanese)
6. Saito M, Soshi S, Fujii K (2003) Effect of hyper- and microgravity on collagen post-translational controls of MC3T3-E1 osteoblasts. J Bone Miner Res 18:1695–1705
7. Maruhashi T, Kii I, Saito M et al (2010) Interaction between periostin and BMP-1 promotes proteolytic activation of lysyl oxidase. J Biol Chem 85:13294–132303
8. Saito M, Soshi S, Tanaka T et al (2003) Intensity-related differences in collagen post-translational modification in MC3T3-E1 osteoblasts after exposure to low and high intensity pulsed ultrasound. Bone 35:644–655
9. Shiraki M, Urano T, Kuroda T et al (2008) The synergistic effect of bone mineral density and methylenetetrahydrofolate reductase (MTHFR) polymorphism (C677T) on fractures. J Bone Miner Metab 26:595–602
10. Shiraki M, Kuroda T, Tanaka S et al (2008) Non-enzymatic collagen cross-links induced by glycoxidation (pentosidine) predicts vertebral fractures. J Bone Miner Metab 26:93–100
11. Tanaka S, Kuroda T, Saito M et al (2011) Urinary pentosidine improves risk classification using fracture risk assessment tools for postmenopausal women. J Bone Miner Res 26: 2778–2784
12. Saito M, Fujii K, Soshi S et al (2006) Reductions in degree of mineralization and enzymatic collagen cross-links and increases in glycation induced pentosidine in the femoral neck cortex in cases of femoral neck fracture. Osteoporos Int 17:986–995
13. Saito M, Fujii K, Marumo K (2006) Degree of mineralization-related collagen crosslinking in the femoral neck cancellous bone in cases of hip fracture and controls. Calcif Tissue Int 79: 160–168
14. Saito M, Marumo K, Soshi S et al (2010) Raloxifene ameliorates detrimental enzymatic and nonenzymatic collagen cross-links and bone strength in rabbits with hyperhomocysteinemia. Osteoporos Int 21:655–666

15. Saito M, Fujii K, Mori Y et al (2006) Role of collagen enzymatic and glycation induced cross-links as a determinant of bone quality in the spontaneously diabetic WBN/Kob rats. Osteoporos Int 17:1514–1523
16. Mitome J, Yamamoto H, Saito M et al (2011) Nonenzymatic cross-linking pentosidine increase in bone collagen and are associated with disorders of bone mineralization in dialysis patients. Calcif Tissue Int 88:521–529
17. Saito M (1999) Age-related changes in biochemical characteristics of collagen from human weight-bearing and non-weightbearing bone. Tokyo Jikeikai Ika Daigaku Zasshi 114:327–337. http://sciencelinks.jp/j-east/article/200010/000020001000A0286989.php (in Japanese)
18. Fujii K, Kajiwara T, Kurosu H (1979) Effect of vitamin B6 deficiency on the crosslink formation of collagen. FEBS Lett 97:193–195
19. Saito M, Marumo K, Ushiku C et al (2011) Effects of alfacalcidol on mechanical properties and collagen cross-links of the femoral diaphysis in glucocorticoid-treated rats. Calcif Tissue Int 88:314–324
20. Saito M, Marumo K, Fujii K et al (1997) Single column high – performance liquid chromatographic – fluorescence detection of immature, mature and senescent cross-links of collagen. Anal Biochem 253:26–32
21. Saito M, Mori S, Mashiba T et al (2008) Collagen maturity, glycation induced-pentosidine, and mineralization are increased following 3-year treatment with incadronate in dogs. Osteoporos Int 19:1343–1354
22. Sanguineti R, Storace D, Monacelli F et al (2008) Pentosidine effects on human osteoblasts in vitro. Ann N Y Acad Sci 1126:166–172
23. Ogawa N, Yamaguchi T, Yano S et al (2007) The combination of high glucose and advanced glycation end-products (AGEs) inhibits the mineralization of osteoblastic MC3T3-E1 cells through glucose-induced increase in the receptor for AGEs. Horm Metab Res 39:871875
24. Garnero P, Borel O, Gineyts E et al (2006) Extracellular post-translational modifications of collagen are major determinants of biomechanical properties of fetal bovine cortical bone. Bone 38:300–309
25. Takahashi M, Oikawa M, Nagano A (2000) Effect of age and menopause on serum concentrations of pentosidine, an advanced glycation end product. J Gerontol A Biol Sci Med Sci 55: M137–M140
26. Odetti P, Rossi S, Monacelli F et al (2005) Advanced glycation end products and bone loss during aging. Ann N Y Acad Sci 1043:710–717
27. Kida Y, Saito T, Soshi S et al (2010) The establishment of non-invasive bone quality: skin auto-fluorescence, urinary excretion, and plasma pentosidine correlate to bone collagen AGEs. Osteoporos Jpn 18:25–28 (Japanese)
28. Nakano M, Kubota M, Owada S et al (2013) The pentosidine concentration in human blood specimens is affected by heating. Amino Acids 44:1451–1456
29. McLean RR, Jacques PF, Selhub J et al (2004) Homocysteine as a predictive factor for hip fracture in older persons. N Engl J Med 350:2042–2049
30. van Meurs JB, Dhonukshe-Rutten RA, Pluijm SM et al (2004) Homocysteine levels and the risk of osteoporotic fracture. N Engl J Med 350:2033–2041
31. Leboff MS, Narweker R, LaCroix A et al (2009) Homocysteine levels and risk of hip fracture in postmenopausal women. J Clin Endocrinol Metab 94:1207–1213
32. McLean RR, Hannan MT (2007) B vitamins, homocysteine, and bone disease: epidemiology and pathophysiology. Curr Osteoporos Rep 5:112–119
33. Yang J, Hu X, Zhang Q et al (2012) Homocysteine level and risk of fracture: a meta-analysis and systematic review. Bone 51:376–382
34. Gineyts E, Munoz F, Bertholon C et al (2010) Urinary levels of pentosidine and risk of fracture in post menopausal women: the OFELY study. Osteoporos Int 21:243–250
35. Vestergaard P (2007) Discrepancies in bone mineral density and fracture risk in patients with type 1 and type 2 diabetes: a meta-analysis. Osteoporos Int 18:427–444

36. Yamamoto M, Yamaguchi T, Yamauchi M et al (2007) Serum pentosidine levels are positively associated with the presence of vertebral fractures in postmenopausal women with type 2 diabetes. J Clin Endocrinol Metab 93:1013–1019
37. Schwartz AV, Garnero P, Hillier TA et al (2009) Health, aging, and body composition study. Pentosidine and increased fracture risk in older adults with type 2 diabetes. J Clin Endocrinol Metab 94:2380–2386
38. Shiraki M, Kuroda T, Shiraki Y et al (2011) Urinary pentosidine and plasma homocysteine levels at baseline predict future fractures in osteoporosis patients under bisphosphonate treatment. J Bone Miner Metab 29:62–70
39. Kuroda T, Tanaka S, Saito M et al (2013) Plasma level of homocysteine associated with severity of vertebral fracture in postmenopausal women. Calcif Tissue Int 93:269–275
40. Saito M, Fujii K, Soshi S et al (2005) Effects of vitamin B6 and vitamin K2 on bone mechanical properties and collagen cross-links in spontaneously diabetic WBN/Kob rats. J Bone Miner Res 20(supple):SU420 (abstract)
41. Nagaoka H, Mochida Y, Atsawasuwan P et al (2008) 1,25(OH)2D3 regulates collagen quality in an osteoblastic cell culture system. Biochem Biophys Res Commun 377:674–678
42. Saito M, Shiraishi A, Ito M et al (2010) Comparison of effects of alfacalcidol and alendronate on mechanical properties and bone collagen cross-links of callus in the fracture repair rat model. Bone 46:1170–1179
43. Saito M, Grynpas MD, Burr DB et al (2015) Treatment with eldecalcitol positively affects mineralization, microdamage, and collagen crosslinks in primate bone. Bone 73:8–15. doi:10.1016/j.bone.2014.11.025
44. Walsh BW, Paul S, Wild RA et al (2000) The effects of hormone replacement therapy and raloxifene on C-reactive protein and homocysteine in healthy postmenopausal women: a randomized, controlled trial. J Clin Endocrinol Metab 85:214–218
45. Mann V, Huber C, Kogianni G et al (2007) The antioxidant effect of estrogen and selective estrogen receptor modulators in the inhibition of osteocyte apoptosis in vitro. Bone 40:674–684
46. Saito M, Marumo K, Kida Y et al (2011) Changes in the contents of enzymatic immature, mature, and non-enzymatic senescent cross-links of collagen after once-weekly treatment with human parathyroid hormone (1–34) for 18 months contribute to improvement of bone strength in ovariectomized monkeys. Osteoporos Int 22:2373–2383

Chapter 4
Assessment of Femoral Geometric Strength in Osteoporosis Using Hip Structure Analysis

Junichi Takada

Abstract Hip structure analysis (HSA) was applied to measure proximal femur geometry and strength using conventional dual-energy X-ray absorptiometry. The structural parameters were cross-sectional area (CSA, index of resistance to forces directed along the long axis), section modulus (index of resistance to bending forces), and buckling ratio (index of cortical stability). HSA has been investigated in racial and gender differences, aging trends, and relations among bone biological makers, body composition, and physical activity and treatment effects by osteoporotic medications. In most of the studies on HSA by antiresorptive drugs (raloxifene, alendronate, risedronate, minodronate, denosumab), the percent change of section modulus was higher than that of bone mineral density (BMD), and the improvements in section modulus are superior in intertrochanter than in femoral neck. On the other hand, teriparatide improved section modulus and BMD; however, the tendency to change in these parameters is different from antiresorptive drugs. The improvement in section modulus was approximately similar in BMD, and the improvement in intertrochanter is not higher than femoral neck. HSA method has some limitations; however, if technological improvements can make them reliable enough for clinical use, geometric measurements may ultimately provide a clearer view of the efficacy of treatment.

Keywords Hip structure analysis • Geometry • Osteoporosis • Dual-energy X-ray absorptiometry

---

J. Takada, M.D., Ph.D. (✉)
Kitago Orthopaedic Clinic, Kitago, 3-8, 5-33, Shiroishi-ku, Sapporo 003-0833, Japan

Department of Orthopaedic Surgery, Sapporo Medical University, Sapporo, Japan
e-mail: jtanaka@kitago-ortho.com

Y. Shimada, N. Miyakoshi (eds.), *Osteoporosis in Orthopedics*,
DOI 10.1007/978-4-431-55778-4_4

4.1 Hip Structure Analysis (HSA)

4.1.1 Limitations of Areal Bone Mineral Density (BMD)

Areal BMD measured by dual-energy X-ray absorptiometry (DXA) is a valuable tool for the evaluation of bone fragility and shows significant correlations between BMD decline and risk of fracture [1–3].

Although patients with fragility fractures typically have lower BMD than unfractured controls, about half of the fractures occurred in women who would not be classified as osteoporosis by BMD criteria [4, 5]. Moreover, BMD may not be the best assessment of treatment efficacy since the fracture reduction after treatment is only partially explained by increased BMD [6–8]. Strength of bone is however governed by structural dimensions and tissue materials properties, neither of which is directly measured in a conventional BMD measurement.

A DXA scanner generates a two-dimensional (2D) projection image of a bone with pixel values expressed in mineral area mass (g/cm^2); the conventional software averages pixel values over selected regions to measure BMD (Fig. 4.1). On the other hand, bone geometry measurements have a more direct relationship with mechanical strength.

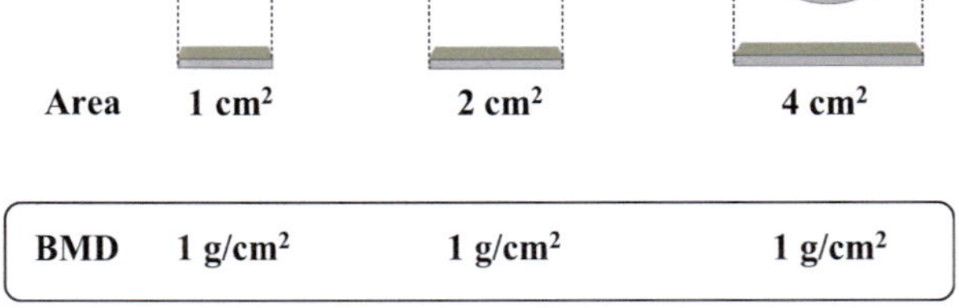

Fig. 4.1 *Limitations of areal bone mineral density*. One of the limitations of areal bone mineral density is not presented bone structure. DXA scanner generates a 2D projection image of a bone with pixel values expressed in mineral area mass (g/cm^2); however, strength of bone is governed by structural dimensions and tissue material properties, neither of which is directly measured in a conventional BMD measurement. *BMC* bone mineral content, *BMD* bone mineral density, *DXA* dual-energy X-ray absorptiometry

4.1.2 Technical Methods

Beck and Ruff have applied the HSA method to measure proximal femur geometry and strength using conventional DXA scans of the hip [9, 10]. The archived DXA images were analyzed using the HSA method which is described in detail in earlier publications [11]. Briefly, DXA scan files were first converted into bone mass images in which pixel values represent bone mass in grams per square centimeter, using an automated program. Structural analysis was then done in image files using a special interactive computer program. The underlying principle of the method is that a line of pixels traversing the bone axis is a projection of the corresponding cross section from which certain geometric properties can be derived.

The scan was performed using a commercially available hip positioner system (HPS; OsteoDyne, Durham, NC, USA) in order to ensure consistent positioning [12]. This device keeps the subject's legs positioned in abduction and internal rotation (15°).

Three measured sites were defined as (1) narrow neck, traversing the narrowest width of the femoral neck; (2) intertrochanter, along the bisector of the shaft and femoral neck axes; and (3) shaft, at a distance of 1.5 times minimum neck width, distal to the intersection of the neck and shaft axes.

4.1.3 Structural Parameters

The structural parameters were as follows [13, 14]:

4.1.3.1 Areal BMD (g/cm^2)

Areal BMD was measured using routine methods. Mean values of BMD from narrow neck region are on the average about 14 % higher than the conventional neck region of interest (ROI) values on the same subjects, although age trends are similar in previous reports [15].

4.1.3.2 Average Cortical Thickness (cm)

Average cortical thickness is an estimate of the mean cortical thickness assuming a circular (narrow neck or shaft) or elliptical (intertrochanter) annulus model of the cross section for use in the estimated buckling ratio. The model assumes that 60 %, 70 %, and 100 % of the measured bone mass is in the cortex for narrow neck, intertrochanter, and shaft, respectively. These methods have the possibility of overestimate of the cortical thickness in the cases having the increase of trabecular bone, especially in narrow neck and intertrochanter regions.

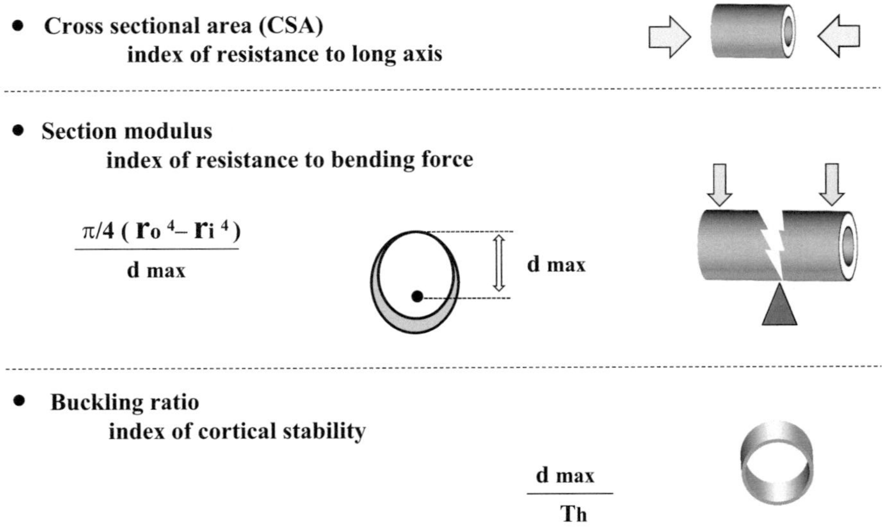

Fig. 4.2 *Structural parameters in HSA*
CSA is an index of resistance to forces directed along the long axis of the bone
Section modulus is an index of resistance to bending forces. Due to limitations of a 2D DXA image, section modulus is only relevant for bending in the plane of the DXA image
Buckling ratio is an index of cortical stability
HSA hip structure analysis, *CSA* cross-sectional area, *DXA* dual-energy X-ray absorptiometry, r_o outer diameter, r_i inner diameter, d_{max} maximum distance from either bone edge to the centroid of the profile, *Th* average cortical thickness

4.1.3.3 Cross-Sectional Area (CSA, cm^2) (Fig. 4.2)

This is defined as the surface area of bone tissue in the cross section after excluding soft tissue (marrow) spaces. CSA is derived from the integral of the bone mass profile and is not equivalent to the total area within the periosteal envelope as widely misinterpreted. CSA is an index of resistance to forces directed along the long axis of the bone.

4.1.3.4 Section Modulus (cm^3) (Fig. 4.2)

This is an index of resistance to bending forces and is calculated as CSMI/d_{max} where CSMI is the cross-sectional moment of inertia and d_{max} is the maximum distance from either bone edge to the centroid of the profile [13, 14]. The CSMI is derived from the integral of the bone mass profile across the bone weighted by the square of distance from the center of mass. Due to limitations of a 2D DXA image, the CSMI and section modulus derived by HSA are only relevant for bending in the plane of the DXA image.

4.1.3.5 Buckling Ratio (Fig. 4.2)

Buckling ratio describes stable configurations of thin-walled tubes subjected to compressive loads and requires an estimate of the cortical thickness. The buckling ratio is computed as the ratio of d_{max} to the estimated mean cortical thickness. Buckling ratio is mainly presented in narrow neck and intertrochanter region, because this parameter in the shaft is not important in meaning.

4.1.3.6 Other Parameters

In addition to these parameters, the HSA program measures neck-shaft angle and femoral neck length. The latter is defined as the distance from the center of the femoral head to the intersection of the neck and shaft axes.

Based on a preceding study, precision error (CV%) for HSA variables at the narrow neck, intertrochanter, and shaft ranges from 0.8 to 4.7 %, with an average of 2.2 % [16, 17].

4.1.4 Methodological Limitations

There are methodological limitations in HSA. DXA scanners are not designed or optimized to measure structural dimensions so that precision was relatively poor. In addition, it is difficult in reproducing the position of the 3D femur in 2D images separated months to years apart, although hip positioner systems are available in clinical use [12]. The use of 2D DXA scans means that the section modulus is assessed only in the scan plane; effects of treatment may be different for bending directions out of the image plane. The HSA method expresses the same data geometrically but assumes a constant tissue mineralization to do so and does not evaluate material strength effects.

The HSA method has these limitations; however, if technological improvements can make them reliable enough for clinical use, geometric measurements may ultimately provide a clearer view of the efficacy of treatment.

4.1.5 Correlations in Structural Parameters Between HSA and Quantitative Computed Tomography (QCT)

Khoo et al. reported the correlations between in structural parameters between HSA and QCT in 237 elderly females (77.6 ± 5.1, mean ± standard deviation) [18]. The correlations with coefficients were 0.45 for endosteal width, 0.46 for subperiosteal width, 0.73 for cross-sectional moment of inertia, 0.75 for buckling ratio, 0.77 for

Table 4.1 Correlations in structural parameters between HSA and QCT

Parameters	*R*
Areal BMD	0.86
CSA	0.90
Cross-sectional moment of inertia	0.73
Section modulus	0.77
Averaged cortical thickness	0.85
Endosteal width	0.45
Subperiosteal width	0.46
Buckling ratio	0.75

The strength index, section modulus, CSA, and buckling ratio showed strong correlations between HSA and QCT. The assumptions underlying the HSA derived from DXA have been substantiated by 3D images obtained by QCT

HSA hip structure analysis, *QCT* quantitative computed tomography, *DXA* dual-energy X-ray absorptiometry, *BMD* bone mineral density, *CSA* cross-sectional area

Paired t-test with *P* values for regression being <0.001 in all cases

Reference [18]

section modulus, 0.85 for averaged cortical thickness, 0.86 for BMD, and 0.90 for cross-sectional area with *P* values for regression being <0.001 in all parameters (Table 4.1). The correlations in endosteal width and subperiosteal width were lower, because of the relatively small range of values. On the other hand, the strength index, section modulus, CSA, and buckling ratio showed strong correlations between HSA and QCT.

These results demonstrated that the assumptions underlying the HSA approach using 2D data derived from DXA have been substantiated by true 3D images obtained by QCT; however, geometrical variables dependent on mass calibration standards, location of neck ROI, and mathematical derivation techniques are different.

4.2 Structural Trends in Aging

4.2.1 Aging Trends in Japanese Women (Fig. 4.3)

The trends in aging into the proximal femur geometry in Japanese women were analyzed using a cross-sectional sample obtained from a clinical sample [17]. The data of BMD was acquired from outpatient clinic for the screening of osteoporosis on 409 Japanese women aged from 50 to 93 years. For the purpose of interpretation of apparent age trends, mean values for women in the 50–59 year age group were used as a reference standard value (100 %), and all expressed means relative to

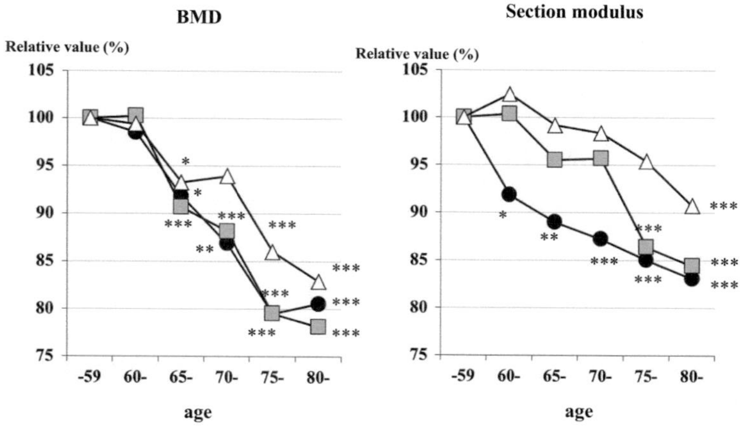

Fig. 4.3 *Aging trends in Japanese women*. The trends in aging into the proximal femur geometry in Japanese women were analyzed using a cross-sectional sample obtained from a clinical sample. Areal bone mineral density (*BMD*) in each femur site appears to decline in the same trends; however, section moduli are quite discordant with those in areal BMD. Δ shaft, □ intertrochanter, ● narrow neck. *$p < 0.05$, **$p < 0.01$, ***$p < 0.001$ vs standard reference (50–59 years of age) (Reference [17])

standard values in 5 year intervals (those over 80 were put in a single group). Sample sizes in each group ranged from 50 to 90 subjects.

Areal BMD in each femur site appears to decline in the same trends. BMD at narrow neck, intertrochanter, and shaft in the oldest group (80+ years) decreased by 19.5 %, 21.8 %, and 17.1 % compared to the standard value, respectively (Fig. 4.3). Measured on the same subjects, section modulus are quite discordant with those in areal BMD. Section modulus at narrow neck decreased age-dependent manner; the oldest group (80+ years) averages 17.0 % less than standard value. In contrast, section modulus at intertrochanter and shaft appears to decline more slowly before 75 years of age; after that, it significantly decreased by 15.6 % in the oldest group (80+ years) at intertrochanter. There are no significant differences between narrow neck and intertrochanter in the group of 75–79 years and 80+ years. On the other hand, section modulus at shaft appears to remain static by 95.4 % until 70–74 years of age and 90.8 % in the group of 80+ years. This was also true in the rate of expansion of subperiosteal diameter which partially explains the reduction in areal BMD and that provides a mechanical explanation for why the apparent decline in section modulus is smaller than the change in BMD.

HSA in Japanese women showed that reduction in geometric strength as reflected by the section modulus was not dependent on decline in BMD. The section modulus is mainly influenced by changes in cortical dimensions. Mathematically, the section modulus is more strongly dependent on subperiosteal diameter than endocortical diameter, so that a greater bone loss at the endocortical surface can be compensated by a smaller increase in subperiosteal diameter. Subperiosteal expansion with age is thought to be a response to bone resorption in the endocortical surface for maintaining bone strength [19]. Indeed, subperiosteal diameters were positively correlated with age at all three regions in this study. Although cortices become progressively thinner through life, geometric strength at the femoral shaft is maintained.

Iki et al. showed the geographical differences in HSA parameters in four areas in Japan [20]. The areal differences were within the range of 10 % between the lowest area (Sanuki) and the highest area (Memuro) with an inverse association in buckling ratio.

4.2.2 The Epidemiology of Hip Fracture and Structural Trends in Japan

The committee for osteoporosis treatment of the Japanese Orthopaedic Association had elucidated the current status of hip fracture incidence in Japan [21]. The number of patients with femoral neck fractures gradually increased with age from 60 to 75 years, and exceeded that with trochanteric fractures before 75 years. In contrast, the number of patients with intertrochanter fracture rapidly increases after 75 years of age, and these figures became inverted thereafter.

The results in a cross-sectional sample of Japanese women show that although BMD declines with age in all regions, the section modulus appears to decline at a slower rate than that of BMD. The changing pattern in the section modulus at narrow neck and intertrochanter in Japan might be consistent with the epidemiological evidence of hip fracture (neck and trochanteric fracture) rates in Japan (Fig. 4.3).

4.2.3 Racial and Gender Differences

The previous reports have investigated gender differences in femoral neck geometry in an aging population and differences in pre- and postmenopausal hip geometry in white and black women [10, 15, 22, 23]. Note that there are some apparent differences in age trends between Japanese and US white women. Rates of bone loss (CSA decline) are actually greater in Japanese while rates of neck expansion (outer diameter) appear to be greater in US whites. The age trend in bending resistance is actually greater in Japanese women while the apparent increase in buckling ratio (toward greater instability) is greater in white women. These differences are reflected in geometric properties like the bone CSA and section modulus which define resistance to axial and bending loads, respectively.

Beck et al. analyzed structural parameters in non-Hispanic white men and women acquired in the Third National Health and Nutrition Examination Survey (NHANES III) [15]. The BMD decline with age in the narrow neck and shaft was similar to that in conventional regions. On the other hand, the section modulus at both the narrow neck and the shaft regions remains nearly constant until the fifth decade in females and then declined at a slower rate than BMD. In males, the narrow neck section modulus declined modestly until the fifth decade and then remained nearly constant whereas the shaft section modulus was static until the fifth decade and then increased steadily. The aging loss of BMD in the hip does not necessarily mean reduced mechanical strength.

Wang et al. measured the structural basis of racial and sex differences in femoral neck fragility in 829 healthy Chinese and 1181 healthy Caucasian subjects aged 18-93 years. For both races, women had a higher fracture risk in bending than men [22].

4.3 Relations Between Bone Biological Makers and Structural Parameters

Takada et al. had clarified the correlations between biochemical marker of bone resorption and structural geometry of the proximal femur in postmenopausal women with osteoporosis [24].

Forty-five postmenopausal women with osteoporosis were measured serum type I collagen cross-linked N-telopeptide (sNTX) as biochemical markers of bone resorption and HSA parameters. The median sNTX at baseline was 15.3 nmol bone collagen equivalent (BCE)/L (reference range for Japanese healthy premenopausal women, 7.5–16.5 nmol BCE/L) [25]. At baseline, sNTX correlated inversely with BMD, CSA, average cortical thickness, and section modulus and positively with buckling ratio in the intertrochanter and shaft (but not the narrow neck) (Table 4.2). These correlations were significant, both crude and adjusted for

Table 4.2 Correlations (Peason's R) between sNTX and HSA parameters

	Narrow neck	Intertrochanter	Shaft
BMD (g/cm^2)	0.056	−0.404**	−0.413**
CSA (cm^2)	0.030	−0.386**	−0.433**
Inner diameter (cm)	−0.064	0.168	0.248
Average cortical thickness (cm)	0.057	−0.370*	−0.378*
Section modulus (cm^3)	−0.177	−0.325*	−0.321*
Buckling ratio	0.036	0.504**	0.390**

sNTX correlated inversely with BMD, CSA, average cortical thickness, and section modulus and positively with buckling ratio in the intertrochanter and shaft (but not the neck). These data indicated that the surrogate markers for hip fracture, among sNTX, BMD, and HSA parameters, showed significant correlations

sNTX serum type I collagen cross-linked N-telopeptide, *HSA* hip structure analysis, *BMD* bone mineral density, *CSA* cross-sectional area

*$p < 0.05$, **$p < 0.01$ adjust for age

Reference [24]

Table 4.3 Correlations (Peason's R) between bone metabolic markers (TRACP-5b, P1NP) and HSA parameters

	TRACP-5b ($n = 201$)	P1NP ($n = 83$)
Narrow neck		
BMD (g/cm^2)	−0.253**	−0.406**
CSA (cm^2)	−0.232**	−0.323*
Average cortical thickness (cm)	−0.250**	−0.394**
Section modulus (cm^3)	−0.090	−0.179
Buckling ratio	0.233**	0.485**
Intertrochanter		
BMD (g/cm^2)	−0.296**	−0.369**
CSA (cm^2)	−0.260**	−0.338*
Average cortical thickness (cm)	−0.254**	−0.357*
Section modulus (cm^3)	−0.190*	−0.290*
Buckling ratio	0.257**	0.404**

TRACP-5b and P1NP were also significantly correlated with HSA parameters in narrow neck and intertrochanter region

HSA hip structure analysis, *TRACP-5b* tartrate resistant acid phosphatase 5b, *P1NP* type 1 procollagen-N-propeptide

*$p < 0.01$, **$p < 0.001$ adjust for age

Reference [26]

age. These data indicated that the surrogate markers for hip fracture, among sNTX, BMD and HSA parameters, showed significant correlations.

The other bone metabolic markers, type 1 procollagen-N-propeptide (P1NP) and tartrate-resistant acid phosphatase 5b (TRACP-5b), were also correlated inversely with BMD, CSA, average cortical thickness, and section modulus and positively with buckling ratio in narrow neck and intertrochanter in another study (Table 4.3) [26].

4.4 Relations Between Body Weight, Body Composition, and HSA Parameters

4.4.1 Body Weight

Longitudinal hip data in 4187 mostly white, elderly women were analyzed whether altered skeletal load should stimulate adaptive increases or decreases in hip geometry [27]. Subjects with increasing load (weight gain >5 % in 3.5 years) lost narrow neck BMD, but section modulus increased markedly. On the other hand, those with declining skeletal loads (weight lost >5 % in 3.5 years) showed the greatest loss of BMD and significant declines in section modulus (Fig. 4.4). These results indicated that mechanical homeostasis in the hip is evident in section modulus but not in BMD.

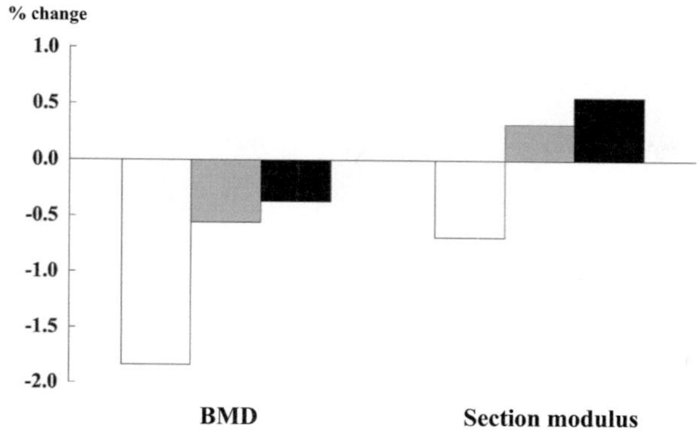

Fig. 4.4 *Changes of body weight and structural parameters in narrow neck.* Subjects with increasing load (weight gain >5 % in 3.5 years) lost bone mineral density (*BMD*), but gained section modulus. On the other hand, those with declining skeletal loads (weight lost >5 % in 3.5 years) showed the greatest loss of BMD and section modulus. □ weight losers, those who lost >5 % in 3.5 years; ▒ static weight, those who changed weight within 5 %; ■ weight gainers, those who gained >5 % in 3.5 years (Reference [27])

4.4.2 Body Composition (Bone Mineral Content (BMC), Lean Mass, Fat Mass)

Takada et al. had reported the first presentation for the relations between the body composition (BMC, lean, fat) and HSA parameters in Japanese women [28]. One hundred eighty-three community-dwelling Japanese women (65.6 years of age) who had a checkup for osteoporosis were measured body composition in lower leg and hip geometry parameters by whole-body scan DXA and HSA, respectively. BMC and lean mass at narrow neck and intertrochanter were positively correlated with BMD, CSA, and section modulus ($r = 0.425$–0.874), and BMC was inversely correlated with buckling ratio ($r = -0.494$, -0.572). On the other hand, fat mass did not show significant correlation with CSA and section modulus (Table 4.4).

The highest quartile (Q4) in lean/fat ratio at narrow neck and intertrochanter was significantly higher in section modulus compared to other quartiles (Q1–3) but not in BMD (Fig. 4.5). These results indicated that the protective effects of body weight in preventing fracture and osteoporosis are mediated by BMC and lean mass, not fat mass.

Table 4.4 Correlations between HSA parameters and body composition (bone mineral content, lean mass, fat mass)

		BMD (g/cm^2)	CSA (cm^2)	Section modulus (cm^3)	Buckling ratio
BMC	Narrow neck	$r = 0.774^*$	$r = 0.839^*$	$r = 0.773^*$	$r = -0.494^*$
	Intertrochanter	$r = 0.836^*$	$r = 0.874^*$	$r = 0.840^*$	$r = -0.572^*$
Lean	Narrow neck	$r = 0.425^*$	$r = 0.555^*$	$r = 0.588^*$	$r = -0.143$
	Intertrochanter	$r = 0.444^*$	$r = 0.562^*$	$r = 0.635^*$	$r = -0.107$
Fat	Narrow neck	$r = 0.125$	$r = 0.061$	$r = -0.023$	$r = -0.126$
	Intertrochanter	$r = 0.184^\#$	$r = 0.102$	$r = 0.066$	$r = -0.259^*$

BMC and lean mass at narrow neck and intertrochanter were positively correlated with BMD, CSA, and section modulus, and BMC were inversely correlated with buckling ratio. Fat mass did not show significant correlation with CSA and section modulus. These results indicated that the protective effects of body weight in preventing fracture and osteoporosis are mediated by BMC and lean mass, not fat mass

BMC bone mineral content, *BMD* bone mineral density, *CSA* cross-sectional area

$^*p < 0.001$, $^\#p < 0.05$

Reference [28]

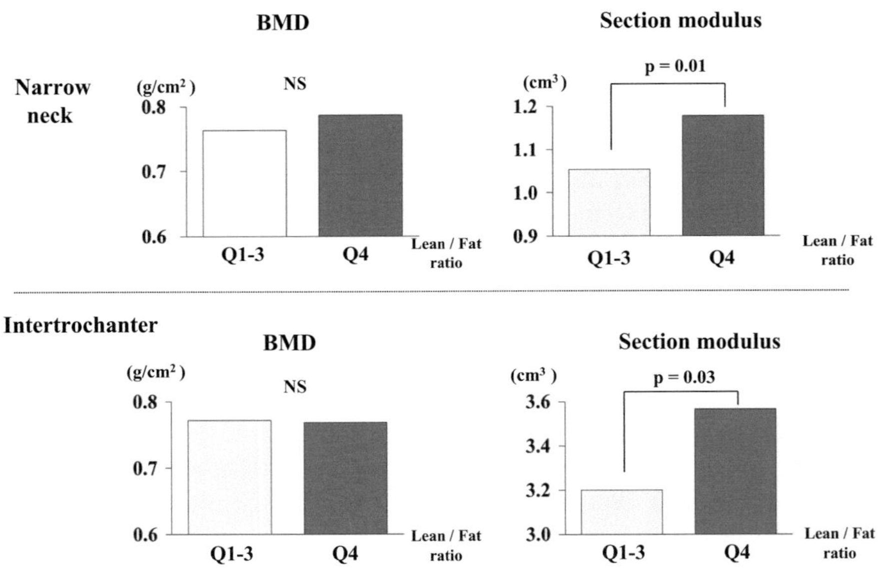

Fig. 4.5 *The comparison of BMD and section modulus between highest (Q4) and other (Q1–3) quartiles in lean/fat ratio*. The highest quartile (Q4) in lean/fat ratio at narrow neck and intertrochanter were significantly higher in section modulus compared to other quartiles (Q1–3), but not in BMD. *BMD* bone mineral density, *NS* not significant (Reference [28])

4.5 Physical Activity and Structural Parameters

Nurzenski et al. investigate the effects of habitual physical activity and dietary calcium intake on femoral geometry in older women. One thousand and eight population-based women (median age, 75 years) were measured in femoral geometry, habitual physical activity, and dietary calcium intake [29]. Physical activity showed a significant dose–response effect on CSA of all hip sites and section modulus at the narrow neck and intertrochanter sites. The subjects with high physical activity (excess of 65.5 kcal/day) and high calcium intake (excess of 1039 mg/day) had had significantly greater CSA and section modulus. Women with high levels of physical activity and calcium intake had significantly greater CSA than women with high physical activity but low calcium intake (Fig. 4.6). Women in the high calcium intake /high physical activity group had a more favorable BMD and geometry than the women with low calcium intake and physical activity.

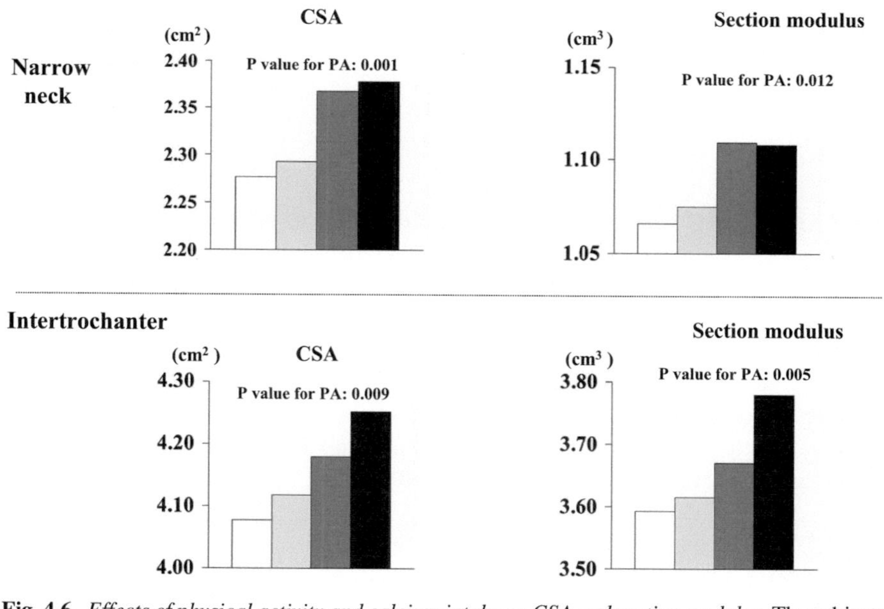

Fig. 4.6 *Effects of physical activity and calcium intake on CSA and section modulus*. The subjects with high physical activity (excess of 65.5 kcal/day) and high calcium intake (excess of 039 mg/day) had had significantly greater CSA and section modulus. Women with high levels of physical activity and calcium intake had significantly greater CSA than women with high physical activity but low calcium intake. *PA* physical activity, *CI* calcium intake, *CSA* cross-sectional area, lower and higher PA $\leq$ 65.5 or >65.5 kcal/day, lower and higher CI $\leq$ 1039 or >1039 mg/day. □ low CI/low PA, □ high CI/low PA, ■ low CI/high PA, ■ high CI/high PA. All of *P* values for CI and for PA × CI interaction were not significant (Reference [29])

4.6 Fracture Risk and Structural Parameters

Postmenopausal women from the Women's Health Initiative were examined whether hip geometry parameters predicted hip fracture [30]. The results indicated that outer diameter and buckling ratio at intertrochanter predict incident hip fracture after accounting for clinical risk factors and BMD with hazard ratios for a one standard deviation increase of 1.61 (95 % confidence interval (CI), 1.25–2.08) for outer diameter and 1.43 (95 % CI, 1.10–1.87) for buckling ratio. However, it is controversial which parameter could predict hip fracture, so that prospective study is necessary.

4.7 Pharmacological Efficacy of Osteoporosis and HSA Parameters

Hip fracture induced greater reduction in morbidity and mortality among the common osteoporotic fracture sites. However, most clinical trials for the efficacy of treatment of osteoporosis are lack for the reduction in hip fracture, because hip fractures are less frequent than vertebral fractures. The geometric measurements may ultimately provide a clearer view of pharmacological efficacy of osteoporosis treatments for hip strength.

4.7.1 SERM (Selective Estrogen Receptor Modulator)

4.7.1.1 MORE (Multiple Outcomes of Raloxifene Evaluation) Study

Uusi-Rasi et al. reported HSA data in hip scans from a subset of the MORE study including 4806 postmenopausal women with osteoporosis [31]. They conclude that raloxifene does not influence periosteal apposition in the proximal femur but significant improvement in resistance to axial and bending stresses (CSA and section modulus, respectively) at all analyzed regions.

4.7.1.2 Outcomes of Raloxifene Effects in Japan

Takada et al. had analyzed that the effects of 2 year treatment with raloxifene on the proximal femoral geometry among 198 Japanese women with osteoporosis by HSA [32]. BMD, CSA, and section modulus at narrow neck significantly increased by 1.27 %, 2.67 %, and 3.90 % at 2 years, respectively. BMD, CSA, and section modulus at intertrochanter significantly increased by 2.55 %, 4.49 %, and 6.60 % at study termination, respectively (Fig. 4.7). The buckling ratio at intertrochanter

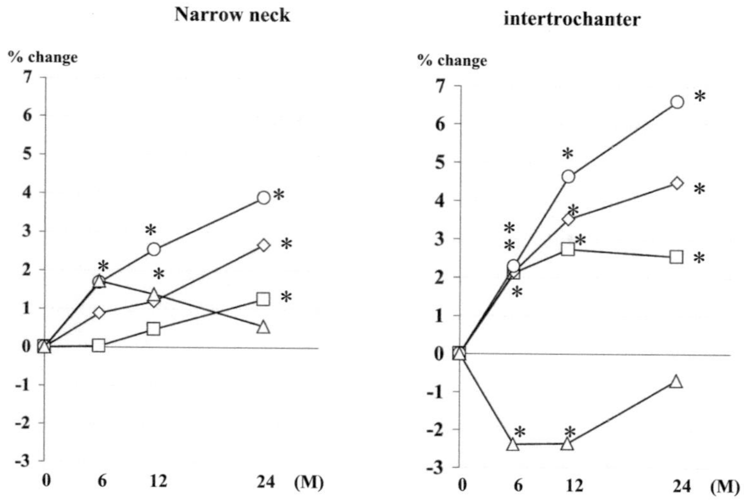

Fig. 4.7 *Effects of 2 year treatment with raloxifene in Japanese osteoporotic women*. BMD, CSA, and section modulus at neck and intertrochanter significantly increased at 2 years. The buckling ratio at intertrochanter significantly decreased at 1 year but differences at 2 years became nonsignificant. *BMD* bone mineral density, *CSA* cross-sectional area, ○ section modulus, ◇ CSA, □ BMD, Δ buckling ratio. *$p < 0.05$ vs baseline (Reference [32])

decreased by 2.36 % at 1 year, but differences at 2 years became nonsignificant. Parameters at shaft were qualitatively similar to those of the narrow neck and intertrochanter.

Raloxifene treatment produced positive changes in CSA and section modulus. These changes were particularly evident at the narrow neck and intertrochanter regions that correspond to common fracture sites. The percent change of section modulus was significantly higher than that of BMD at 2 years in all three regions. These data indicated that Japanese osteoporotic women on raloxifene therapy have significant improvements of both BMD and geometry in proximal femur.

These Japanese results were generally consistent with the larger MORE study of raloxifene effects on a mostly (95.7 %) white population of postmenopausal women with osteoporosis with one notable difference [31, 32]. In both studies, significant improvements (reduction) in buckling ratios were evident at the narrow neck and intertrochanter regions at early time points, but differences declined with time. In the MORE study, a 2 % lower buckling ratio remained significant at 3 years, but in Japanese study, the buckling ratios were no longer significant after 2 years of treatment. A clinical trial by Greenspan et al. evaluated the effects of estrogen replacement therapy on femur geometry and showed positive effects on CSA and section modulus that were comparable to those of the present study [33]. Interestingly, after 3 years of estrogen treatment, there were no apparent differences from baseline in buckling ratio at the narrow neck, intertrochanter, and shaft regions. Treatments followed for longer periods seem to initially reduce the buckling ratio, but with continued expansion, the effect seems to moderate with time [31, 34, 35].

4.7.2 Bisphosphonate

4.7.2.1 Alendronate and Risedronate in Caucasians

Bonnick et al. reported that treatment with once-weekly alendronate or risedronate resulted in significant improvements in HSA parameters in 947 Caucasian patients with osteoporosis in the Fosamax Actonel Comparison Trial (FACT) [36]. Two years of treatment with either alendronate or risedronate resulted in statistically significant improvements from baseline in most geometric parameters at narrow neck, intertrochanter, and shaft, and the largest treatment effects were seen at the intertrochanter. The greater treatment effects were seen with alendronate compared with risedronate at all three regions.

4.7.2.2 Alendronate and Risedronate in Japanese

The doses of bisphosphonates for Japanese patients are half of those applied to Caucasians (alendronate 70 vs 35 mg/week and risedronate 35 vs 17.5 mg/week in Caucasians vs Japanese, respectively). These dosages seemed to be associated with race differences [37, 38]. Takada et al. had previously reported the effects of 1 year treatment of either alendronate or risedronate on the proximal femoral geometry among Japanese women with osteoporosis by HSA [39].

In alendronate treatment group, BMD, CSA, and section modulus significantly increased by 0.81 %, 1.35 %, and 2.23 % at narrow neck and increased by 2.19 %, 2.28 %, and 2.85 % at intertrochanter, respectively (Fig. 4.8). Buckling ratio at

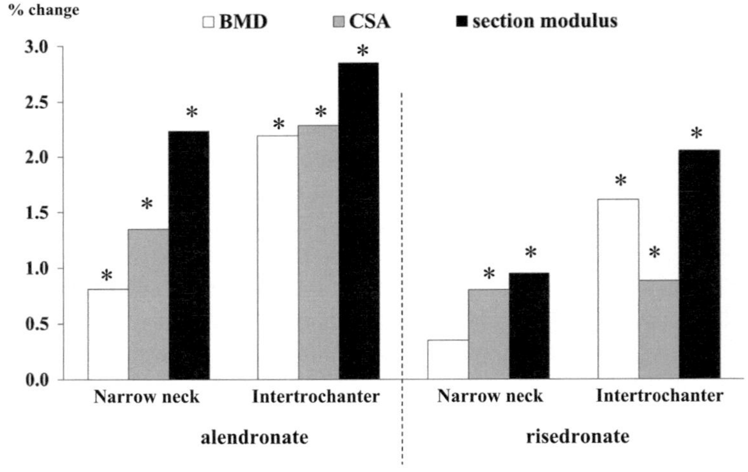

Fig. 4.8 *Effects of 1 year treatment of either alendronate or risedronate in Japanese women with osteoporosis*. CSA and section modulus at narrow neck and intertrochanter significantly increased in either alendronate or risedronate treatment group. *BMD* bone mineral density, *CSA* cross-sectional area. *$p < 0.05$ vs baseline (Reference [39])

intertrochanter significantly decreased by 2.50 %. CSA and section modulus at shaft significantly increased.

In risedronate treatment group, CSA and section modulus at narrow neck significantly increased by 0.80 % and 0.95 %, respectively. BMD, CSA, and section modulus at intertrochanter significantly increased by 1.61 %, 0.88 %, and 2.05 %, respectively (Fig. 4.8), and buckling ratio significantly decreased by 1.53 %. BMD, CSA, and section modulus at shaft also significantly increased.

In addition, the comparisons of the percent changes of parameters between alendronate and risedronate showed that statistically significant differences were seen for section modulus in narrow neck and CSA in intertrochanter (not direct comparison) [39]. The other parameters did not show significant difference; however, alendronate shows a greater improvement in several parameters compared with risedronate. Both alendronate and risedronate treatment over 1 year resulted in improvement in HSA parameters with consistently greater effects seen with alendronate than risedronate. These consistent trends of efficacy in Japanese data are approximately similar in FACT study in mostly Caucasians [36].

4.7.2.3 Minodronate

Ito et al. reported minodronic acid hydrate, new bisphosphonates developed in Japan, on the geometry of the proximal femur in 103 Japanese postmenopausal patients with osteoporosis [40]. The results showed a significant increase in cortical thickness, CSA, and section modulus and a significant reduction in buckling ratio in narrow neck, intertrochanter, and shaft. These findings indicated that minodronic acid hydrate reduces endocortical bone resorption, leading to increased cortical thickness and improved bone strength index.

4.7.3 Denosumab

Beck et al. reported the effects for hip geometry in denosumab 60 mg 6 monthly (human monoclonal antibody against receptor activator of nuclear factor-kappa B ligand) in postmenopausal women with low BMD for 24 months [34]. Denosumab improved geometric parameters (cortical thickness, outer diameter, endocortical diameter) and strength indices (CSA, section modulus) compared with placebo, and denosumab effects were greater than alendronate at the intertrochanteric and shaft sites (Fig. 4.9). These results indicated that denosumab treatment may lead to improved bone mechanical properties compared to placebo and alendronate.

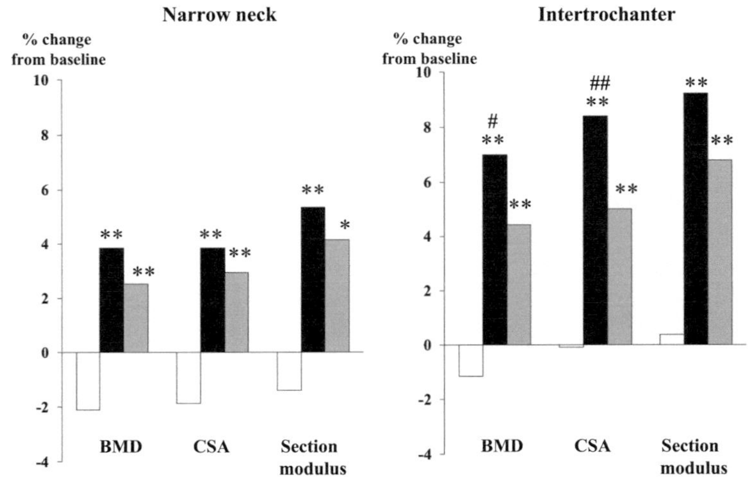

Fig. 4.9 *Effects of denosumab in postmenopausal women.* Denosumab improved BMD and strength indices (CSA, section modulus) compared with placebo at narrow neck, and intertrochanter and denosumab effects were greater than alendronate at the intertrochanter. *BMD* bone mineral density, *CSA* cross-sectional area. $*p < 0.01$, $**p < 0.001$ vs baseline, $\#p < 0.05$, $\#\#p < 0.01$ vs alendronate. □ placebo, ■ denosumab, ▨ alendronate (Reference [34])

4.7.4 Changing Patterns in Parameters by Antiresorptive Drugs

In most of the studies on HSA by antiresorptive drugs, the percent change of section modulus was higher than that of BMD in all three regions. These results might suggest the clinical outcomes that the reduction of fracture rate is not fully explained by increased BMD. The baseline values of section modulus at all regions are greater than that of BMD, and the percent changes of section modulus are also greater than that of BMD; therefore, small increasing of absolute value in section modulus did not lead to the greater increasing of percent changes.

The changing trends of HSA parameters were generally consistent with alendronate and risedronate in FACT study in most Caucasians, minodronic acid study, alendronate, risedronate, and raloxifene study in Japanese (Table 4.5). These changes were particularly evident at the intertrochanter region, that is, BMD, CSA, and section modulus showed significant improvements in bisphosphonates and raloxifene treatment. CSA and section modulus at narrow neck also showed significant increase in all of treatment groups. The tendency to change in the other parameters is approximately similar in bisphosphonates and raloxifene treatment groups.

If geometric parameters better explain osteoporotic fragility than BMD, bisphosphonates and raloxifene clearly change geometry toward improved strength at the narrow neck and intertrochanteric regions in Japanese women with osteoporosis.

Table 4.5 Comparison of changing trends of HSA parameters in alendronate, risedronate, minodronate, and raloxifene

	Alendronate (70 mg/week)	Risedronate (35 mg/week)	Alendronate (35 mg/week)	Risedronate (17.5 mg/week)	Minodronate (1 mg/day)	Raloxifene (60 mg/day)
Report [reference]	Bonnick [36]	Bonnick [36]	Takada [39]	Takada [39]	Ito [40]	Takada [32]
Narrow neck						
BMD	↑	↑	↑	NS	↑	↑
CSA	↑	↑	↑	↑	↑	↑
Section modulus	↑	↑	↑	↑	↑	↑
Buckling ratio	↓	NS	NS	NS	↓	NS
Intertrochanter						
BMD	↑	↑	↑	↑	↑	↑
CSA	↑	↑	↑	↑	↑	↑
Section modulus	↑	↑	↑	↑	↑	↑
Buckling ratio	↓	↓	↓	↓	↓	NS

The changing trends of HSA parameters were particularly evident at intertrochanter region, that is, BMD, CSA, and section modulus showed significant improvements in bisphosphonates and raloxifene treatment

BMD bone mineral density, *CSA* cross-sectional area, *NS* not significant, ↑ significant increase from baseline, ↓ significant decrease from baseline

Reference [39]

4.7.5 Antiresorptive Drug (SERM or Bisphosphonate) Plus Active Vitamin D_3 (Eldecalcitol)

Patients in most randomized clinical trials for the evaluations of the effects of antiresorptive drugs were treated with supplemental calcium and vitamin D, because a vitamin D deficiency seems a common health issue among elderly individuals, especially among those with osteoporosis [41–44]. Based on the above evidence, the concomitant use of antiresorptive drugs with active vitamin D is a popular strategy for treating osteoporosis in Japan [45] because active, not native, vitamin D is covered for this purpose by Japanese health insurance. Eldecalcitol is a novel active vitamin D3 analogue with a hydroxypropyloxy group at the 2β position of 1α, 25-dihydroxyvitamin D3. It significantly increases BMD at the lumbar spine and total hip and decreases bone resorption markers and the incidence of both vertebral and non-vertebral (wrist) fractures compared with alfacalcidol [46–48].

Takada et al. have analyzed the effects of the concomitant use of antiresorptive drugs plus eldecalcitol on the geometric parameters in 203 postmenopausal patients who had been given eldecalcitol (0.75 μg/day) with bisphosphonate [alendronate (35 mg/week), 65 cases; risedronate (17.5 mg/week), 17 cases; minodronate (50 mg/month), 46 cases; ibandronate (1 mg/month, intravenous), five cases] or SERM [raloxifene (60 mg/day), 52 cases; bazedoxifene (20 mg/day), 18 cases] for 12 months with medication possession ratio over 80 % [26]. The concomitant use of bisphosphonate or SERM plus eldecalcitol significantly improved the strength parameters at 6 months, and these improvements continued at 12 months.

Bisphosphonate plus eldecalcitol treatment group significantly improved by 1.92 %, 2.55 %, and 3.24 % in BMD, CSA, and section modulus at narrow neck, respectively, and 3.17 %, 3.65 %, 4.49 %, and −4.30 % in BMD, CSA, section modulus, and buckling ratio at intertrochanter, respectively (Fig. 4.10). SERM plus eldecalcitol treatment group also significantly improved by 2.35 % and 2.32 % in BMD and CSA at narrow neck, respectively, and 2.40 %, 3.79 % and −2.91 % in CSA, section modulus, and buckling ratio at intertrochanter, respectively.

Alendronate plus eldecalcitol treatment group showed early (6 months) improvement in strength parameters compared to alendronate treatment group (not direct comparison). These results indicated that the concomitant use of bisphosphonate plus eldecalcitol might be recommended for the patients with hip fracture risk [26, 39].

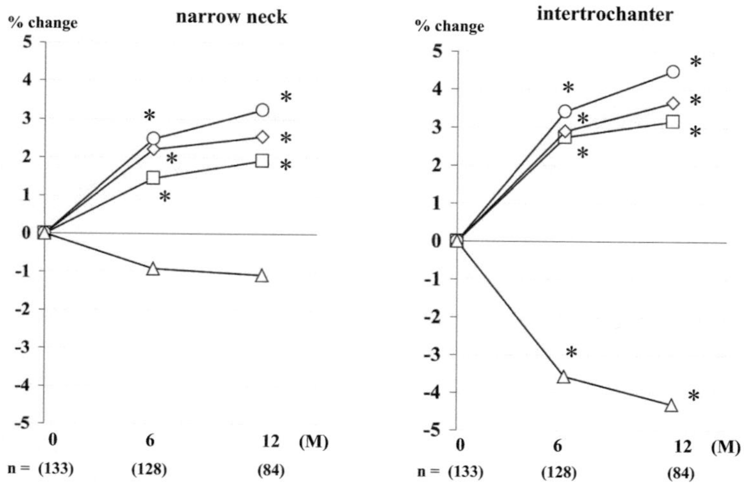

Fig. 4.10 *Effects of the concomitant use of bisphosphonate plus eldecalcitol on HSA parameters in Japanese women with osteoporosis.* BMD, CSA, and section modulus at neck and intertrochanter significantly increased at 6 months. The buckling ratio at intertrochanter significantly decreased at 6 months. *BMD* bone mineral density, *CSA* cross-sectional area, ○ section modulus, ◇ CSA, □ BMD, Δ buckling ratio. *$p < 0.05$ vs baseline (Reference [26])

4.7.6 *Teriparatide*

4.7.6.1 Daily (20 μg/day)

Uusi-Rasi et al. evaluated effects of teriparatide (20 μg/day) among a subset 558 postmenopausal women enrolled in the Fracture Prevention Trial [49]. At the narrow neck, teriparatide increased bone mass and improved bone geometric strength (CSA, section modulus, buckling ratio) compared to the placebo group. The changes at the intertrochanteric region were comparable to those at the narrow neck although the changes were slightly smaller. These data indicated that teriparatide treatment improved axial and bending strength and increased cortical thickness and stability at the femoral neck and intertrochanteric region.

4.7.6.2 Weekly (56.5 μg/week)

Weekly administration of teriparatide is available for the treatment of osteoporosis in Japan [50]. Sone et al. reported the effects of once-weekly teriparatide for 72 weeks on hip geometry in 209 postmenopausal osteoporotic women [51].

Once-weekly teriparatide showed significantly higher BMD, cortical thickness, CSA, and section modulus and lower buckling ratio at both the narrow neck and intertrochanter regions compare to placebo. There was no significant improvement in geometric parameters at the shaft. These results indicated that once-weekly teriparatide improved hip geometry and strength in Japanese patients with osteoporosis.

4.7.7 Differences Between Antiresorptive Drugs and Teriparatide

Antiresorptive drugs (BP, SERM, denosumab) and bone formation drug (teriparatide) improved on hip geometry; however, there are differences in the trends for changing parameters.

First, the percent change of section modulus was higher than that of BMD in all three regions in antiresorptive drugs; however, teriparatide did not show these patters. Second, these changes were particularly evident at the intertrochanter region in antiresorptive drugs, but not in teriparatide.

References

1. Schott AM, Cormier C, Hans D, Favier F, Hausherr E, Dargent-Molina P, Delmas PD, Ribot C, Sebert JL, Breart G, Meunier PJ for EPIDOS Group (1998) How hip and whole-body bone mineral density predict hip fracture in elderly women: the EPIDOS Prospective Study. Osteoporos Int 8:247–254
2. Kanis JA (2002) Diagnosis of osteoporosis and assessment of fracture risk. Lancet 359:1929–1936
3. Miller PD (2003) Bone mass measurements. Clin Geriatr Med 19:281–297
4. Schuit SCE, van der Klift M, Weel AEAM, de Laet CEDH, Burger H, Seeman E, Hofman A, Uitterlinden AG, van Leeuwen JP, Pols HA (2004) Fracture incidence and association with bone mineral density in elderly men and women: the Rotterdam Study. Bone 34:195–202
5. Siris ES, Chen YT, Abbott TA, Barrett-Connor E, Miller PD, Wehren LE, Berger ML (2004) Bone mineral density thresholds for pharmacological intervention to prevent fracture. Arch Intern Med 164:1108–1112
6. Li Z, Meredith MP, Hoseyni MS (2001) A method to assess the proportion of treatment effect explained by a surrogate endpoint. Stat Med 20:3175–3188
7. Cummings SR, Karpf DB, Harris F, Genant HK, Ensrud K, LaCroix AZ, Dennis M, Black DM (2002) Improvement in spine bone density and reduction in risk of vertebral fractures during treatment with antiresorptive drugs. Am J Med 112:281–289
8. Sarkar S, Mitlak BH, Wong M, Stock JL, Black DM, Harper KD (2002) Relationships between bone mineral density and incident vertebral fracture risk with raloxifene therapy. J Bone Miner Res 17:1–10
9. Beck TJ, Ruff CB, Warden KE, Scott WW Jr, Rao GU (1990) Predicting femoral neck strength from bone mineral data: a structural approach. Invest Radiol 25:6–18
10. Beck TJ, Ruff CB, Scott WW Jr, Plato CC, Tobin JD, Quan CA (1992) Sex differences in geometry of the femoral neck with aging: a structural analysis of bone mineral data. Calcif Tissue Int 50:24–29
11. Beck T (2003) Measuring the structural strength of bones with dual-energy X-ray absorptiometry: principles, technical limitations, and future possibilities. Osteoporos Int 14(Suppl 5): S81–S88

12. Hans D, Duboeuf F, Schott AM, Horn S, Avioli LV, Drezner MK, Meunier PJ (1997) Effects of a new positioner on the precision of hip bone mineral density measurements. J Bone Miner Res 12:1289–1294
13. Ruff CB, Hayes WC (1983) Cross-sectional geometry of Pecos Pueblo femora and tibiae – a biomechanical investigation. I. Method and general patterns of variation. Am J Phys Anthropol 60:359–381
14. Melton LJ III, Beck TJ, Amin S, Khosla S, Achenbach SJ, Oberg AL, Riggs BL (2005) Contributions of bone density and structure to fracture risk assessment in men and women. Osteoporos Int 16:460–467
15. Beck TJ, Looker AC, Ruff CB (2000) Structural trends in the aging femoral neck and proximal shaft: analysis of the Third National Health and Nutrition Examination Survey dual-energy X-ray absorptiometry data. J Bone Miner Res 15:2297–2304
16. Nelson DA, Barondess DA, Hendrix SL, Beck TJ (2000) Cross-sectional geometry, bone strength, and bone mass in the proximal femur in black and white postmenopausal women. J Bone Miner Res 15:1992–1997
17. Takada J, Beck TJ, Iba K, Yamashita T (2007) Structural trends in the aging proximal femur in Japanese postmenopausal women. Bone 41:97–102
18. Khoo BCC, Brown K, Zhu K, Pollock M, Wilson KE, Price RI, Prince RL (2012) Differences in structural geometrical outcomes at the neck of the proximal femur using two-dimensional DXA-derived projection (APEX) and three-dimensional QCT-derived (BIT QCT) techniques. Osteoporos Int 23:1393–1398
19. Seeman E (2003) Periosteal bone formation – a neglected determinant of bone strength. N Engl J Med 349:320–323
20. Iki M, DongMei N, Tamaki J, Sato Y, Kagamimori S, Kagawa Y, Yoneshima H, for the Japanese Population-based Osteoporosis (JPOS) Study Group (2011) Age-specific reference values of hip geometric indices from a representative sample of the Japanese female population: Japanese Population-based Osteoporosis (JPOS) Study. Osteoporos Int 22:1987–1996
21. Committee for Osteoporosis Treatment of The Japanese Orthopaedic Association (2004) Nationwide survey of hip fractures in Japan. J Orthop Sci 9:1–5
22. Wang XF, Duan Y, Beck TJ, Seeman E (2005) Varying contributions of growth and ageing to racial and sex differences in femoral neck structure and strength in old age. Bone 36:978–986
23. Beck TJ, Ruff CB, Bissessur K (1993) Age-related changes in female femoral neck geometry: implications for bone strength. Calcif Tissue Int 53(Suppl 1):S41–S46
24. Takada J, Iba K, Yoshizaki T, Yamashita T (2012) Correlation between a bone resorption marker and structural geometry of the proximal femur in osteoporotic women treated with raloxifene. J Orthop Surg 20:209–213
25. Nishizawa Y, Nakamura T, Ohta H, Kushida K, Gorai I, Shiraki M, Fukunaga M, Hosoi T, Miki T, Chaki O, Ichimura S, Nakatsuka K, Miura M, Committee on the Guidelines for the Use of Biochemical Markers of Bone Turnover in Osteoporosis Japan Osteoporosis Society (2004) Guidelines for the use of biochemical markers of bone turnover in osteoporosis. J Bone Miner Metab 23:97–104
26. Takada J, Ikeda S, Kusanagi T, Mizuno S, Wada H, Iba K, Sasaki K, Kanaya K, Yoshizaki T, Yamashita T (2014) Evaluation of structural geometry at proximal femur in osteoporotic women treated by eldecalcitol with either raloxifene or bisphosphonate (Japanese). Osteoporos Jpn 22(Suppl 1):338
27. Beck TJ, Oreskovic TL, Stone KL, Ruff CB, Ensrud K, Nevitt MC, Genant HK, Cummings SR (2001) Structural adaptation to changing skeletal load in the progression toward hip fragility: the study of osteoporotic fractures. J Bone Miner Res 16:1108–1119
28. Takada J, Iba K, Sasaki K, Kanaya K, Douke T, Yoshizaki T, Yamashita T (2013) Lean mass but not fat mass is associated with hip geometry in Japanese women. BoneKEy 10:s104
29. Nurzenski MK, Briffa NK, Price RI, Khoo BCC, Devine A, Beck TJ, Prince RL (2007) Geometric indices of bone strength are associated with physical activity and dietary calcium intake in healthy older women. J Bone Miner Res 22:416–424

30. LaCroix AZ, Beck TJ, Cauley JA, Lewis CE, Bassford T, Jackson R, Wu G, Chen Z (2010) Hip structural geometry and incidence of hip fracture in postmenopausal women: what does it add to conventional bone mineral density? Osteoporos Int 21:919–929
31. Uusi-Rasi K, Beck TJ, Semanick LM, Daphtary MM, Crans GG (2006) Structural effects of raloxifene on the proximal femur: results from the multiple outcomes of raloxifene evaluation trial. Osteoporos Int 17:575–586
32. Takada J, Miki T, Imanishi Y, Nakatsuka K, Wada H, Naka H, Yoshizaki T, Iba K, Beck TJ, Yamashita T (2010) Effects of raloxifene treatment on the structural geometry of the proximal femur in Japanese women with osteoporosis. J Bone Miner Metab 28:561–567
33. Greenspan SL, Beck TJ, Resnick NM, Bhattacharya R, Parker RA (2005) Effect of hormone replacement, alendronate, or combination therapy on hip structure geometry: a 3-year, double blind, placebo-controlled clinical trial. J Bone Miner Res 20:1525–1532
34. Beck TJ, Lewiecki EM, Miller PD, Felsenberg D, Liu Y, Ding B, Libanati C (2008) Effects of denosumab on the geometry of the proximal femur in postmenopausal women in comparison with alendronate. J Clin Densitom 11:351–359
35. Chen Z, Beck TJ, Cauley JA, Lewis CE, LaCroix A, Bassford T, Wu G, Sherrill D, Going S (2008) Hormone therapy improves femur geometry among ethnically diverse postmenopausal participants in the Women's Health Initiative hormone intervention trials. J Bone Miner Res 23:1935–1945
36. Bonnick SL, Beck TJ, Cosman F, Hochberg MC, Wang H, de Papp AE (2009) DXA-based hip structural analysis of once-weekly bisphosphonate-treated postmenopausal women with low bone mass. Osteoporos Int 20:911–921
37. Uchida S, Taniguchi T, Shimizu T, Kakikawa T, Okuyama K, Okaniwa M, Arizono H, Nagata K, Santora AC, Shiraki M, Fukunaga M, Tomomitsu T, Ohashi Y, Nakamura T (2005) Therapeutic effects of alendronate 35 mg once weekly and 5 mg once daily in Japanese patients with osteoporosis: a double-blind, randomized study. J Bone Miner Metab 23:382–388
38. Kishimoto H, Fukunaga M, Kushida K, Shiraki M, Itabashi A, Nawata H, Nakamura T, Ohta H, Takaoka K, Ohashi Y, for the Risedronate Phase III Research Group (2006) Efficacy and tolerability of once-weekly administration of 17.5 mg risedronate in Japanese patients with involutional osteoporosis: a comparison with 2.5-mg once-daily dosage regimen. J Bone Miner Metab 24:405–413
39. Takada J, Katahira G, Iba K, Yoshizaki T, Yamashita T (2011) Hip structure analysis of bisphosphonate-treated Japanese postmenopausal women with osteoporosis. J Bone Miner Metab 29:458–468
40. Ito M, Sone T, Fukunaga M (2010) Effect of minodronic acid hydrate on hip geometry in Japanese women with postmenopausal osteoporosis. J Bone Miner Metab 28:334–341
41. Ettinger B, Black DM, Mitlak BH, Knickerbocker RK, Nickelsen T, Genant HK, Christiansen C, Delmas PD, Zanchetta JR, Stakkestad J, Glüer CC, Krueger K, Cohen FJ, Eckert S, Ensrud KE, Avioli LV, Lips P, Cummings SR (1999) Reduction of vertebral fracture risk in postmenopausal women with osteoporosis treated with raloxifene: results from a 3-year randomized clinical trial. JAMA 282:637–645
42. Harris ST, Watts NB, Genant HK, McKeever CD, Hangartner T, Keller M, Chesnut CH 3rd, Brown J, Eriksen EF, Hoseyni MS, Axelrod DW, Miller PD (1999) Effects of risedronate treatment on vertebral and nonvertebral fractures in women with postmenopausal osteoporosis: a randomized controlled trial. JAMA 282:1344–1352
43. Matsumoto T, Hagino H, Shiraki M, Fukunaga M, Nakano T, Takaoka K, Morii H, Ohashi Y, Nakamura T (2009) Effect of daily oral minodronate on vertebral fractures in Japanese postmenopausal women with established osteoporosis: a randomized placebo-controlled double-blind study. Osteoporos Int 20:1429–1437
44. Hagino H, Shiraki M, Fukunaga M, Nakano T, Takaoka K, Ohashi Y, Nakamura T, Matsumoto T (2012) Three years of treatment with minodronate in patients with postmenopausal osteoporosis. J Bone Miner Metab 30:439–446

45. Orimo H, Nakamura T, Fukunaga M, Ohta H, Hosoi T, Uemura Y, Kuroda T, Miyakawa N, Ohashi Y, Shiraki M (2011) Effects of alendronate plus alfacalcidol in osteoporosis patients with a high risk of fracture: the Japanese Osteoporosis Intervention Trial (JOINT) – 02. Curr Med Res Opin 27:1273–1284
46. Matsumoto T, Miki T, Hagino H, Sugimoto T, Okamoto S, Hirota T, Tanigawara Y, Hayashi Y, Fukunaga M, Shiraki M, Nakamura T (2005) A new active vitamin D, ED-71, increases bone mass in osteoporotic patients under vitamin D supplementation: a randomized, double-blind, placebo-controlled clinical trial. J Clin Endocrinol Metab 90:5031–5036
47. Matsumoto T, Ito M, Hayashi Y, Hirota T, Tanigawara Y, Sone T, Fukunaga M, Shiraki M, Nakamura T (2011) A new active vitamin D3 analog, eldecalcitol, prevents the risk of osteoporotic fractures: a randomized, active comparator, double-blind study. Bone 49:605–612
48. Nakamura T, Takano T, Fukunaga M, Shiraki M, Matsumoto T (2013) Eldecalcitol is more effective for the prevention of osteoporotic fractures than alfacalcidol. J Bone Miner Metab 31:417–422
49. Uusi-Rasi K, Semanick LM, Zanchetta JR, Bogado CE, Eriksen EF, Sato M, Beck TJ (2005) Effects of teriparatide [rhPTH (1–34)] treatment on structural geometry of the proximal femur in elderly osteoporotic women. Bone 36:948–958
50. Nakamura T, Sugimoto T, Nakano T, Kishimoto H, Ito M, Fukunaga M, Hagino H, Sone T, Yoshikawa H, Nishizawa Y, Fujita T, Shiraki M (2012) Randomized Teriparatide [human parathyroid hormone (PTH) 1–34] Once-Weekly Efficacy Research (TOWER) trial for examining the reduction in new vertebral fractures in subjects with primary osteoporosis and high fracture risk. J Clin Endocrinol Metab 97:3097–3106
51. Sone T, Ito M, Fukunaga M, Tomomitsu T, Sugimoto T, Shiraki M, Yoshimura T, Nakamura T (2014) The effects of once-weekly teriparatide on hip geometry assessed by hip structural analysis in postmenopausal osteoporotic women with high fracture risk. Bone 64:75–81

Chapter 5
Vertebral Strength Changes as Assessed by Finite Element Analysis

Taro Mawatari, Satoshi Ikemura, and Yukihide Iwamoto

Abstract Currently available surrogate markers of osteoporosis including areal bone mineral density (aBMD) measured by dual energy absorptiometry (DXA), bone turnover markers (BTMs), and fracture risk assessment tool (FRAX®) are limited for the use as targets, because those values are not directly reflecting bone strength. Because directly measuring the strength of any bone in a living human subject is not feasible, the combination of finite element analysis (FEA) and clinical computed tomography (CT) is an alternative and powerful technique for noninvasive assessment of whole bone strength. While there are several limitations including the radiation exposure, FEA has the potential to improve clinical assessment of osteoporosis. In this chapter, methodology and recent advances of FEA in this field including treatment efficacy assessment and fracture risk assessment are presented.

Keywords Strength • Finite element analysis • Osteoporosis

5.1 Introduction

Osteoporosis is a disease characterized by decreased bone strength predisposing an individual to an increased susceptibility for fracture. Despite that fracture reduction is the primary target for the treatment of osteoporosis, treatment of osteoporosis is

---

This work was supported in part by JSPS KAKENHI (Grant No. 24592269).

T. Mawatari (✉)
Department of Orthopaedic Surgery, Hamanomachi Hospital, 3-3-1 Nagahama, Chuo-ku, Fukuoka 810-8539, Japan

Department of Orthopaedic Surgery, Graduate School of Medical Sciences, Kyushu University, Fukuoka, Japan
e-mail: mawtaro@gmail.com

S. Ikemura
Department of Orthopaedic Surgery, Hamanomachi Hospital, 3-3-1 Nagahama, Chuo-ku, Fukuoka 810-8539, Japan

Y. Iwamoto
Department of Orthopaedic Surgery, Graduate School of Medical Sciences, Kyushu University, Fukuoka, Japan

Y. Shimada, N. Miyakoshi (eds.), *Osteoporosis in Orthopedics*,
DOI 10.1007/978-4-431-55778-4_5

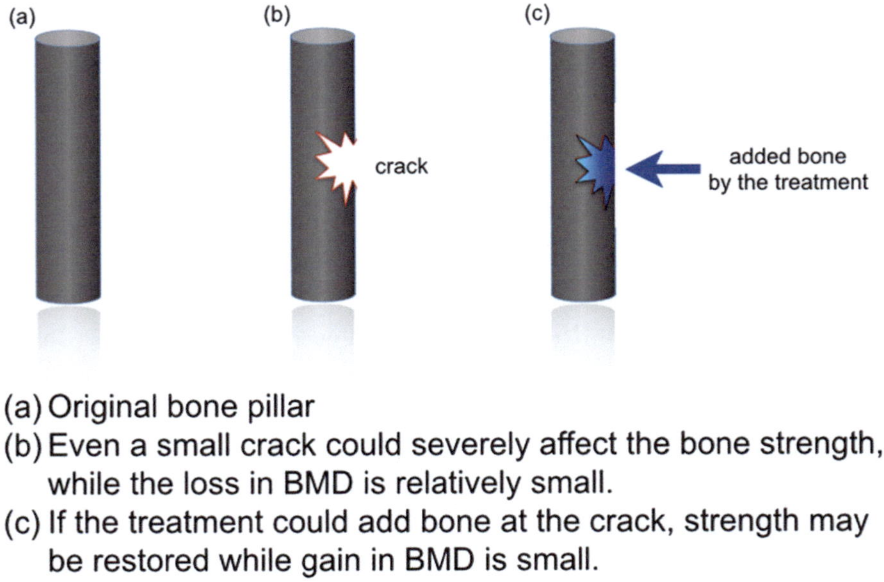

Fig. 5.1 Schematic representation why small loss in BMD could result in big loss in mechanical strength of the whole bone and why small gain in BMD could contribute to big gain in strength. (**a**) Original bone pillar. (**b**) Even a small crack could severely affect the bone strength, while the loss in BMD is relatively small. (**c**) If the treatment could add bone at the crack, strength may be restored while gain in BMD is small

usually initiated based on BMD and fracture risk, considering clinical risk factors for fracture. And the response to treatment is monitored by periodically measuring BMD and sometimes BTMs.

However, most of those who sustain fragile fractures are not in fact osteoporotic as classified by DXA measurement of areal BMD. Treatment-induced increases in areal BMD do not fully explain the known efficacy of osteoporosis drug treatments; why do small changes in areal BMD are associated with large reduction in fracture risk? Because of its two-dimensional nature, DXA is unable to distinguish between differential changes in cortical and trabecular bone and is confounded at the hip and spine by variable bone depth in the anterior–posterior direction and at the spine by formation of osteophytes and aortic calcification [1].

Furthermore, BMD literally shows the bone volume divided by the tissue volume. Figure 5.1 represents a bone pillar with a crack. While the volume of decreased bone at the crack is small compared with the whole pillar, in other words, decrease in BMD is small, we could easily assume that the strength of the pillar is severely deteriorated by the small crack. On the other hand, if the treatment could add bone at the crack, small increase in BMD may result in big gain for the strength of the whole bone. Like this schema, mechanical integrity of the bone depends on the distribution of the bone which areal BMD by DXA cannot account for.

BTMs reflect the pharmacological responses to osteoporosis therapies and are taking an increasingly important role in patient management; however, there are no consensus views to characterize high and normal bone turnover. For some analyses, the premenopausal reference range has been used to define a normal range, but there is a wide overlap between pre- and postmenopausal women, and a large overlap between those who will fracture compared with those that remain fracture free. The poor predictive value of BTMs in fracture risk suggests that absolute values for BTMs are not suited as treatment targets, at least with current technologies, while the change in BTMs would be useful as an index of compliance shortly after the onset of treatment [2].

The FRAX® tool has been developed by the World Health Organization (WHO) to evaluate fracture risk of individual patients from studying population-based cohorts from Europe, North America, Asia, and Australia. The FRAX® algorithms give the 10-year probability of fracture, however, unable to detect the impact of treatment on fracture risk [2].

As such, treatment has no clear consensus goal for BMD, BTMs, or fracture risk up until now. So understandably, the US Food and Drug Administration (FDA) still requires evidence for fracture risk reduction over 3 years as compared to placebo for registration of treatments for postmenopausal osteoporosis – a prohibitively expensive, and perhaps unethical, place for patients, clinical investigators, and industry research and development to be put at this time [3].

Given these limitations, there is a substantial interest in developing improved means for clinical assessment of bone strength. In this sense, finite element analysis is one of the best candidates up until now. The FEA technique is successful primarily because it biomechanically integrates all of the 3-dimensional geometry and density information within the CT scan. Promising data suggest that a more trustworthy surrogate marker of bone strength, such as FEA, could possibly substitute for fracture endpoints [1, 4].

5.2 Finite Element Analysis for Osteoporosis

FEA is a powerful numerical technique widely used by engineers and scientists for understanding the mechanics of physical systems. Engineers employ FEA to simulate how a physical system will respond to the expected loading conditions with an advantage of being applicable to solids of irregular geometry that contain heterogeneous material properties. Practical applications of FEA include structural analysis of various buildings, crash analysis of automobiles, aerodynamic analysis of airplanes, fluid flow analysis in channels and pipes, and so on. FEA in this osteoporosis field was first applied to live patients in a clinical research study in the early 1990s and used since then in many orthopedic biomechanical studies. With advances in the imaging modality and the processing power of computers, FEA has become more accessible and as such is becoming an increasingly popular tool to address questions about structure–function relationships in the bone field. FEA has

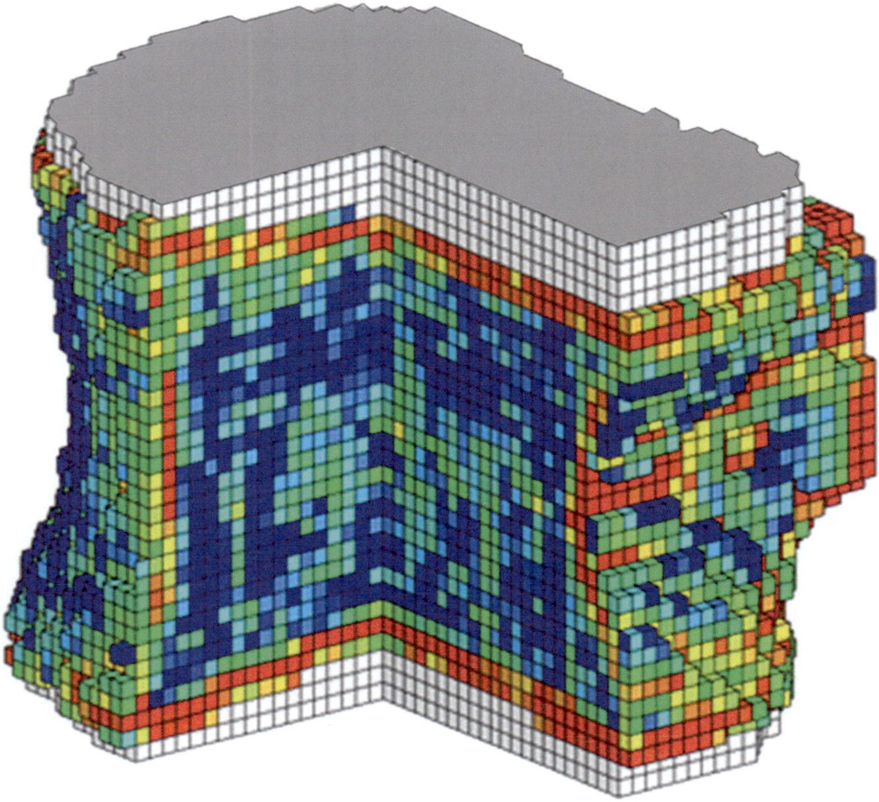

Fig. 5.2 Voxel-based FE model or a whole vertebral body from QCT scan, with individual finite elements color-coded according to their local material strength values

been used for various parts of the body including skeletal sites at high risk of osteoporotic fractures: the spine, hip, wrist, or more microscopically trabecular column, or individual trabeculae.

Typical analytical procedures of voxel-based FE analysis of CT scans of vertebra are as follows:

Step 1: Modeling

Firstly, subject-specific CT-based finite element model (Fig. 5.2) is generated by converting the QCT (quantitative computed tomography) scans. Each vertebra image is rotated into a standard coordinate system, thresholded, calibrated, and converted into an isopropic $1 \times 1 \times 1$-mm voxel-type finite element mesh using 8-noded brick elements with material properties derived directly from the calibrated mineral values in each element. More specifically, gray-scale Hounsfield unit data in the standard DICOM (Digital Imaging and Communications in Medicine)-formatted CT image is converted into calibrated values of BMD. Such material property–density relations are typically derived from cadaver experiments,

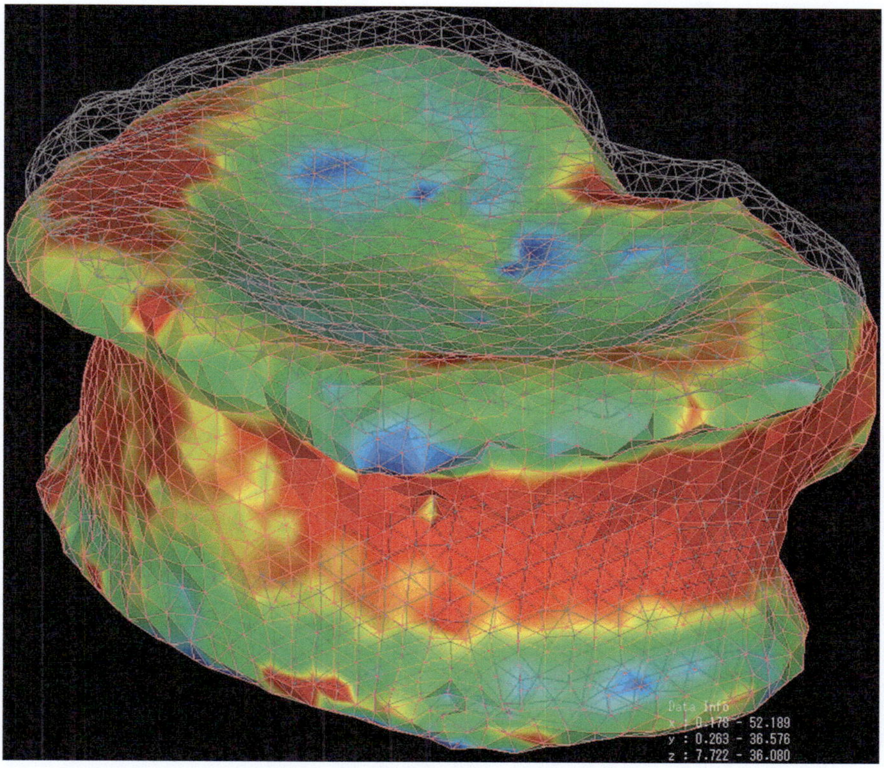

Fig. 5.3 FE model of a whole vertebral body from QCT scan, structured with tetrahedral elements. The cortical shell was modeled by using triangular plates with a thickness of 0.4 mm

adjusted to account for side artifacts, and elastic anisotropy of the bone was accounted for by assuming fixed ratios of the various elastic constants with respect to the longitudinal modulus. Material failure of the bone is modeled by assigning an elastic–perfectly plastic von Mises failure criterion to the bone [5, 6].

The finite elements themselves can be hexahedral-shaped replicas or scaled versions of the voxels, can be tetrahedral or curved, and can employ either linear or quadratic nodal-displacement formulation [1].

In order to take cortical shell into consideration, one approach would be the use of the thin element (Fig. 5.3) and another would be high-resolution image-based FEA. The former has inherent limitations since the cortical shell does not have a uniform thickness and has a porous structure. The latter may be able to account for microarchitecture; however, such high-resolution in vivo imaging in routine practice raises concerns about radiation dosage [1].

Step 2: Boundary and Loading Conditions

Secondly, boundary and loading conditions are applied to the model. When the model simulates an in vitro compressive-strength test, a thin layer of polymethylmethacrylate (PMMA) is virtually placed at the ends of each model vertebra to simulate test conditions commonly used in compressive-strength testing of cadaver vertebrae. In addition, another loading condition could be used to assess the bending structural behavior of the vertebra [5, 6].

Step 3: Calculation and Interpretation of the Outcome
Finally, nonlinear FEA is performed on models to compute strength, defined as the total reaction force generated at an imposed displacement equivalent to an overall vertebral compressive strain of 2 % (applied displacement divided by height). These techniques have been shown to provide excellent predictions of vertebral compressive strength [7]. When nonlinear finite element analysis is used, spatial distribution of failed bone material and bone damage within the whole bone can also be assessed, which can provide insight into the type of fracture to be expected under the prescribed loading conditions.

To assess compressive strength changes associated with changes only in the trabecular compartment, trabecular strength values could be calculated by removing the outer 2 mm of the bone from the model (which includes the thin cortical shell and adjacent trabecular bone) and recomputing strength for the remaining trabecular compartment. While it is impossible to directly calculate the strength associated with the cortical bone, the strength for the peripheral compartment could be estimated by subtracting the trabecular compartment strength from the whole vertebral compressive strength [6].

Alternatively, Imai et al. defined vertebral fracture as being at least one element failed, which occurs when the minimum principal strain of the first element was less than −10,000 microstrain, during application of uniaxial compressive load with a uniform distribution and a uniform load increment. They analyzed the yield load, the fracture load, the sites where elements failed, and the distribution of minimum principal strain [8].

5.3 Validation Study

Before applying this new technique to human clinical study, cadaver validation is required.

Crawford et al. found that vertebral strength and stiffness from in vitro mechanical testing using 13 vertebral specimens were positively correlated with FEA-predicted strength and stiffness ($r^2 = 0.86$ $P < 0.0001$, $r^2 = 0.82$ $P < 0.0001$, respectively) [7].

Imai et al. verified their method using a quasi-static uniaxial compression test of 12 thoracolumbar vertebral specimens. The FEA-predicted yield loads, fracture loads, and minimum principal strains were significantly correlated with those measured in cadaver study ($r = 0.949$ $P < 0.0001$, $r = 0.978$ $P < 0.0001$, $r = 0.838$ $P < 0.0001$, respectively) [8].

As such, reported cadaver studies have consistently shown that FEA of CT scans provides excellent predictions of vertebral compressive strength. Because of its projective and scalar nature, the performance of BMD in predicting bone strength depended on loading mode and was significantly inferior to FEA. The positive results of these biomechanical studies in vitro provided solid ground for its use in cross-sectional or prospective clinical studies [4].

5.4 FE Strength vs. aBMD

When comparing FE-estimated strength and aBMD by DXA, Mawatari et al. reported that baseline values of FE strength were poorly correlated with baseline values of aBMD ($R^2 = 0.39$, $P = 0.0002$) [6]. Moreover, the weak correlation has reported between individual changes in aBMD by DXA and individual change in FE strength.

Several studies indicate that the decrement in strength is relatively large compared with that in BMD [5, 6]. On the contrary, the increment in strength in response to treatment is relatively large, whereas the increment in BMD is modest. So evaluation of osteoporosis by BMD may underestimate the change in strength.

The available evidence indicates that treatment effects can be detected earlier and with greater statistical power (lower P values) by FEA because of improved statistical sensitivity [1].

5.5 FEA Using HR-pQCT

While QCT-based FEA represents a promising mechanistic alternative to densitometric techniques in accurately estimating the strength of the bone and predicting osteoporotic fracture risk, the voxel size often used for the current FE model was not small enough to explicitly capture such details as trabecular thickness, spacing, and connectivity or the true geometry of the cortical shell.

While a clinical CT is able to scan the human spine with minimum resolution of 150–350 μm, the voxel size is not high enough for taking individual trabecular structures or thin cortical shell into account. Several studies tried to use μCT and HR-pQCT images in combination with FE technique. High-resolution CT as the imaging technique requires a high X-ray dose of ~3 mSv but offers the possibility to generate high-resolution models as well as analyze the bone structure of a central fracture site, the spine. A lower effective dose would be possible if dedicated peripheral CT was used. This technique allows for a better image quality, but only at peripheral sites such as the forearm [9].

Dall'Ara has reported the HR-pQCT-based μFE and QCT-based nonlinear homogenized voxel-based FE for the same set of cadaveric spines [10]. The HR-pQCT ($0.082 \times 0.082 \times 0.082$ mm^3 voxel size) images were segmented after the application of a Laplace–Hamming filter with a fixed 40 % threshold, and the voxels were then directly converted to hexahedral elements. This model is able to account for trabecular microstructure, but due to the high amount of time and resources needed to run the μFE, only linear analysis was feasible for large samples. Linear μFE models were solved with ParFE on a Cray XT3 using 256 CPUs in parallel. While both HR-pQCT-based μFE and QCT-based FE predicted material properties better than aBMD, the latter provided reasonable quantitative estimations of the experimental mechanical properties without fitting the model parameters [10].

When the image resolution is improved to 82 μm, no benefits were found for prediction of any vertebral mechanical property using densitometric variables, and a significant improvement was only seen only for prediction of stiffness using linear μFE.

In vivo image voxel size for the human spine of 82 μm with a reasonable radiation dose is not expected in the close future [10].

5.6 Treatment Efficacy Assessment

5.6.1 Alendronate vs. Teriparatide for Postmenopausal Osteoporosis [5]

Both antiresorptives including alendronate (ALN) and anabolic agent such as teriparatide (TPTD) are reported to increase aBMD and reduce fracture risk, while underlying mechanisms on bone remodeling are opposite. Keaveny et al. have demonstrated the effect of TPTD and ALN on 3rd lumbar vertebral bone strength by comparative study using the FE modeling of QCT scans. Also trabecular strength values were calculated by removing the outer 2 mm of bone from the model and recomputing strength for the remaining trabecular compartment.

In an 18-month active comparator study of 53 patients ($N = 28$ TPTD 20 μg/day; $N = 25$ ALN 10 mg/day), both treatments had positive effects on vertebral compressive strength. At 18 months, the median percentage increase for TPTD was 5.7-fold greater from baseline compared with ALN, 21.1 % versus 3.7 %. Both treatments also increased the strength–density ratio from baseline, but the median percentage increases were three to five times larger for the TPTD group (6.01 % versus 2.15 %, $p = 0.002$). Comparison of change in the FEA vertebral compressive strength versus the change in aBMD indicated that DXA did not capture well the changes in biomechanical properties that occurred with treatment and that, in general, the relation between BMD changes and FEA strength changes depended on treatment. They concluded that both TPTD and ALN increased vertebral strength, while larger increases in the strength–density ratio were also observed for TPTD, and these were primarily attributed to preferential increases in trabecular strength. This is the first study that compares two approved treatments for osteoporosis on FE-derived biomechanical measurements of the spine in a clinical setting.

5.6.2 Alendronate for Rheumatoid Arthritis [6]

Osteoporosis occurs more frequently in patients with rheumatoid arthritis (RA) than in otherwise healthy individuals. Treatment with antiresorptive agents such as ALN is the generally accepted recommendation for prevention and treatment of osteoporosis in RA patients who are receiving glucocorticoids; significant reductions in the risk of incident radiographic vertebral fractures have been found with ALN treatment. However, the biomechanical mechanisms by which ALN treatment alters vertebral strength in RA and the relative effect of such treatment on the cortical versus the trabecular compartment remain unclear. A prospective randomized clinical trial was undertaken to compare strength changes, measured using FEA, in rheumatoid arthritis (RA) patients who were treated with ALN versus those who were not. Nonlinear finite element analysis was performed on the CT scans of L_3 vertebra ($n = 29$) to compute an estimate of compressive strength and to assess strength changes associated with changes in the trabecular compartment and the outer 2 mm of bone (peripheral compartment).

As a result, vertebral strength was significantly decreased from baseline in the control group (median change −10.6 %; $P = 0.008$) but was maintained in the ALN group (median change +0.4 %; $P = 0.55$), with a significant difference between the two groups ($P < 0.01$). Strength decreased more rapidly within the trabecular bone, and ALN treatment was much more effective in the peripheral than the trabecular compartment. Mawatari et al. concluded that patients with RA can lose a substantial amount of vertebral strength over a relatively short period of time, and this loss can be prevented by ALN, primarily via its positive effect on the outer 2 mm of vertebral bone.

5.6.3 Alendronate for Postmenopausal Osteoporosis [11]

Imai et al. analyzed vertebral strength in 104 postmenopausal Japanese women in vivo using QCT-based nonlinear FE model with 2-mm tetrahedral elements and 2-mm triangular plates on the outer surface of the cortical shell and explored the discriminatory power for vertebral fracture cross-sectionally. They also prospectively assessed the effects of ALN by this technique in 33 patients with postmenopausal osteoporosis who were treated with ALN for 1 year.

On the age- and body weight-adjusted logistic regression, estimated 2nd lumbar vertebral strength had stronger discriminatory power for vertebral fracture (OR per SD change: 6.71) than aBMD and vBMD. Calculated vertebral fracture threshold was 1.95 kN with 75.9 % sensitivity and 78.7 % specificity. ALN effects were detected on vertebral strength at 3 months (+10.2 % from baseline). At 1 year, the density of the inner cancellous bone increased by 8.3 %, while the density of the juxtacortical areas increased by 13.6 %.

They concluded that QCT-based nonlinear FEM had higher discriminatory power for vertebral fracture than BMD and detected ALN effects as early as 3 months. ALN altered density distribution and decreased the area with a high fracture risk, resulting in increased vertebral strength.

5.6.4 Ibandronate for Postmenopausal Osteoporosis [12]

This 1-year randomized, double-blind, placebo-controlled study investigated the effects of once-monthly oral ibandronate (IBN) on both the hip and spine in postmenopausal osteoporosis by 3D techniques of QCT and FEA and the 2D techniques of DXA and hip structure analysis (HSA). Women aged from 55 to 80 years old with BMD T-score −2.0 or less to −5.0 or greater were randomized 1:1 to receive oral IBN 150 mg ($n=47$) or placebo ($n=46$) once monthly for 12 months.

IBN increased vertebral, peripheral, and trabecular strength and anterior and posterior bending stiffness vs. placebo [7.1 % ($P<0.001$), 7.8 % ($P<0.001$), 5.6 % ($P=0.023$), and 6.3 % ($P<0.001$), respectively], while lumbar spine aBMD increased more with IBN than placebo [4.3 % ($P<0.001$)]. FE-derived hip strength to density ratio and femoral strength, as well as total hip QCT BMD and DXA aBMD, also increased with IBN vs. placebo. HSA-estimated femoral narrow sectional area and moment of inertia and outer diameter increased with IBN vs. placebo. Lewiecki et al. concluded that once-monthly oral IBN for 12 months improved hip and spine BMD measured by QCT and DXA and strength estimated by FEA of QCT scans.

5.6.5 Teriparatide for Postmenopausal Osteoporosis [9]

Changes in DXA-based areal BMD explain only ~30 % of the anti-fracture efficacy of TPTD. However, monitoring of osteoporosis based solely on DXA is insufficient to assess anti-fracture efficacy. Graeff et al. assessed the feasibility of using nonlinear FE analysis to monitor TPTD treatment and the additional information gained in comparison with DXA. FE models based on high-resolution CT (HRCT) of T_{12} with an in-plane voxel size of 156 or 188 μm were evaluated after 0, 6, 12, and 24 months of TPTD treatment (20 μg/day) in 44 postmenopausal women with established osteoporosis participating in the EUROFORS study. FE-based strength and stiffness calculations for three loading models, including compression, bending, and combined compression and bending, were compared with volumetric BMD and apparent bone volume fraction, as well as DXA-based areal BMD of the lumbar spine. Significant improvements in all analyzed variables as early as 6 months after TPTD treatment were found.

The observed increases after 2-year treatment of TPTD were in the order of 10 % for a BMD, 20 % for vBMD, and up to 30 % for FE variables. This is in good agreement with results from the FACT trial, where Keaveny et al. showed close to 20 % increase in compression and bending stiffness after 18 months of TPTD treatment. The authors also compared the linear and nonlinear model used for the compression test, and both models resulted in similar responses to treatment. Furthermore, stiffness and strength in the nonlinear model were well correlated.

5.6.6 Risedronate vs. Teriparatide for Glucocorticoid-Induced Osteoporosis in Men [13]

The long-term use of glucocorticoid (GC) is the most common cause of secondary osteoporosis; however, the data on GC-induced osteoporosis in men are scare. Due to GCs' primary effect of a profound inhibition of osteoblastic bone-forming activity, a need exists for therapies that can substantially improve bone formation and the microarchitecture status of patients with GIO. Along with such therapies, more sensitive diagnostic and evaluation methods beyond aBMD by DXA, such as vBMD by QCT, assessment of trabecular microarchitecture with high-resolution QCT, and strength using FEA should be applied.

Glüer et al. performed a randomized, open-label trial in men who have taken GC for $\geq$3 months and had an aBMD T-score ≤ -1.5 SD. Subjects received 20 μg/day TPTD ($n = 45$) or 35 mg/week risedronate (RIS) ($n = 47$) for 18 months.

QCT scans of L_1–L_3 (pixel sizes of 0.6 mm) and HRQCT scans of Th_{12} (pixel sizes of 156 or 188 μm) were obtained at months 0, 6, and 18. Regarding the evaluation of bone strength, FE analyses with axial compression, anterior bending, and axial torsion were conducted.

BMD increased for both groups; however, observed bone volume and tissue mineral density were different in these groups. Bone volume was increased and tissue mineral density was reduced under TPTD reflecting apposition of not yet fully mineralized bone, whereas tissue mineral density was increased and bone structure was maintained under RIS due to reduction of bone turnover. Statistically significant increases in vertebral strength were observed for both treatment groups and all three loading modes, with statistically significant larger increase in the TPTD group. In conclusion, TPTD showed larger improvements in spinal BMD, microstructure, and FE-estimated strength than RIS.

5.6.7 Add or Switch to Teriparatide for Postmenopausal Osteoporosis [14]

In patients previously treated with antiresorptive drugs, two approaches are available when initiating TPTD: stopping the antiresorptive agent when TPTD is initiated (the Switch approach) or continuing the antiresorptive agent when TPTD is initiated (the Add approach).

Randomized prospective open-label study was conducted to assess the effects of adding versus switching to TPTD 20 μg/day in patients pretreated with ALN 70 mg/week ($n=91$) or RLX 60 mg/day ($n=77$) for at least 18 months. QCT scans of L_1 and hip were performed at baseline, 6 and 18 months to assess changes in vBMD and strength for simulated compression overload and femoral strength for simulated sideways fall by nonlinear finite element analysis.

At the spine, median vBMD and strength increased from baseline in all groups (13.2–17.5 %, $p<0.01$); there were no significant differences between the Add and Switch groups. In the RLX stratum, hip vBMD and strength increased at 6 and 18 months in the Add group but only at 18 months in the Switch group (Strength, Month 18: 2.7 % Add group, $p<0.01$, and 3.4 % Switch group, $p<0.05$). In the ALN stratum, hip vBMD increased in the Add but not in the Switch group (0.9 % versus −0.5 % at 6 months and 2.2 % versus 0.0 % at 18 months, both $p<0.004$ group difference). At 18 months, hip strength increased in the Add group (2.7 %, $p<0.01$) but not in the Switch group (0 %); however, the difference between groups was not significant ($p=0.076$).

Cosman et al. concluded that adding or switching to TPTD conferred similar benefits on spine strength in postmenopausal women with osteoporosis pretreated with ALN or RLX. Increases in hip strength were more variable. In RLX-treated women, strength increased more quickly in the Add group; in ALN-treated women, a significant increase in strength compared with baseline was seen only in the Add group.

5.6.8 *Denosumab for Postmenopausal Osteoporosis [15]*

Denosumab (DMAB) is a fully human monoclonal antibody that inhibits receptor activator of NF-kB ligand (RANKL), a key modulator of osteoclast formation, function, and survival. In the phase 3 Fracture Reduction Evaluation of Anti-RANKL antibody Denosumab in Osteoporosis Every 6 Months (FREEDOM) study of 7808 postmenopausal women with osteoporosis showed that DMAB reduced the risk of hip and new vertebral fracture over 36 months compared with placebo by 40 % and 68 %, respectively.

To gain further insight into the observed clinical efficacy of DMAB in reducing the risk of hip and spine fractures, in a subset of subjects in the FREEDOM study ($n=48$ placebo; $n=51$ DMAB), Keaveny et al. applied FEA to the hip and spine QCT scans to noninvasively assess changes in hip and spine strength associated with DMAB treatment over 36 months.

Hip strength as estimated by FEA increased significantly compared with baseline by 5.3 % at 12 months ($p<0.0001$) and progressively over time, reaching 8.6 % at 36 months ($p<0.0001$ compared with baseline and 12 months) in the women treated with DMAB. In contrast, hip strength did not change at 12 months and decreased −5.6 % at 36 months compared with baseline ($p < 0.0001$) in the women treated with placebo. Similar changes were observed at the spine: strength increased by 18.2 % at 36 months for the DMAB group ($p < 0.0001$) and decreased by −4.2 % for the placebo groups ($p = 0.002$). At 36 months, hip and spine strength increased for the DMAB group compared with the placebo group by 14.3 and 22.4 %, respectively. Further analysis indicated that strength associated with the trabecular bone was lost at the hip and spine in the placebo group, whereas strength associated with both the trabecular and cortical bone improved in the DMAB group.

5.6.9 *Odanacatib for Postmenopausal Osteoporosis [16]*

Odanacatib (ODN) is a highly selective and reversible oral inhibitor of the collagenase cathepsin K that is secreted by osteoclast. ODN reduces bone resorption without reducing osteoclast number and hence appears to preserve bone formation. In a phase 2 trial of women with low areal BMD, it has already been demonstrated that bone resorption markers remained reduced in women treated with ODN 50 mg once weekly for 5 years, while bone formation markers initially reduced and returned to near baseline levels with 2 years of continued therapy. In the phase 2 trial extension, continuous treatment with ODN for 5 years resulted in mean increases in a BMD from baseline of 11.9 % at the lumbar spine.

In this randomized, double-blind, international, 2-year, phase 3 trial comparing ODN 50 mg once weekly with placebo in postmenopausal women, Brixen et al. used BTMs, QCT, and FEA to assess bone density, geometry, and strength at the spine and hip.

Bone resorption marker C-telopeptide of type 1 collagen was significantly lower with ODN ($n = 109$) vs. placebo ($n = 105$) at 6 months and 2 years ($p < 0.001$), whereas bone formation marker procollagen 1 N-terminal peptide initially decreased with ODN group but by 2 years did not differ from placebo.

After 6 months, ODN-treated women had greater increase in trabecular vBMD and estimated compressive strength at the spine and vBMD and estimated strength at the hip ($p < 0.001$). Significantly greater gain was seen in ODN group compared with placebo at 2 years in aBMD at the spine and femoral neck (+3.5 % $p < 0.001$, +3.8 % $p < 0.001$, respectively), trabecular vBMD at L_1 and femoral neck (+11.5 % $p < 0.001$, +3.3 % $p < 0.001$), and FE-estimated compressive strength at the spine and hip (+14.3 % $p < 0.001$, +5.6 % $p < 0.001$, respectively).

The results of their study suggest that ODN decreased bone resorption, maintained bone formation, increased areal and volumetric BMD, and increased estimated bone strength at both the hip and spine.

5.6.10 Teriparatide for Adult Osteogenesis Imperfecta [17]

Osteogenesis imperfecta (OI) is caused by mutations in the genes encoding type 1 collagen, and fractures and skeletal deformity are frequently observed in their childhood, but fracture risk remains high in adulthood. Currently, few treatment options are available, and bone anabolic therapies have not been tested in clinical trials for the treatment of OI. Orwoll et al. evaluated 79 adult patients with OI who received 20 μg/day TPTD ($n = 38$, 40.8 ± 12.9 years old) or placebo ($n = 40$, 41.2 ± 10.1 years old) for 18 months in a randomized, double-blind, placebo-controlled trial with the vertebral areal BMD by DXA, vertebral volumetric BMD by QCT, and vertebral strength by FEA. Compared with the placebo group, the TPTD group showed increased vertebral aBMD (6.1 % ± 1.0 % vs. 2.8 % ± 1.0 % change from baseline; $P < 0.05$) and total hip aBMD (2.6 % ± 1.0 % vs. –2.4 % ± 1.0 % change; $P < 0.001$). Vertebral vBMD and strength improved with TPTD therapy (18 % ± 6 % and 15 % ± 3 % change, respectively) but declined with placebo (−5.0 % ± 6 % and −2.0 % ± 3 % change; $P < 0.05$ for both comparisons). A milder form of OI (type I) patients exhibited robust BMD increases with TPTD; however, there was no observed benefit for those with severe forms of OI (type III/IV). They concluded that TPTD therapy significantly increased aBMD at the hip and spine and estimated vertebral strength in adults with a mild form of OI (type I).

5.6.11 Blosozumab for Postmenopausal Osteoporosis [18]

Blosozumab is a humanized monoclonal antibody targeted to inhibit sclerostin and promote new bone. To determine the effects of subcutaneous blosozumab treatment on noninvasive estimates of spine and hip strength, Keaveny et al. performed a FEA on QCT images in postmenopausal women with low areal BMD (lumbar spine T-score −3.5 to −2.0). These 42 women, mean age 62 years, were a subgroup of patients enrolled in a double-blind, placebo-controlled, randomized, multicenter, 1-year, phase II dosing study of four treatment groups: placebo, blosozumab 180 mg every 4 weeks, blosozumab 180 mg every 2 weeks, or blosozumab 270 mg every 2 weeks. After confirming uniformity of the groups at baseline, they found for the placebo group that neither spine nor hip strength changed significantly from baseline. By contrast, in the treated groups, there were statistically significant increases in both spine and hip strength, at both 24 and 52 weeks. These effects were substantial in the highest dose group; blosozumab increased spine and hip strength compared to baseline by up to 37.0 and 12.6 % at Week 52.

At both the spine and hip, these strength changes were associated with statistically significant increases in volumetric BMD of both the trabecular and cortical compartments. Other than mild injection site reactions that were more frequent with blosozumab than placebo, adverse events were similar across all groups. They concluded that blosozumab increased FE-estimated spine and hip strength in the phase II study, displaying a statistically significant positive dose response at both sites.

5.7 Fracture Risk Assessment

5.7.1 Structural Determinants of Vertebral Fracture Risk [19]

It is unclear whether the association of aBMD with vertebral fracture risk depends on bone density per se, bone macro- or microstructure, overall bone strength, or spine load/bone strength ratios. Melton III et al. studied 40 women with a clinically diagnosed vertebral fracture caused by moderate trauma (mean age, 78.6 ± 9.0 year) and compared them with 40 controls with no osteoporotic fracture (mean age, 70.9 ± 6.8 year) from an age-stratified sample of Rochester, MN. Lumbar spine vBMD and geometry were assessed by central QCT, whereas microstructure was evaluated by HR-pQCT at the ultradistal radius. Vertebral failure load (~strength) was estimated from voxel-based FEA, and the factor of risk (ø) was determined as the ratio of applied spine loads to failure load.

While estimated axial compressive force on L_3 was similar in vertebral fracture cases and controls (e.g., for 90° forward flexion, 2639 versus 2706 N; age-adjusted $p = 0.173$), fracture cases had inferior values for most bone density and structure variables. Bone strength measures were also reduced, and the factor of risk was 35–37 % greater (worse) among women with a vertebral fracture. By age-adjusted logistic regression, relative risks for the strongest fracture predictor in each of the five main variable categories were bone density (total lumbar spine vBMD: OR per SD change, 2.2; 95 % CI, 1.1–4.3), bone geometry (vertebral apparent cortical thickness: OR, 2.1; 95 % CI, 1.1–4.1), bone microstructure (none significant); bone strength ("cortical" [outer 2 mm] compressive strength: OR, 2.5; 95 % CI, 1.3–4.8), and factor of risk (ø for 90° forward flexion/overall vertebral compressive strength: OR, 3.2; 95 % CI, 1.4–7.5). Finally, authors concluded that vertebral fractures are more strongly associated with specific bone density, structure, and strength parameters than with areal BMD, while all of these variables are correlated.

5.7.2 Prediction of New Clinical Vertebral Fractures in Elderly Men [20]

In order to compare vertebral strength, as estimated by FEA of CT scans against aBMD by DXA for prospectively assessing the risk of new clinical vertebral fractures, Wang et al. conducted a case–cohort analysis of 306 men aged 65 years and older observed over an average of 6.5 years. This cohort included 63 men who developed new clinically identified vertebral fractures and 243 men who did not.

They found that, for the risk of new clinical vertebral fracture, the age-adjusted hazard ratio per standard deviation change for aBMD (3.2; 95 % confidence interval [CI], 2.0–5.2) was significantly lower ($p < 0.005$) than for strength (7.2; 95 % CI, 3.6–14.1), numerically lower than for vBMD (5.7; 95 % CI, 3.1–10.3), and similar for the load-to-strength ratio (3.0; 95 % CI, 2.1–4.3). After also adjusting for race, body mass index (BMI), clinical center, and aBMD, all these hazard ratios remained highly statistically significant, particularly those for strength (8.5; 95 % CI, 3.6–20.1) and vBMD (9.4; 95 % CI, 4.1–21.6). The area under the curve for areal BMD (AUC = 0.76) was significantly lower than for strength (AUC = 0.83, $p = 0.02$), volumetric BMD (AUC = 0.82, $p = 0.05$), and the load-to-strength ratio (AUC = 0.82, $p = 0.05$). They concluded that, compared to aBMD by DXA, vertebral compressive strength and vBMD consistently improved vertebral fracture risk assessment in this cohort of elderly men.

5.7.3 Assessment of Incident Spine and Hip Fractures in Women and Men [21]

FEA-derived strength estimates have been validated in cadaver studies and clinically validated for prediction of incident clinical spine and hip fractures in men and incident hip fractures in women. Associations have also been shown in women between FEA and both prevalent spine fractures and any prevalent osteoporotic fracture. However, FEA methodology has not yet validated for prediction of incident spine fractures in women. Further, although clinical guidelines for interpreting BMD are well established (e.g., $T \leq -2.5$ for defining osteoporosis), such guidelines remain to be validated for FEA-derived measures of strength.

Kopperdahl et al. performed a 5-year case–control study of 1110 women and men over the age of 65 years. They found that for incident radiographically confirmed spine fractures ($n = 167$) out of 843 subjects in Spine arm, the age-adjusted odds ratio for FEA-estimated vertebral strength was significant for women (2.8, 95 % confidence interval [CI] 1.8-4.3) and men (2.2, 95 % CI 1.5-3.2). For incident hip fractures ($n = 171$) out of 1408 subjects in Hip arm, the age-adjusted odds ratio for femoral strength was significant for women (4.2, 95 % CI 2.6-6.9) and men (3.5, 95 % CI 2.3-5.3) and remained significant after adjusting for femoral neck aBMD in women and for total hip aBMD in both sexes; fracture classification improved for women by combining femoral strength with femoral neck aBMD ($p = 0.002$).

For both sexes, the probabilities of spine and hip fractures were similarly high at the BMD-based interventional thresholds for osteoporosis and at corresponding preestablished thresholds for "fragile bone strength" (spine: women 4500 N, men 6500 N; hip: women 3000 N, men 3500 N). Because it is well established that individuals over the age of 65 years who have osteoporosis at the hip or spine by BMD criteria should be considered at high risk of fracture, authors think that these results should indicate that individuals who have fragile bone strength at the hip or spine should also be considered at high risk of fracture.

5.8 Limitations of FEA

Despite the sophistication of the analysis technique, there are several limitations of FEA in this field.

One clinical challenge with QCT-based FE analysis is the actual need for a CT scan and the associated cost and radiation exposure. With continuing advances in CT technology, development of lower-radiation scanning techniques is anticipated. Alternatively, the use of retrospective analysis of preexisting CT exams including CT colonography and CT angiography with phantomless calibration technique has been proposed [1].

Several investigators have reported that glucocorticoid treatment might alter bone metabolism to the extent that the bone becomes more fragile and can break at higher bone mass values than are seen in postmenopausal women [6]. Also patients with diabetes, chronic obstructive pulmonary disease, and chronic kidney disease are reported to have more fragile bone than estimated by BMD. Material property or strength–density relationship of the bone may be different under various conditions including disease and treatments; however, tuning material properties for a given data set may well achieve higher correlations to the actual strength but disregard the universality sought for a better surrogate of bone strength [4].

The other important limitation is that submillimeter bone quality factors – such as collagen cross-linking [22], mineral crystal structure, microdamage, or resorption space-induced stress raisers – are not described by clinical CT exams. However, the role of any such factors on clinical fracture risk assessment is not fully understood. At present, there is no clear consensus on the biomechanical effects of such bone quality effects or bone quality effects associated with pharmaceutical intervention, and such bone quality effects are not considered in current FE models and remain an area of ongoing research [1].

5.9 Perspectives

Considering the cumulated evidence from the published validation studies, it is concluded that FEA of CT scans provide the most reliable surrogates of bone strength and could be used as targets for the treatment of osteoporosis when considering goal-directed approach.

FEA-derived strength estimates have been used to show the effect of various pharmacological interventions as described above. As a FDA-approved approach to monitor treatment effects [15], this method has became already an indispensable measure for newly developed agents aside from stochastic approach in large-scale clinical trials.

Furthermore, FEA of CT scans have shown to predict new incident hip and spine fractures and to differentiate those with or without prevalent fractures. FEA has also been used to study effects of aging and long-duration space flight on bone strength and estimate changes in strength [1].

Given the advantages discussed in this chapter, FEA of CT scans would provide unique clinical insight and have a profound impact on the management of osteoporosis.

References

1. Keaveny TM (2010) Biomechanical computed tomography-noninvasive bone strength analysis using clinical computed tomography scans. Ann N Y Acad Sci 1192:57–65. doi:10.1111/j.1749-6632.2009.05348.x
2. Kanis JA, McCloskey E, Branco J, Brandi ML, Dennison E, Devogelaer JP, Ferrari S, Kaufman JM, Papapoulos S, Reginster JY, Rizzoli R (2014) Goal-directed treatment of osteoporosis in Europe. Osteoporos Int 25(11):2533–2543. doi:10.1007/s00198-014-2787-1
3. Jacques RM, Boonen S, Cosman F, Reid IR, Bauer DC, Black DM, Eastell R (2012) Relationship of changes in total hip bone mineral density to vertebral and nonvertebral fracture risk in women with postmenopausal osteoporosis treated with once-yearly zoledronic acid 5 mg: the HORIZON-Pivotal Fracture Trial (PFT). J Bone Miner Res 27(8):1627–1634. doi:10.1002/jbmr.1644
4. Zysset PK, Dall'ara E, Varga P, Pahr DH (2013) Finite element analysis for prediction of bone strength. Bonekey Rep 2:386. doi:10.1038/bonekey.2013.120
5. Keaveny TM, Donley DW, Hoffmann PF, Mitlak BH, Glass EV, San Martin JA (2007) Effects of teriparatide and alendronate on vertebral strength as assessed by finite element modeling of QCT scans in women with osteoporosis. J Bone Miner Res 22(1):149–157. doi:10.1359/jbmr.061011
6. Mawatari T, Miura H, Hamai S, Shuto T, Nakashima Y, Okazaki K, Kinukawa N, Sakai S, Hoffmann PF, Iwamoto Y, Keaveny TM (2008) Vertebral strength changes in rheumatoid arthritis patients treated with alendronate, as assessed by finite element analysis of clinical computed tomography scans: a prospective randomized clinical trial. Arthritis Rheum 58 (11):3340–3349. doi:10.1002/art.23988
7. Crawford RP, Cann CE, Keaveny TM (2003) Finite element models predict in vitro vertebral body compressive strength better than quantitative computed tomography. Bone 33 (4):744–750. doi:10.1016/s8756-3282(03)00210-2
8. Imai K, Ohnishi I, Bessho M, Nakamura K (2006) Nonlinear finite element model predicts vertebral bone strength and fracture site. Spine 31(16):1789–1794
9. Graeff C, Chevalier Y, Charlebois M, Varga P, Pahr D, Nickelsen TN, Morlock MM, Gluer CC, Zysset PK (2009) Improvements in vertebral body strength under teriparatide treatment assessed in vivo by finite element analysis: results from the EUROFORS study. J Bone Miner Res 24(10):1672–1680. doi:10.1359/jbmr.090416
10. Dall'Ara E, Pahr D, Varga P, Kainberger F, Zysset P (2012) QCT-based finite element models predict human vertebral strength in vitro significantly better than simulated DEXA. Osteoporos Int 23(2):563–572. doi:10.1007/s00198-011-1568-3
11. Imai K, Ohnishi I, Yamamoto S, Nakamura K (2009) Assessment of vertebral fracture risk and therapeutic effects of alendronate in postmenopausal women using a quantitative computed

tomography-based nonlinear finite element method. Osteoporos Int 20:801–810. doi:10.1007/s00198-008-0750-8
12. Lewiecki EM, Keaveny TM, Kopperdahl DL, Genant HK, Engelke K, Fuerst T, Kivitz A, Davies RY, Fitzpatrick LA (2009) Once-monthly oral ibandronate improves biomechanical determinants of bone strength in women with postmenopausal osteoporosis. J Clin Endocrinol Metab 94(1):171–180. doi:10.1210/jc.2008-1807
13. Gluer CC, Marin F, Ringe JD, Hawkins F, Moricke R, Papaioannu N, Farahmand P, Minisola S, Martinez G, Nolla JM, Niedhart C, Guanabens N, Nuti R, Martin-Mola E, Thomasius F, Kapetanos G, Pena J, Graeff C, Petto H, Sanz B, Reisinger A, Zysset PK (2013) Comparative effects of teriparatide and risedronate in glucocorticoid-induced osteoporosis in men: 18-month results of the EuroGIOPs trial. J Bone Miner Res 28(6):1355–1368. doi:10.1002/jbmr.1870
14. Cosman F, Keaveny TM, Kopperdahl D, Wermers RA, Wan X, Krohn KD, Krege JH (2013) Hip and spine strength effects of adding versus switching to teriparatide in postmenopausal women with osteoporosis treated with prior alendronate or raloxifene. J Bone Miner Res 28 (6):1328–1336. doi:10.1002/jbmr.1853
15. Keaveny TM, McClung MR, Genant HK, Zanchetta JR, Kendler D, Brown JP, Goemaere S, Recknor C, Brandi ML, Eastell R, Kopperdahl DL, Engelke K, Fuerst T, Radcliffe HS, Libanati C (2014) Femoral and vertebral strength improvements in postmenopausal women with osteoporosis treated with denosumab. J Bone Miner Res 29(1):158–165. doi:10.1002/jbmr.2024
16. Brixen K, Chapurlat R, Cheung AM, Keaveny TM, Fuerst T, Engelke K, Recker R, Dardzinski B, Verbruggen N, Ather S, Rosenberg E, de Papp AE (2013) Bone density, turnover, and estimated strength in postmenopausal women treated with odanacatib: a randomized trial. J Clin Endocrinol Metab 98(2):571–580. doi:10.1210/jc.2012-2972
17. Orwoll ES, Shapiro J, Veith S, Wang Y, Lapidus J, Vanek C, Reeder JL, Keaveny TM, Lee DC, Mullins MA, Nagamani SC, Lee B (2014) Evaluation of teriparatide treatment in adults with osteogenesis imperfecta. J Clin Invest 124(2):491–498. doi:10.1172/JCI71101
18. Keaveny T, Myers S, Chiang A, Alam J, Robins D, Krege J, Sipos A, Mitlak B, Benson C (2013) Effects of blosozumab on estimated spine and hip strength in postmenopausal women with low bone mineral density: finite element analysis of a phase-II dosing study. J Bone Miner Res 28(Suppl 1). Available at http://www.asbmr.org/education/AbstractDetail?aid=7214d65b-b1c1-4ad1-bd87-23206e3630cb. Accessed 30 June 2015
19. Melton LJ 3rd, Riggs BL, Keaveny TM, Achenbach SJ, Hoffmann PF, Camp JJ, Rouleau PA, Bouxsein ML, Amin S, Atkinson EJ, Robb RA, Khosla S (2007) Structural determinants of vertebral fracture risk. J Bone Miner Res 22(12):1885–1892. doi:10.1359/jbmr.070728
20. Wang X, Sanyal A, Cawthon PM, Palermo L, Jekir M, Christensen J, Ensrud KE, Cummings SR, Orwoll E, Black DM, Osteoporotic Fractures in Men Research G, Keaveny TM (2012) Prediction of new clinical vertebral fractures in elderly men using finite element analysis of CT scans. J Bone Miner Res 27(4):808–816. doi:10.1002/jbmr.1539
21. Kopperdahl DL, Aspelund T, Hoffmann PF, Sigurdsson S, Siggeirsdottir K, Harris TB, Gudnason V, Keaveny TM (2014) Assessment of incident spine and hip fractures in women and men using finite element analysis of CT scans. J Bone Miner Res 29(3):570–580. doi:10.1002/jbmr.2069
22. Saito M, Marumo K (2010) Collagen cross-links as a determinant of bone quality: a possible explanation for bone fragility in aging, osteoporosis, and diabetes melitus. Osteoporos Int 21 (2):195–214. doi:10.1007/s00198-009-1066-z

Part II
Factors Affecting Osteoporosis

Chapter 6
The Geometry of Lower Extremity and Atypical Femoral Fractures

Muneaki Ishijima, Yoshitomo Saita, Haruka Kaneko, Mayuko Kinoshita, and Kazuo Kaneko

Abstract Osteoporosis is a systemic skeletal disease that is characterized by low bone mass and the structural deterioration of bone tissue leading to bone fragility and an increased risk of fracture. Fractures, most notably of the hip, are associated with significant morbidity and mortality. From a patient's perspective, a hip fracture and the subsequent loss of mobility and autonomy often represent a major drop in the quality of life.

Although it had been thought to be a natural part of the aging process in women, osteoporosis is no longer considered age or sex dependent, and it is largely preventable due to the remarkable progress in the scientific understanding of its causes, diagnosis, and treatment. Bone strength primarily reflects the integration of bone density and bone quality. The treatment of osteoporosis seeks to increase the bone mass and, hopefully, to improve bone quality, resulting in the strengthening of the bone structure. As bone is a remodeling organ and because of recent developments in the field of bone biology, we have recently become able to increase bone mass and bone strength by modulating the bone remodeling processes. However, the goal of therapy is fracture prevention.

The bisphosphonates (BPs), a class of antiresorptive agents, are the current cornerstone of osteoporosis treatment and prevention. These nitrogen-containing compounds bind to the bone surface. Treatment with bisphosphonates reduces the rate of bone resorption, increases bone mineral density, and improves trabecular connectivity. These resultant effects serve to improve bone strength and reduce the risk of fracture. Denosumab, a fully human monoclonal antibody against the receptor activator of nuclear factor-κB ligand (RANKL), prevents the interaction of RANKL with RANK, its receptor, on osteoclasts and their precursors, thereby blocking the formation, function, and survival of osteoclasts. At the moment, these anti-bone-resorbing agents are only drugs that can reduce the incidence of osteoporotic hip fragility fractures in osteoporotic patients. However, treatments with

M. Ishijima, M.D., Ph.D. (✉) • Y. Saita, M.D., Ph.D. • H. Kaneko, M.D., Ph.D.
M. Kinoshita, M.D. • K. Kaneko, M.D., Ph.D.
Department of Medicine for Orthopaedics and Motor Organ, Juntendo University Graduate School of Medicine, 2-1-1, Hongo, Bunkyo-ku, Tokyo 113-8421, Japan
e-mail: ishijima@juntendo.ac.jp

Y. Shimada, N. Miyakoshi (eds.), *Osteoporosis in Orthopedics*,
DOI 10.1007/978-4-431-55778-4_6

these agents must be continued for 3–4 years in order to reduce the risk of both vertebral and non-vertebral fractures in osteoporotic women.

In spite of their clinical benefits, the long-term treatment with BPs has raised questions regarding their associations with rare but serious adverse events, including atypical femoral fractures (AFFs). Currently, the long-term use of BPs is considered to be linked to the occurrence of AFFs. Although the evidence had been controversial regarding the association between the occurrence of AFFs and the use of BPs, more recent studies with radiographic adjudication have supported that an association exists. However, the pathogenesis of AFFs is still not completely understood.

AFFs are characterized by unique radiographic features, such as a transverse fracture line, a periosteal callus formation at the fracture site and little or no comminution, and also by unique clinical features, such as prodromal pain and bilaterality, that resemble stress fractures or reactions. Based upon new information, an American Society for Bone and Mineral Research (ASBMR) task force reported the original case definition to highlight the unusual radiographic features that distinguish AFFs from ordinary osteoporotic typical femoral fractures (TFFs) and to provide more precise guidance on what is meant by transverse orientation. The epidemiological evidence for a relationship between BP use and AFFs has become more compelling. While AFFs appear to be more common in patients who have been exposed to the long-term use of BPs, every series includes patients who have not been treated with BPs, which suggests the possible presence of AFF "background factors" in osteoporosis patients. The majority of studies have found a significant association with glucocorticoid (GC) use or duration of use. Although the relative risks of AFFs are very high in patients who use BPs, ranging from 2.1 to 128, the absolute risk is extremely low, ranging from 3.2 to 50 cases per 100,000 person-years. Thus, these fractures are rare, particularly when considered against the incidence of common osteoporotic fractures of all types and of ordinary TFFs, all of which have been proven to decrease with BP therapy. In addition, increasing reports have suggested an association between denosumab and AFFs. Therefore, it becomes more important to know the "risk factors" and/or the "background factors" of AFF to treat patients with osteoporosis who are susceptible to osteoporotic fractures.

We previously reported that the incidence of AFFs in the Japanese population was similar to that in Caucasians and that the taking of BPs and GCs and the presence of collagen diseases were the risk factors for developing AFFs. We also reported that fracture sites of AFFs are associated with the standing lower limb alignment and that lower limb alignment is suggested to be one of the risk factors for AFFs. In this section, we focus on the epidemiology, pathology, and risk factors of AFFs and especially on the involvement of the geometry of the lower extremities as one of the risk factors of AFFs.

Keywords Atypical femoral fracture • Anti-bone-resorptive drugs • Bisphosphonate • Denosumab • Geometry

6.1 Introduction

Osteoporosis is a systemic skeletal disease characterized by low bone mass and the structural deterioration of bone tissue leading to bone fragility and the increased risk of fracture. Fractures, most notably of the hip, are associated with significant morbidity and mortality. From a patient's perspective, a fracture of the hip, and the subsequent loss of mobility and autonomy, often represents a major drop in quality of life [1].

Although it had been thought to be a natural part of the aging process in women, osteoporosis is no longer considered to be age or sex dependent. It is largely preventable due to the remarkable progress in the scientific understanding of its causes, diagnosis, and treatment. Bone strength primarily reflects the integration of bone density and bone quality. The treatment of osteoporosis is to increase the bone mass and, hopefully, to improve the bone quality, resulting in the strengthening of the bone structure. As the bone is an organ that is constantly remodeling and because of recent developments in the field of bone biology, we have recently become able to increase bone mass and strength by modulating the bone remodeling processes with newly developed medications.

Due to the recent advantages of molecular biology in the field of bone biology, several medications for osteoporosis have been developed, which modulate bone metabolism and reduce the occurrence of osteoporotic fragility fractures in patients with osteoporosis. Medications for osteoporosis fall into two classes: antiresorptive drugs, which slow down bone resorption, and anabolic drugs, which stimulate bone formation. Currently, several approved treatment options exist for the management of osteoporosis that effectively reduce the risk of vertebral, non-vertebral, and hip fractures. Bisphosphonates (BPs) are an analog of the naturally occurring pyrophosphates and are one of the representative antiresorptive drugs for bone resorption. The development of BPs was a milestone in this field, as the large-scale clinical trials for patients with osteoporosis clearly showed that BPs were able to suppress the loss of bone volume and, largely as a result, reduce the incidence of vertebral and non-vertebral fractures [2]. However, it has been speculated that BP therapy may be associated with some unfavorable effects. BPs inhibit the function of osteoclasts and induce apoptosis, resulting in the suppression of the bone turnover rate [3]. The prolonged use of BP therapy has been suggested to cause the accumulation of microdamage in the bone, reduce the heterogeneity of the organic matrix and mineral properties [4], increase the levels of advanced glycation end products [5], and promote the deterioration of bone quality. These effects of BPs, especially of long-term BP use, have been speculated to be related to the occurrence of atypical femoral fractures (AFFs) [6]. However, AFFs have also been known to occur in patients who do not have a history of therapeutic BP use [7–11]. Furthermore, other types of antiresorptive medications, such as denosumab, which is a fully human monoclonal antibody against the receptor activator of nuclear factor-κB ligand (RANKL), a cytokine that is essential for the formation, function, and survival of osteoclasts, have been reported to be associated with the occurrence of AFFs [12, 13]. As the goal of therapy is fracture prevention, the development of drugs alone is not enough to prevent the occurrence of osteoporotic fragility fractures. Long-term treatment, in addition to the treatment adherence and the evaluation of aspects of calcium metabolism, such as the vitamin D status and intestinal calcium absorption capability, is also important to the successful prevention of fragility fractures [12, 13]. Therefore, the risk factors for the development of AFFs include not only the taking of BPs but also various other factors that affect the bone metabolism, bone remodeling processes, and bone quality. Recently, the geometry of the lower extremities has been revealed to be another factor that is associated with the occurrence of AFFs [8, 9, 11, 14].

In this section, we summarize the "background factors" of AFF in addition to summarizing the epidemiology, risk factors, and pathology of AFFs.

6.2 The Characteristics of Patients with AFFs and the History of the Definition of AFF

BPs are highly effective for reducing the incidence of both vertebral and non-vertebral osteoporotic fragility fractures. However, it has been speculated that patients who undergo long-term treatment with BPs show an increased incidence of spontaneous nonspinal fractures. The first report of these cases was published in 2005 with nine cases of nonspinal fractures [15]. In this report, the authors suggested the possibility of an association between nontypical nonspinal fractures and long-term BP use, especially administration of alendronate, which may over-suppress bone turnover, resulting in an impaired ability to repair skeletal microfractures and increased skeletal fragility.

6.2.1 The American Society for Bone and Mineral Research (ASBMR) Task Force Report, 1st Edition

In 2010, the ASBMR task force summarized the characteristics of 310 patients with AFFs from the published literature [6]. The task force carefully reviewed the available information for AFFs, shedding light on what is actually known and what is not known about AFFs, and examined their potential relationship with BPs. Based on the information, the task force provided a provisional case definition of AFFs that will facilitate subsequent studies on the same condition.

AFFs are observed most commonly in the proximal one-third of the femoral shaft but may occur anywhere along the femoral diaphysis from just distal to the lesser trochanter to proximal to the supracondylar flare of the distal femoral metaphysis. The fracture usually occurs as a result of no or minimal trauma, equivalent to a fall from a standing height or less. The fracture may be complete, extending across the entire femoral shaft, often with the formation of a medial spike. Complete atypical femoral fractures are generally transverse, although they may have a short oblique configuration, and are not comminuted. Alternatively, the fracture may be incomplete and manifested by a transverse radiolucent line in the lateral cortex. Both complete and incomplete fractures are commonly associated with a periosteal stress reaction and the thickening of the lateral cortex at the fracture site (abnormalities that are indicative of a stress fracture). In addition, there may be a generalized bilateral thickening of both the medial and lateral cortices. Both complete and incomplete atypical fractures may be bilateral. The fractures may display delayed healing. There are often prodromal symptoms such as a pain in the groin or thigh lesions. AFFs may be associated with a variety of comorbid conditions and the use of pharmaceutical agents. The diagnosis of AFFs should specifically exclude fractures of the femoral neck, intertrochanteric fractures with spiral subtrochanteric extension, pathologic fractures associated with local primary or metastatic bone tumors, and periprosthetic fractures. Although AFFs have been reported most prominently in individuals who have been treated with BPs, they are also reported in individuals who have no history of BP exposure. AFF patients are predominantly female and younger than the patients with typical osteoporotic femoral fractures.

The task force defined the major and minor features for complete and incomplete atypical fractures of the femur to assist in case identification and reporting (Table 6.1). All of the major features should be present in order to designate a

Table 6.1 2010 ASBMR Task Force Case Definition of AFFs[a] [6]

Major features[b]
Located anywhere along the femur from just distal to the lesser trochanter to just proximal to the supracondylar flare
Associated with no trauma or minimal trauma, as in a fall from a standing height or less
Transverse or short oblique configuration
Noncomminuted
Complete fractures extend through both cortices and may be associated with a medial spike; incomplete fractures involve only the lateral cortex
Minor features
Localized periosteal reaction of the lateral cortex[c]
Generalized increase in cortical thickness of the diaphysis
Prodromal symptoms such as dull or aching pain in the groin or thigh
Bilateral fractures and symptoms
Delayed healing
Comorbid conditions (e.g., vitamin D deficiency, RA, hypophosphatasia)
Use of pharmaceutical agents (e.g., BPs, GCs, PPIs)

[a]Specifically excluded are fractures of the femoral neck, intertrochanteric fractures with spiral subtrochanteric extension, pathologic fractures associated with primary or metastatic bone tumors, and periprosthetic fractures

[b]All major features are required to satisfy the case definition of atypical femoral fracture. None of the minor features are required but sometimes have been associated with these fractures

[c]Often referred to in the literature as beaking or flaring

fracture as atypical and distinguish it from more common hip fractures (i.e., femoral neck, intertrochanteric). Minor features have often been described in association with AFFs but may or may not be present in individual patients. Prodromal thigh or groin pain is observed in approximately 70 % of the reported cases. Bilateral complete fractures and/or bilateral radiographic abnormalities, including cortical reactions, existed in approximately one-third of the cases. Regarding the treatment of AFFs, delayed healing was observed in one quarter of the reported cases. Thirty-four percent of the patients with AFFs were using corticosteroids at the time of the fracture.

Based on these previous results, the task force summarized that AFFs are rare, particularly when considered in the context of the millions of patients who have taken BPs and also when compared with typical and common femoral neck and intertrochanteric fractures (Fig. 6.1). The task force also emphasized that while BPs

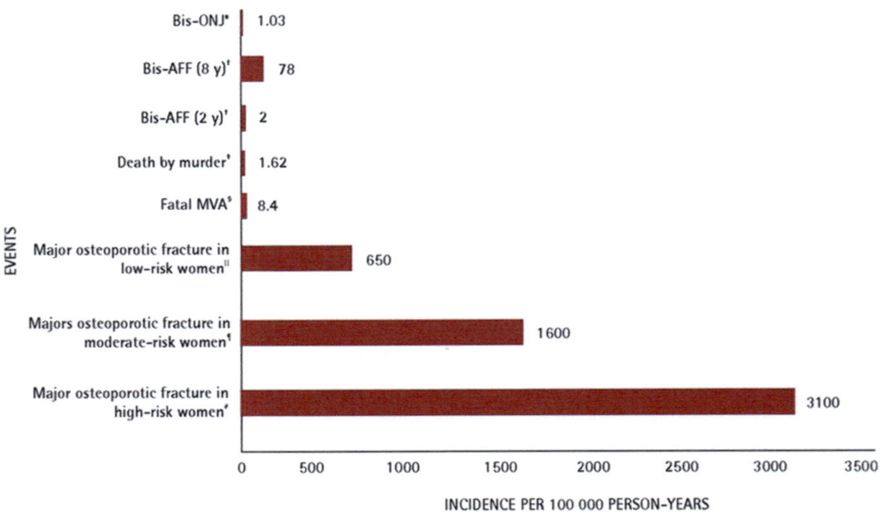

Fig. 6.1 Risks of major osteoporotic fracture and other rare events. *Bis-AFF* bisphosphonate-associated atypical subtrochanteric and diaphyseal femur fracture, *Bis-ONJ* bisphosphonate-associated osteonecrosis of the jaw, *BMD* bone mineral density, *FN* femoral neck, *FRAX* fracture risk assessment tool, *MVA* motor vehicle accident. *[16] (Reprinted with permission from the college of family physicians of Canada [17]) (†: Data from Dell R, Greene D, Ott SM, Silverman S, Eisemon E, Funahashi T, et al. A retrospective analysis of all atypical femur fractures seen in a large California HMO from the years 2007 to 2009 [abstract]. J Bone Miner Res 2010:25; ‡: Data from Statistics Canada, Homicide offences, number and rate, by province and territory. Ottawa: Statistics Canada; 2011; §: Data from Transport Canada. 2007 casualty rates. Ottawa: Transport Canada 2010; ‖: The 10-year risk of major osteoporotic fracture in a low-risk woman by Canadian FRAX (65-year-old woman, weighing 60 kg with a height of 168 cm; BMD FN T-score –1.2); ¶: The 10-year risk of major osteoporotic fracture in a moderate-risk woman by Canadian FRAX (65-year-old woman weighing 60 kg with a height of 168 cm; parent hip fracture history; BMD FN T-score -2.0); #: The 10-year risk of major osteoporotic fracture in a high-risk woman by Canadian FRAX (65-year-old woman weighing 60 kg with a height of 168 cm; parent hip fracture history; previous fracture; BMD FN T-score -2.6))

are important drugs for the prevention of common osteoporotic fractures, the occurrence of AFFs is a matter of concern, and that there is an urgent need for to assist in identifying the patients who are at particular risk of developing AFFs and to guide decision-making regarding the duration of BP therapy. Physicians and patients should be made aware of the possibility of AFFs and of the potential for bilaterality. Given the relative rarity of AFFs (Fig. 6.1) [17], the task force emphasized the facilitation of future research, especially with regard to case reporting based on the case definition that is established.

6.2.2 The ASBMR Task Force Report, 2nd Edition

Following the publication of the first edition of the ASBMR task force report in 2010, several studies were published on the epidemiology of AFFs, their risk factors, and their relationship with the use of BPs. The ASBMR reconvened the task force at the 2012 Annual Meeting of the ASBMR. The first goal of the task force was to review the major studies that had been published since the original task force report in 2010, with a focus on studies that addressed three major aspects of AFFS: their epidemiology, pathogenesis, and medical management. The second

Table 6.2 ASBMR Task Force 2013 Revised Case Definition of AFFs [18]

To satisfy the case definition of AFF, the fracture must be located along the femoral diaphysis from just distal to the lesser trochanter to just proximal to the supracondylar flare
In addition, at least four of five major features must be present. None of the minor features are required but have sometimes been associated with these fractures
Major features[a]
The fracture is associated with minimal or no trauma, as in a fall from a standing height or less
The fracture line originates at the lateral cortex and is substantially transverse in its orientation, although it may become oblique as it progresses medially across the femur
Complete fractures extend through both cortices and may be associated with a medial spike; incomplete fractures involve only the lateral cortex
The fracture is noncomminuted **or minimally comminuted**
Localized periosteal or endosteal thickening of the lateral cortex is present at the fracture site ("beaking" or "flaring")
Minor features
Generalized increase in cortical thickness of the **femoral diaphyses**
Unilateral or bilateral prodromal symptoms such as dull or aching pain in the groin or thigh
Bilateral **incomplete or complete femoral diaphysis fractures**
Delayed **fracture** healing

Changes from the 2010 ASBMR Task Force Case Definition of AFFs are in bold
ASBMR American Society for Bone and Mineral Research, *AFF* atypical femur fracture
[a]Excludes fractures of the femoral neck, intertrochanteric fractures with spiral subtrochanteric extension, periprosthetic fractures, and pathological fractures associated with primary or metastatic bone tumors and miscellaneous bone diseases (e.g., Paget's disease, fibrous dysplasia)

goal was to assess whether the information in the reviewed studies provided data that could be used to refine the original case definition. Following these processes, the task force published the 2nd edition of the ASBMR task force report on the AFFs (Table 6.2) [18].

The reports were revised to more clearly delineate the features that distinguish AFFs from ordinary osteoporotic femoral fractures. New epidemiologic studies, many of which incorporated radiographic reviews and provided new information on the incidence of AFFs and the association with BPs, and new data on the pathogenesis and management of AFFs were reviewed and summarized in the second report. The features linking AFFs to comorbid conditions and medication exposures, including BPs and GCs, were removed, because it was deemed more appropriate for studies to seek these associations than to include them in the case definition.

6.3 Epidemiology

There are two types of published epidemiologic studies on AFFs: large registry-based cohort studies to demonstrate the incidence of subtrochanteric fractures (STs) and femoral shaft fractures (FSs) and studies in which AFFs were categorized based on radiographic findings. In the first type of studies, the overall incidence of STs and FSs was evaluated in registry-based cohort studies using a large database, such as the International Classification of Diseases (ICD) codes [19–22]. The studies lacked radiographic adjudication in differentiating the STs and FSs from the typical osteoporotic femur fractures from AFFs. The studies demonstrated that the age-adjusted rates for hip fractures decreased by 31.6 % from 1996 to 2006, while the number of STs and FSs increased by 31.2 % [23]. The rate of STs and FSs among overall hip fractures increased, and the incidence of STs and FSs in females was between 10 and 35 per 100,000 person-years. Although this trend indirectly suggests a relationship between the increased use of BPs and the incidence of AFFs, the actual risk could not be estimated from these types of studies. Therefore, while the large database-based studies are helpful for estimating the incidence of AFFs, it is hard to determine the actual number of AFFs from these studies.

In the second type of studies, AFFs were determined and categorized based on the reviewing of radiographs [11, 24–33]. Thirty-two percent of the overall STs and FSs treated at the Hospital for Special Surgery in New York from 2000 to 2007 were AFFs [29]. In Australia, 13 % of 152 patients with STs and FSs were AFFs [27]. In the Netherlands, 16 % (10/63) of STs and FSs were AFF [28]. In the reviewing of 1234 radiographs of STs and FSs that occurred in Sweden in 2008, approximately 5 % were found to be AFFs [32]. Among 3515 patients with femoral fractures in the United Kingdom, 27 AFFs were identified, which represented 0.8 % of all hip fractures and 7 % of FSs [33]. In Japan, we identified 14 AFF cases among

402 STs and FSs (3.5 %) by reviewing the radiographs of 2238 hip and FS fractures [10].

Based on these radiographic adjudication studies and large database studies, the incidence of AFFs is estimated to be between 0.3 and 11 per 100,000 person-years. Similarly, in the United States, the incidence of AFFs among the femur fractures in females over 50 years of age and males over of 65 years of age between 1996 and 2009 was 5.9 per 100,000 person-years [34]. In Switzerland, the incidence rate of AFFs was 3.2 per 100,000 person-years [31].

6.4 Risk Factors

Several case–control studies with radiographic adjudication have compared typical osteoporotic fractures with AFFs [10, 27, 31, 32, 34, 35]. In Australia, 152 femoral fractures (not including hip fractures), which occurred in 152 patients (mean age 78 years) from June 2003 to May 2008, were reviewed [27]. Twenty of the 152 fractures (13 %) were classified as AFFs, and 17 of the 20 AFF patients (85 %) were BP users, while three of 132 patients with typical femoral fractures (2.3 %) were taking BPs. The relative risk of an AFF patient being on a BP was 37.4 (95 % CI, 12.9–113.3; $p < 0.001$). AFFs were also associated with other factors, such as a history of a low-energy fracture (odds ratio (OR), 3.2; 95 % CI, 2.1–17.1; $p < 0.001$), the use of glucocorticoid (GCs) for more than 6 months (OR, 5.2; 95 % CI, 1.3–31.0; $p = 0.01$), active rheumatoid arthritis (OR, 16.5; 95 % CI, 1.4–142.3; $p < 0.001$), and a serum level of 25-hydroxyvitamin D of less than 16 ng/ml (40 nmol/l) (OR, 3.5; 95 % CI, 1.7–18.7; $p < 0.001$).

In Sweden, when 1234 radiographs of 1271 female patients with STs and FSs were reviewed, 59 patients showed AFFs [32]. As 78 % of the AFF patients and 10 % of the controls had received BPs, the multivariable-adjusted OR was 33.3 (95 % CI, 14.3–77.8). The duration of BP use influenced the risk (OR per 100 daily doses, 1.3; 95 % CI, 1.1–1.6). After drug withdrawal, the risk diminished by 70 % per year after the last use (OR, 0.28; 95 % CI, 0.21–0.38).

In the United States, when the 22 typical FS fractures and the 75 AFFs were reviewed, the adjusted OR of ever taking OR in patients with AFFs vs. non-atypical FSs was 2.11 (95 % CI, 0.99–4.49) [34]. The ORs for exposure to GCs and PPIs did not differ significantly between the groups.

In Switzerland, the fracture of 39 of 477 patients with STs and FSs, who were older than 50 years of age between 1999 and 2010, and who were hospitalized at a single university medical center, was identified as AFFs [31]. Eighty-two percent of the patients with AFFs had been treated with BPs, while 6 % of the patients with typical femoral fractures had been treated with BPs (OR, 66.9; 95 % CI, 27.1–165.1). While the OR for AFFs in patients who had used BPs for less than 2 years was 35.1 (95 % CI, 10.0–123.6), the ORs for AFFs in patients who had used BPs for 2–5 years, 2–9 years, and more than 9 years were 46.9 (14.2–154.4), 117.1 (34.2–401.7), and 175.7 (30.0–1027.6), respectively.

In New Zealand, there were six AFFs among 65 typical femoral fractures (TFFs) [35]. Half of the patients (50 %) with AFFs used BPs at the time of the fracture, while 23 % of the patients with TFFs used BPs (OR, 5.5; 95 % CI, 0.97–31; $p = 0.07$). In addition, the OR for exposure to GCs was 4.9 (95 % CI, 0.74–32.7; $p = 0.13$).

In Japan, we conducted a case–control study in which ten patients with AFFs were compared with 30 patients with low-energy typical STs and FSs [10]. In the AFFs group, 90 % of the patients used BPs, whereas 14.3 % of the patients in the TFFs group used BPs. A fracture location-, age-, and gender-matched (1:3) case–control study revealed that the administration of BPs and GCs and the presence of a collagen disease (CD) were risk factors for the development of AFFs (OR: 36.0 [95 % CI, 3.8–342.2], 13.0 [2.3–74.1], and 9.0 [1.6–50.3], respectively).

In a prospective study of the Healthy Bones Program in Kaiser, Southern California, 142 patients with AFFs were found among all of the femur fractures form 2007 to 2011, in 1,835,116 patients who were older than 45 years of age [26]. One hundred twenty-eight of 142 patients with AFFs (90 %) were BP users. The occurrence of AFFs was not correlated with the duration of use (5.5 years), age (69.3 years of age), or bone density (T-score, −2.1). As 188,814 patients used BPs, the age-adjusted incidence rates for AFF were 1.78/per 100,000/person-years (95 % CI, 1.5–2.0) with 0.1–1.9 years of exposure and increased to 113.1/per 100,000/person-years (95 % CI, 69.3–156.8) with 8–9.9 years of exposure. The incidence of AFFs increased with a longer duration of BP use.

According to these studies, the incidence of AFFs is higher in patients taking BPs, and a longer duration of BP use was related to an elevated risk of developing AFFs. Consistent with these results, the systematic review and meta-analysis examining the association of BPs with AFFs showed that the adjusted relative risk (RR), based on case–control studies with radiographic adjudication, was 11.12 (95 % CI, 2.68–46.18) [36]. These findings indicate that BP use seems to be a risk factor for AFFs and that the risk seems to increase in line with the duration of BP use.

The adherence to oral BPs of 522,287 new BP users was followed among all Medicare fee-for-service female beneficiaries in the United States from 2006 to 2010 [37]. The age-adjusted incidence rates for intertrochanteric fractures (ITs) and femoral neck fractures (FNs) among the highly compliant beneficiaries were significantly lower than those among less compliant users (adjusted hazard ratio [HR] = 0.69; 95 % CI, 0.66–0.73). On the other hand, HR of STs and FSs for the highly compliant users vs. the less compliant users became significant after 2 years of follow-up (HR = 1.51; 95 % CI, 1.06–2.15) and reached the highest risk level in the fifth year (HR = 4.06; 95 % CI, 1.47–11.19).

In addition to these studies, several other studies have indicated an association between GC use and AFFs [10, 26, 27, 31], while other reports did not indicate an association [32, 34]. Female gender and a younger age are also considered to be significant risk factors for AFFs [19, 38].

6.5 Pathogenesis

The mechanisms underlying the development of AFFs have not been fully understood. The characteristics of the radiological features of AFFs, such as focal hypertrophy of the lateral cortex, periosteal and endosteal callus formation, and the transverse fracture line at the lateral cortex, suggest that fatigue damage accumulates within the bone cortex over long period of time and that AFFs are stress or insufficiency fractures. A concentration of mechanical stress on the bone leads to the formation of microcracks, which heal by bone remodeling via the initiation of osteoclastic bone resorption, followed by osteoblastic bone formation to replace new bone. The pathogenesis of BP-associated fractures seems to be related to the alterations of this tissue repair process as a result of the continuous suppression of the bone turnover rate [39].

The reduction of process of the bone turnover by BP treatment alters the bone mineral and matrix properties. BP therapy causes an increase in advanced glycation end products of the extracellular bone matrix, deteriorating the mechanical properties of the bone [5]. Prolonged BP therapy causes the accumulation of microdamage to bone and reduces the heterogeneity of the organic matrix and mineral properties [4]. These changes reduce the bone repair ability, which results in the accumulation of local microdamage especially at the site of maximum mechanical force.

Several reports have investigated the histology of the AFF patients. The ASBMR task force summarized them in 2010 [6]. Most of the histological analyses involved the performance of transiliac bone biopsies on samples from the patients with BP-associated AFFs, which revealed the reduced or absent populations of osteoclasts and osteoblasts, suggesting that a relationship existed between these phenomena and BPs. In contrast to the transiliac bone biopsies, a small number of femoral bone biopsies reports have been conducted. The histomorphometric analysis of a biopsy from the femur of an AFF patient revealed a normal lamellar bone texture, no evidence of adynamic bone, and no impairment of the mineralization, suggesting that there was no association between the AFFs and the over-suppression of bone turnover caused by BP use [40]. However, another study reported (based on a histological analysis of femur biopsies from eight patients with AFFs) that AFFs appeared to consist of a microcrack at the lateral cortex with its main direction perpendicular to the long axis of the bone [41]. The surrounding bone showed the signs of remodeling, mainly represented by the presence of osteoclasts, resorption cavities, and woven bone facing the crack. However, half (4/8) of the AFFs consisted mainly of empty lacunae in osteocyte lacunae. These results suggested that the impaired healing of the cracks, in spite of increased remodeling of the adjacent bone, was related to the development of AFFs in BP users.

Based on these studies, the pathophysiology of AFFs is suggested to be related to the impairment of the bone repair process, where microcracks need to be remodeled to new bone, due to a long-term decrease in bone turnover caused by the

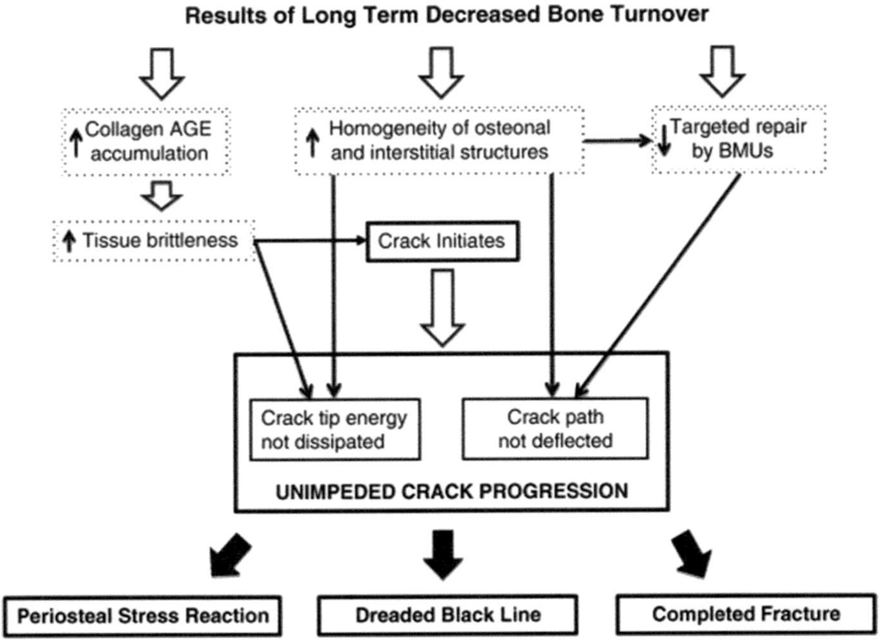

Fig. 6.2 Flow diagram of pathophysiological steps leading from suppression of bone turnover to atypical femoral fracture. *AGEs* advanced glycation end products, *BP* bisphosphonate exposure, *BMU* bone metabolic unit, *AFF* atypical femoral fracture (Reprinted with permission from the Elsevier [42])

suppression of the osteoclast function by antiresorptive agents, such as BPs and, presumably, denosumab (Fig. 6.2) [42].

6.6 Femoral Geometry and the Biomechanical Considerations of the Lower Limb

A "stress fracture" implies the abnormal and excessive loading of a normal bone, while an "insufficiency fracture" implies the normal loading of an abnormal or deficient bone. Bones subjected to repetitive loading that overwhelms the body's capacity for repair are at risk of developing a stress fracture. Thus, stress fractures which result from repetitive mechanical loading on the bone are common overuse injuries in physically active individuals, such as athletes. A stress fracture results from repetitive application of stress of lower strength than that required to fracture bone in a single load. While stress fractures can affect almost any bone, the vast majority of these fractures occur in the lower extremities. As the vague symptoms may lead to delayed diagnosis and an increased risk of major complications, the early detection of high-risk stress fractures, such as the tension side of the femoral neck, the tarsal navicular, and the base of the fifth metatarsal, is important [43]. Stress fractures, which most commonly occur in the tibia, constitute about 10 % of all sport-related injuries [44]. Stress fractures of the femur are relatively uncommon, and the data from the literature suggest that they constitute less than 5–10 % of all sport-related stress fractures [45–47]. Stress fractures of the femoral shaft are especially rare but they do occur in the proximal third of the femur [48–50]. In addition, most of the cases of the stress fractures of the femoral shaft occur in the medial side of the femora [51–53].

Stress is produced in the femur whenever it is subjected to a loading force. The femur is subjected to forces produced by the body's weight several times during normal physiological activity. The femur is exposed both under tension and compression. The femur may be subjected to weight-bearing force below the lesser trochanter in the medial cortex. The femur is usually subjected to a lower force below the lesser trochanter in the lateral cortex (immediately opposite the medial cortex). Bending forces, rather than compressive or torsional forces, are considered to be important in the pathogenesis of the majority of stress fractures [54]. With regard to bending forces, two critical factors exist: (1) the geometric distribution of bone mass, rather than bone mass itself, and (2) the collagen composition of the bone. The bone mass is controlled, at least in part, by bone remodeling. The most widely accepted theory about the development of stress fractures is based on an imbalance in this process. The frequency of the magnitude of load and the number of repetitions are factors that define the fatigue process. Repetitive stress causes periosteal resorption that occurs at a faster rate than bone formation. The cortex, as a result, is weakened and becomes fractured, a process called microdamage. This microdamage within the bone develops with each loading cycle. The bone is unable to adapt to this stress in moderate and high doses of exercise. As a result, cumulative microdamage results in cracks in the bone that act as stress raisers and which allows for the development of fractures. These fractures may be incomplete, complete, nondisplaced, or displaced. Hormonal disorders and nutritional deficiency may impair the normal response of the bone to stress. Certain characteristics of the lower extremities also may influence the stress response of bone by altering the transfer of load to the femur, such as inequality in leg length, coxa vara, and cavus feet [55]. Overall, stress injury to the bone represents a spectrum of diseases, from bone stress reactions to stress fractures, which may initially be subclinical.

A case report demonstrates the initial development of a periosteal callus and the eventual appearance of a transverse cortical fracture in the region of periosteal thickening termed the "dreaded black line" [56]. This pattern is typical of the development of a stress fracture. Based on the evidence of periosteal and endosteal callus, and on the appearance of a transverse cortical fracture prior to the overt fracture, the current consensus of the task force is that AFFs are stress or insufficiency fractures that develop over time. However, AFFs differ from exercise-induced femoral stress fractures in some respects.

The initiation of exercise-induced femoral stress fractures usually occurs on the medial cortex of the femur, in the proximal one-third of the femoral diaphysis, which results in a more oblique fracture surface than is observed in AFFs [57]. In contrast, the initiation of AFFs occurs on the lateral cortex, between the lesser trochanter and the femoral condyles, and results in a smooth transverse surface, which is more characteristic of a brittle material. The lateral cortex of the femur is known to sustain high levels of tensile stress due to bending [58, 59]. Based on these data, it has been suggested that the tensile stress of the lateral cortex of the femur may precipitate the damage in this location, especially in people with lower limb geometry that could exacerbate that effect, such as bowed femur and Asian race.

The geometry of the hip and proximal femur determines, in part, the stresses that are experienced on the lateral aspect of the femoral cortex. In addition, AFFs occur not only in BP users but also in BP-naïve individuals. Thus, the pathophysiology of AFFs cannot be entirely explained by BP usage. The increased tensile stress on the lateral cortex would explain the subtrochanteric and diaphyseal distribution of AFFs.

While AFF can occur anywhere in the femoral bone from just beneath the lesser trochanter to the femoral shaft [6, 18], it remains unclear how the fracture site of an AFF is determined [28, 31, 34, 60]. The patterns in the radiological findings of AFFs, such as cortical thickening, beaking, and flaring of the lateral cortex of the femoral shafts, suggest that this type of fracture is caused by tensile failures of the lateral cortex of the femoral shaft [6, 15]. In addition to these radiological features, bilateral fractures are one of the important clinical characteristics of patients with AFFs [6, 28, 61]. In most cases of bilateral AFFs, the fractures occur in the same anatomical location [28]. This suggests that in the AFFs, individual factor(s), in addition to the other abovementioned factors, may affect the fracture sites. These clinical features suggest that AFFs, as least in part, develop due to the fatigue failure mechanisms that are observed in a stress fracture and which are related to bone tissue properties that become altered as a result of microdamage accumulation as well as altered adaptations to mechanical forces, which may be related to BP, and probably denosumab, treatment, and/or other conditions that can cause bone fragility.

Although long-term antiresorptive therapy may affect bone repair and its mechanical properties and also increase the susceptibility of the bone to stress fracture, the systemic bone changes caused by antiresorptive drugs cannot explain both the specific location where the onset of an AFF takes place and the recurrence of AFFs in a specific femoral region, namely, the lateral cortex of the femoral shaft. A possible explanation for AFFs may reside in the daily mechanical environment of the femoral shaft. Aamodt et al. directly measured the tensile strains in a single location of the lateral femoral shaft in two patients [62]. Theoretical investigations, using a synthetic femur to mimic walking, reported that femoral strain patterns were characterized by combined bending and torsion [63]. Martelli et al. hypothesized that the typical strain patterns in the femoral shaft were activity type dependent and that some of them created a more favorable condition for AFFs in the lateral cortex. The authors focused on the typical strain patterns in the femoral shaft during activities of daily living and reported the three-dimensional in vivo tensile and compressive strain distributions in the femoral shaft during different daily activities [59]. In this study, the cortical strain in the femoral shaft was studied by combining

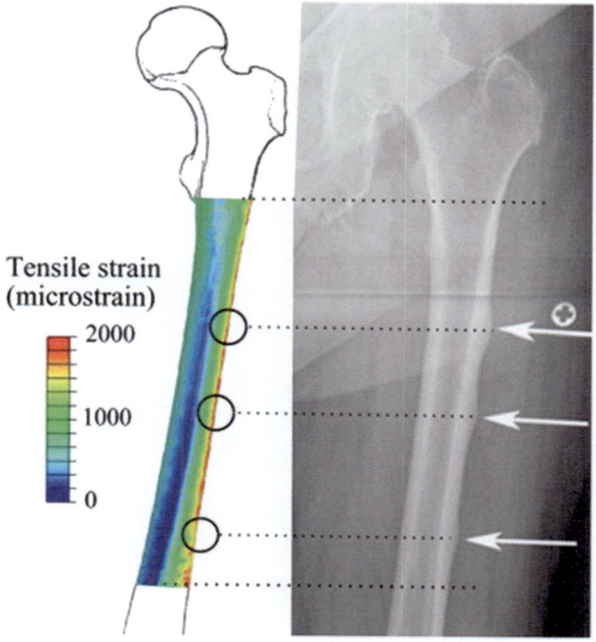

Fig. 6.3 Comparison of the tensile strain pattern during an intermediate frame of walking (*left*) with typical AFFs onset locations arrowed in an X-ray view (*right*) [64] (Reprinted with permission from the HSS Journal [59])

experimental motion data and models of femoral elasticity and forces. The lateral aspect of the femur was subjected to tensile strains during all of the investigated activities. There was an association between typical locations for AFFs and tensile strains in the femoral shaft while walking (Fig. 6.3). Both strain intensity and orientation in the transverse plane were activity dependent, and walking showed the highest average tensile strains in correspondence with the location of onset of commonly observed AFFs. The lateral femoral shaft was subjected to peak tensile loads during most of the walking stance phase, whereas the peak tensile strain was slightly rotated anteriorly during stair descent. The results of this study suggest that the location of the onset of AFF is associated with physiological strain distribution during daily activities and that the tensile loads in the lateral femoral shaft are to be attributed to the hip abduction moment. The lateral femoral shaft is subjected to tensile strains during a variety of physical activities and walking induces the highest tensile strain levels (Fig. 6.4). The hip abduction moment is a strong predictor of the tensile strains in the lateral femoral shaft during walking and stair ascent, but not during general activities. The lateral aspect of the femoral shaft was loaded in tension during every studied activity. The result of the multi-parametric linear regression analysis means that 46–60 % of the tensile strain variance in the lateral femoral shaft can be explained by the whole body dynamics, whereas the remaining 40–54 % of the strain variance is likely to be attributed to other unexplained factors.

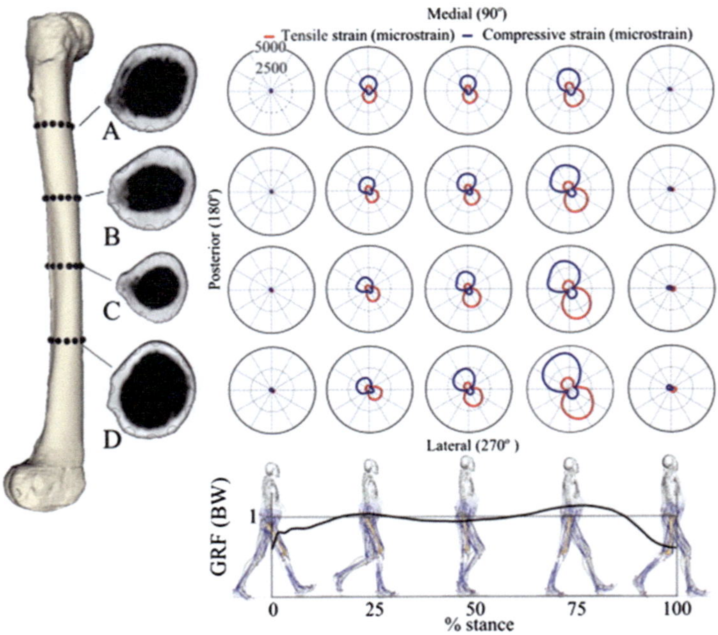

Fig. 6.4 Cortical tensile and compressive strain patterns in four transversal section of the femoral shaft at five time intervals during the stance phase of walking (Reprinted with permission from the Elsevier [59])

Therefore, the combination of tensile loads, in addition to the increased bone fragility that may be associated with long-term antiresorptive therapy, may be an important cofactors in creating a favorable environment for AFFs.

Nine consecutive elderly patients who were treated for low-energy diaphyseal femoral fractures between 2005 and 2010 at Akita University in Japan were retrospectively reviewed and the femoral curvature was suggested to be associated with the occurrence of AFFs [8]. Low energy was defined as a fall from standing height or less. As three of nine patients showed the opposite side of low-energy diaphyseal femoral fractures within a few years, a total of 12 femurs in nine patients were investigated in this report. All patients were female with a mean age at the time of first injury of 75.6 years (range 71–86 years). All nine patients used the medication for the treatment of osteoporosis at the time of fracture. BPs were used by eight of the patients, while the remaining patient used raloxifene. The mean duration of drug administration was 3.6 years. The curvature of the femur was measured with anteroposterior (AP) and lateral views as the angles between two linear lines drawn along the proximal and distal portion of the femoral shaft. The angle on the AP view was identified as angle A, while that on the lateral view was identified as angle B (Fig. 6.5). The femoral curvatures, defined by angles A and B, were significantly larger in the low-energy fracture group than in the control group (Table 6.3), suggesting that increased femoral curvature might be an important causative factor for low-energy diaphyseal femoral fractures.

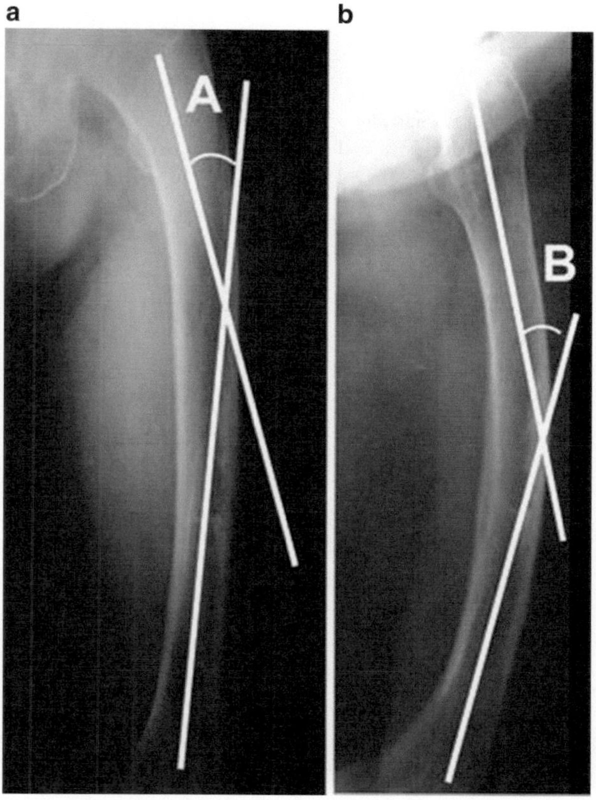

Fig. 6.5 Involvement of the femoral curvature for the atypical femoral fractures (AFFs). For the measurement of femoral curvature, two lines along the proximal and distal portions of the femoral shaft were drawn on anteroposterior (**a**) and lateral (**b**) X-rays. Angle *A* is defined as the angle between the two lines on the anteroposterior view and angle *B* as that on the lateral view (Reprinted with permission from the Springer [8])

Table 6.3 Comparisons of femoral curvature between the low-energy diaphyseal femoral fracture group and the control group [8]

(°)	AFFs ($n = 7$)	Control ($n = 24$)	p
Angle A	12.6	4.6	0.002
Angle B	19.9	11.8	0.001

Thirteen cases of stress fractures of the bowed femoral shaft (SBF) were reviewed retrospectively among elderly Japanese patients [9]. All of the patients were females with a median age at injury of 77.0 years (range 67–88 years), who were able to walk independently before the injury and who met the AFF diagnostic criteria. Six of the 13 cases of AFFs showed a bowing deformity of the femur and used BPs, while one of the seven cases in which the bowing deformity was absent used BPs. The remaining six cases did not use BPs, showing that AFFs can occur in patients without using BPs. Based on the results of this study, the authors demonstrated the concept of the AFF criteria, as shown in Fig. 6.6. However, further study is required to fully reveal the pathophysiology of AFFs (e.g., whether there are cases of SBF who do not meet the radiographic definition of AFFs as defined by ASBMR task force) (Table 6.2) [18].

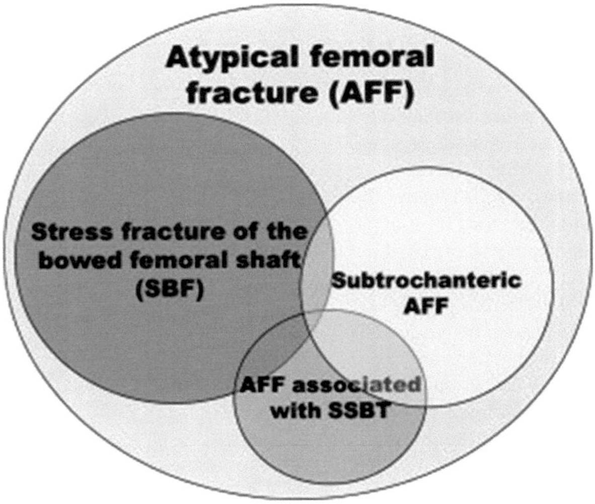

Fig. 6.6 New concept of atypical femoral fracture (AFF) in terms of mechanics. Stress fractures of the bowed femoral shaft should be considered a novel subtype of AFF (Reprinted with permission from the Elsevier [65])

The authors also analyzed the stress concentration in the femoral shaft using the CT-based finite element method (CT/FEM) in the patients with AFFs or a history of AFFs who had a bowing deformity of the femur ($n = 4$) and control patients with thigh pain without AFFs or a history of AFFs ($n = 14$). All patients with either AFFs or a history of AFFs with a bowing deformity of the femur showed a marked concentration of diffuse stress on the anterolateral surface, while there were no significant findings in 13 of the 14 patients in the control group. However, the remaining patient in the control group showed a marked concentration of diffuse stress on the anterolateral surface with radiographic evidence of a bowing deformity and a focally thickened lateral cortex, similar to that which was observed in the bowed AFF group. When these patients were reclassified as either SBF ($n = 5$) or non-SBF ($n = 13$), the femoral bowing of the patients with SBF was significantly more severe in comparison to that of non-SBF patients (lateral, $p = 0.0015$; anterior, $p = 0.0022$). While no significant differences in bone mineral density or bone metabolic markers were found between the SBF and non-SBF patients, the maximum principal stress (MPS) and the tensile stress–strength ratio (TSSR) in the femoral shaft were significantly higher in SBF patients than in non-SBF patients ($p = 0.0031$ for MPS and $p = 0.0022$ for TSSR). These data suggest that the tensile stress to the femoral shaft in AFFs occurs due to the bowing deformity.

In addition to the curvature of the femora, other risk factors must also be present for AFFs to occur because (1) only a small percentage (0.002–0.1 %) of osteoporotic patients taking BPs develop AFFs (Fig. 6.1) and (2) AFFs sometimes occur in patients who are not on long-term therapy. Hagen et al. hypothesized that it is possible that patients who develop AFFs have an anatomic biomechanical predisposition to the condition. They hypothesized that patients on chronic BP therapy who sustain AFFs or display radiographic characteristics consistent with a stress fracture or "lateral cortical beaking" are more likely to display varus proximal

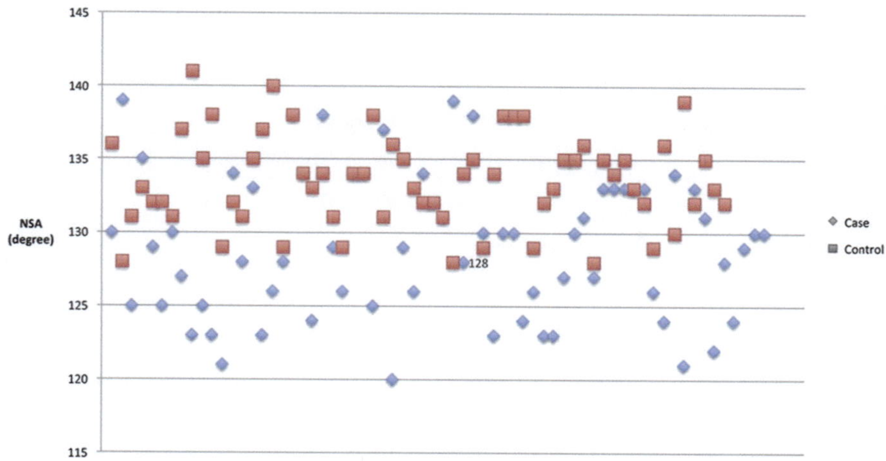

Fig. 6.7 Plot of neck-shaft angles (NSA) in the case group [atypical femoral fracture (AFF)] and the control group (asymptomatic patient) [14]

femoral anatomy than exposure-matched controls [14]. To clarify this hypothesis, the authors conducted a multicenter retrospective case–control study of patients from six institutions in the United States.

A series of 111 patients, who had been treated for complete or incomplete AFFs, was identified and designated as the case group, and a control group was established which consisted of 33 patients who had no history of fracture or prodromal thigh or hip pain. Thus, 144 patients were included in the analysis, and the radiographs of 255 hips were available for measurement. The neck-shaft angle was defined as the angle formed by the intersection of a line down the center of the femoral neck and a line through the center of the femoral shaft. The mean neck-shaft angle in the case group (129.5°) was significantly lower than that in the controls (133.8°; $p < 0.001$) (Fig. 6.7). The mean neck-shaft angle on the pathologic sides(s) in the case group (129.9°) was also significantly lower than the mean angle in the control group ($p < 0.001$). The lowest recorded neck-shaft angles were 128° in the control group and 118° in the case group. Fifty-three (48 %) of the patients in the case group had a neck-shaft angle of <128° on the pathologic side (Fig. 6.7).

The proximal femoral strength is decreased with a varus mechanical axis [66]. Biomechanical studies have shown that trochanteric and femoral shaft fractures are more common in patients with low neck-shaft angles [67]. Koh et al. reviewed the radiographs of 48 patients with AFFs and found that the fractures were clustered in the lateral cortex at the region of maximal tensile loading (Fig. 6.8) [58]. Based on the results of this study and the previous studies, the author noted an association between the proximal femoral geometry and the presence of AFFs.

A case–control study was conducted to identify the radiographic markers for fracture predisposition that could potentially aid in the safer uses of medication [69]. Fifty-three AFF patients with 63 femora radiographs were identified. The

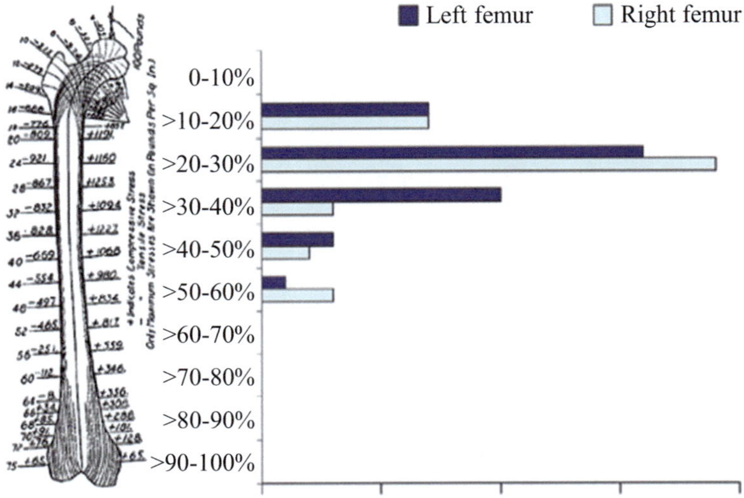

Fig. 6.8 Graph (*right*) shows the concentration of lesions (similar for both femurs) at 20–30 % of the femoral length from the greater trochanter, which corresponds to the region of highest tensile stress, as illustrated on the femoral sketch by Koch (*left*) [68] (Reprinted with permission from the Singapore Medical Journal [58])

radiographic measurements of the AFF group were compared with 43 no-femoral-fracture (NFF) patients with 80 femora radiographs and 64 intertrochanteric femur fracture (IFF) patients with 79 femora films (Fig. 6.9). The mean duration of BP use was nearly 8 years in both the AFF (7.9 years) and NFF (7.7 years) patient groups ($p = 0.7$). The pre-fracture radiographs of 53 BP users who developed AFFs were compared with those of 43 asymptomatic chronic BP users and 64 intertrochanteric fracture patients. The BP users who developed fractures had wider varus pre-fracture neck-shaft angles (NSA), a shorter hip-axis length (HAL), and narrower center-edge (CE) angles (Table 6.4). A weak correlation between NSA and HAL was observed in the bisphosphonate groups (AFF + NFF) ($r = 0.34$, $p < 0.01$). When NSA and HAL were compared in patients who developed fractures, the fractures tended to cluster in the area of the varus NSA with a shorter HAL (Fig. 6.10). A logistic regression model analysis revealed a significant association between NSA, CE angle, and BMI with the development of a fracture. An ROC curve analysis (area under curve = 0.67 [95 % CI = 0.56–0.79]) revealed that an NSA of <128.3° yielded a 69 % sensitivity and 63 % specificity for the predicted development of a complete or incomplete AFF. Based on these results, this study suggests that the varus angle of the femoral neck and a narrow CE angle were associated with the development of AFFs in long-term BP users.

In addition to these radiological features, the bilateral fractures are one of the clinical characteristics of patients with AFFs. In most cases, bilateral AFFs occur in the same anatomical location (Fig. 6.11), suggesting that individual factor(s) determines the fracture sites of AFFs. We hypothesized that the fracture site of an AFF is associated with the weight-bearing alignment of the lower limb. We analyzed the

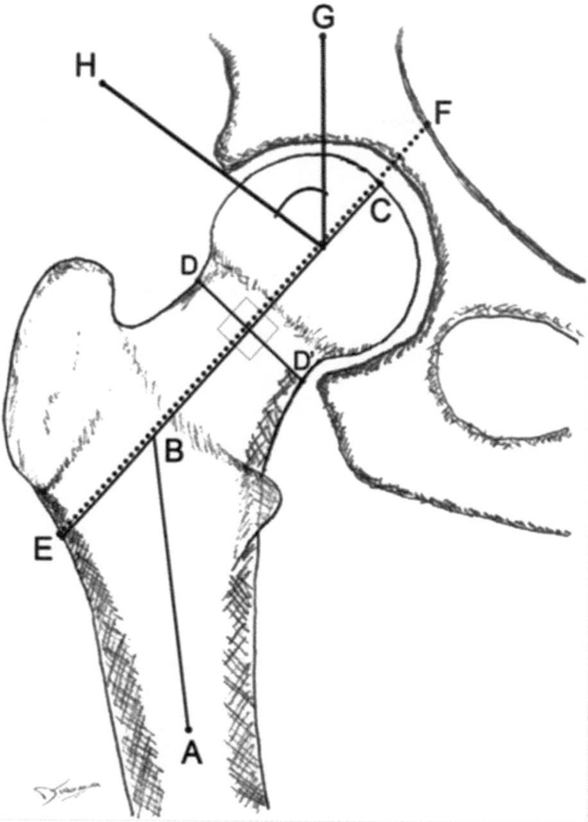

Fig. 6.9 Geometric hip measurements. The neck-shaft angle (NSA) was measured as the angle formed by ABC. AB, radiographic center of the diaphysis; BC, radiographic center of the femoral neck, drawn perpendicular to the narrowest portion, defined by the line DD'. The hip-axis length (HAL) (denoted EF) was measured as the distance from the greater trochanter to the inner pelvic brim along the neck-shaft axis line, perpendicularly bisecting segment DD'. The center-edge (CE) angle was measured by drawing a vertical line down to the center of the femoral head (G), with an angle completed by the extension of a line tangential to the lateral edge of the acetabular roof (H) (Reprinted with permission from the Elsevier [69])

Table 6.4 Radiographic measurement means as well as differences between group means [69]

	AFF	NFF	ITF	Mean difference (AFF vs NFF)	Mean difference (AFF vs ITF)	*p*
Neck-shaft angle (°)	126.4 (6.6)[a, b]	130.3 (5.8)	131.1 (5.6)	3.9 (0.9–7.0)	4.7 (1.9–7.4)	<0.001
Hip-axis length (mm)	120.3 (11.7)[c, d]	127.3 (12.4)	128.2 (13.4)	7.0 (0.6–13.5)	7.9 (2.1–13.8)	0.004
Center-edge angle (°)	42.6 (6.2)[e]	45.1 (4.8)	45.8 (5.0)	2.6 (0.1–5.3)	3.2 (−0.8–5.7)	0.007

AFF atypical femoral fracture patients, *NFF* no-femoral-fracture patients, *ITF* intertrochanteric fracture patients unless otherwise noted. There was no statistical difference in Tukey pairwise post-hoc comparisons at a $p \leq 0.05$ significance level

[a]AFF vs. NFF pairwise comparison, $p < 0.01$

[b]AFF vs. ITF pairwise comparison, $p < 0.001$

[c]AFF vs. NFF pairwise comparison, $p < 0.05$

[d]AFF vs. ITF pairwise comparison, $p < 0.01$

[e]AFF vs. ITF pairwise comparison, $p < 0.01$

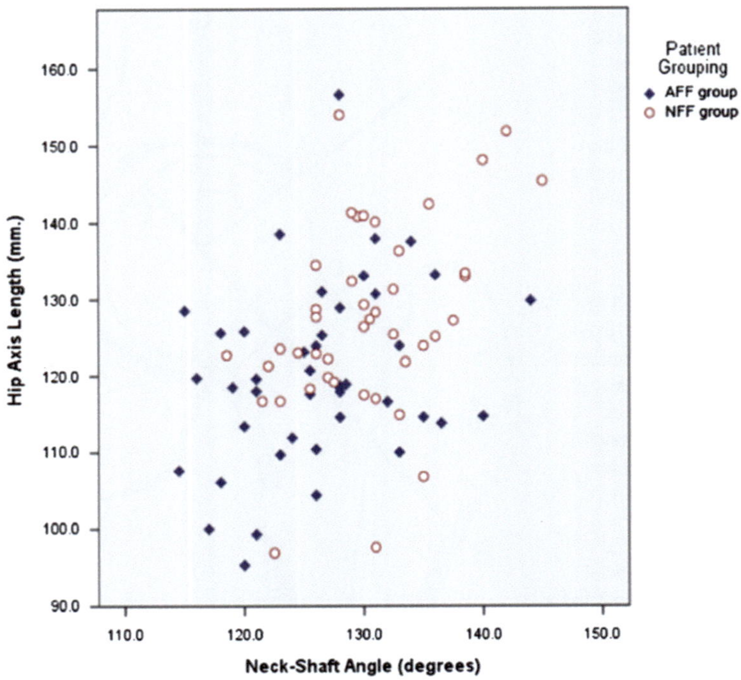

Fig. 6.10 Hip-axis length (HAL) versus neck-shaft angle in chronic bisphosphonate users. Among all bisphosphonate (BP) users, NSA (X-axis) versus HAL (Y-axis) was plotted independently for patients who developed either complete or incomplete atypical femur fracture (AFF group; diamond) and those who had not fractured (NFF group; circle). Patients with femora which fractured tended to cluster having both shorter HAL and narrower NSA. Femora which had obtuse NSA and with larger HAL tended not to fracture (Reprinted with permission from the Elsevier [69])

standing alignment of the lower limb in patients with AFFs and typical femoral fractures (TFFs).

We retrospectively reviewed the patient admission records of the orthopedic wards of six hospitals associated with our university in Japan between 2005 and 2010 [10]. We reviewed the radiographs of all patients with hip fractures ($n = 2238$, femoral neck fractures, intertrochanteric fractures, and subtrochanteric fractures) and diaphyseal femoral fractures treated at these hospitals. Between 2005 and 2010, a total of ten AFF patients were observed. As four patients had AFFs on both sides, 14 AFFs were found to have occurred. With regard to the number of TFFs, 142 patients with TFFs were treated in the university hospital, one of the six hospitals included in this study, during this period. In 44 (28 were either FNs or ITs, six were STs, and the remaining ten were diaphyseal fracture [D]) of the 142 patients with TFF, the radiographs of the lower limb were taken for the purpose of examining lower limb alignment.

To measure the site of the AFFs in the femur, we measured both the femoral full length [A] and the length from the proximal end of the femur to the location of the

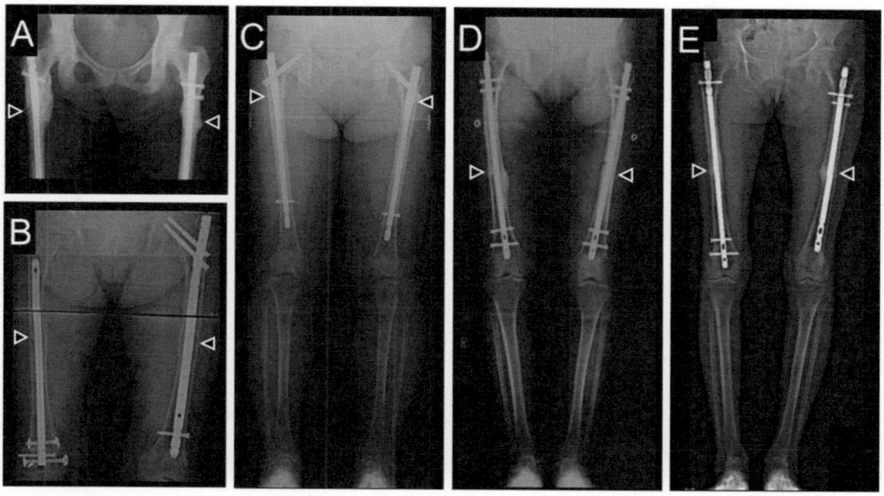

Fig. 6.11 Symmetrical fracture sites in the femora in the patients with bilateral atypical femoral fractures (AFFs). Radiographs of bilateral atypical subtrochanteric femoral fractures (**A** and **C**) and bilateral atypical diaphyseal fractures (**B**, **D**, and **E**) are shown. Panels **C**, **D**, and **E** are images of weight-bearing full-length radiographs of the patients with bilateral AFFs. The *closed arrowheads* indicate the fracture sites. The fracture sites were symmetrical in the femora in the patients with bilateral AFFs (Reprinted with permission from the Elsevier [11])

lateral cortex of the AFF [B]. The femoral full length was measured from the top of the femoral head to the distal end of the medial femoral condyle. The ratio of [B]/[A] was used as a measure of the fracture site in the femur (Fig. 6.12).

To examine the weight-bearing alignment of the lower limb, standing radiographs of the lower limbs were obtained in the patients with both AFFs and TFFs. The standing femorotibial angle (FTA) was measured in the anteroposterior view, as previously described [70, 71]. The FTA is the lateral angle of the intersection between the femoral axis and the tibial axis on an anteroposterior radiograph (Fig. 6.13) [72]. In patients with normal findings, the large joints of the lower limb are aligned on a straight line that represents the mechanical longitudinal axis of the leg, the Mikulicz line (Fig. 6.13). This line stretches from the hip joint (the center of the head of the femur) through the knee joint (the intercondylar eminence of the tibia) and down to the center of the ankle (the ankle mortise, the forklike grip between the medial and lateral malleoli). In the tibial shaft, the mechanical and anatomical axes coincide; however, the femoral shaft diverges at an angle of 2–6°, resulting in an FTA of 174–178° in a leg with a normal axial alignment [73]. The 95 % confidence interval (CI) of the mean value and the 95 % prediction interval of the standing FTA of a Japanese general population over 40 years of age calculated based on the findings of the population-based cohort study ($n = 5860$) were 175.1–178.0° and 168.6–184.6°, respectively [74].

The average fracture site in the femur was 39.5 % (SD, 15.8 %). While there was no correlation between the fracture site and the FTA in the patients with typical

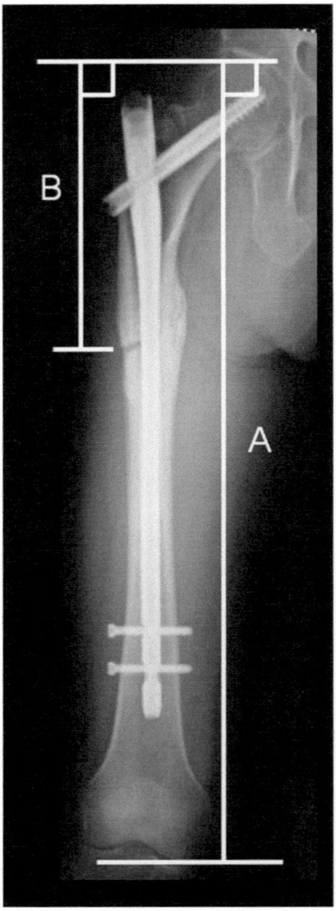

Fig. 6.12 Measurement of the fracture site in the femur on a radiograph. In order to measure the site of the AFFs in the femur, we measured both the femoral full length [**A**] and the length from the proximal end of the femur to the location of lateral cortex of the AFF [**B**]. The femoral full length was measured from the top of the femoral head to the distal end of the medial femoral condyle. The ratio of [**B**]/[**A**] was used as the fracture site in the femur (Reprinted with permission from the Elsevier [11])

subtrochanteric and diaphyseal fractures, there was a positive correlation between the fracture sites of the AFFs and the standing FTA ($r = 0.82$, 95 % CI; 0.49–0.94, Fig. 6.14). To further examine the effect of lower limb alignment on AFFs, the patients with AFFs were divided into subgroups depending on the fracture site (STs [$n = 7$] and Ds [$n = 6$]) and their FTAs were compared with the FTAs of the TFF patients. No significant differences in the FTA were observed between the subgroups of the patients with TFFs (Fig. 6.15). The mean FTA of the TFF patients with hip fracture, STs, and Ds was within the 95 % CI for the FTA of the Japanese general population [74] (Fig. 6.15). In contrast, the mean FTA in the AFF patients was outside of the 95 % CI of the FTA of the Japanese general population. The mean FTA in patients with atypical STs (172.8°) was smaller, while the mean FTA in patients with atypical Ds (183.3°) was larger than the 95 % CI of FTA of the Japanese general population. No significant differences in FTA were observed between the subgroups of the patients with TFFs (Fig. 6.15). The FTA of the patients with atypical Ds was significantly larger than that of those with typical

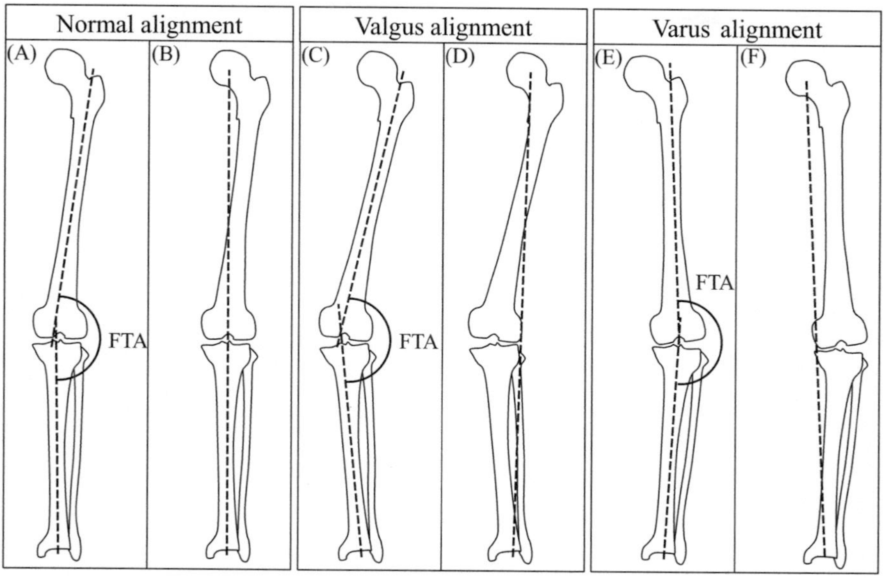

Fig. 6.13 The FTA and mechanical axis of the lower limb. The femorotibial angle (FTA) is the lateral angle between the axis of the femoral shaft and that of the tibial shaft (**A**, **C**, and **E**). The mechanical axis is indicated by *dotted lines* in panels **B**, **D**, and **F**. **A** and **B**, normal alignment; **C** and **D**, valgus alignment; **E** and **F**, varus alignment. In patients with a normal alignment, the mechanical axis passes through the center of knee joint (**B**). In patients with a valgus alignment, the FTA becomes smaller (**C**) and the mechanical axis passes through the lateral side of the knee joint (**D**). In patients with a varus alignment, the FTA becomes larger (**E**) and the mechanical axis passes through the medial side of the knee joint (**F**). The amount of mechanical force passed to the lateral cortex of the femur changes depending on the alignment of the lower limb (Reprinted with permission from the Elsevier [11])

hip and femoral fractures and atypical STs. No significant differences in FTA were observed between the subgroups of the patients with TFFs (Fig. 6.15).

Schematic diagrams of the tensile stress loading on the lateral cortex of the femur in varus and valgus lower limb alignments are shown in Fig. 6.13. Therefore, mechanical alterations due to the lateral bowing of the femur, as shown in the other studies [8, 65], and the femoral neck-shaft angle [14], and/or genu varus alignment, as shown in our study [11], may increase the bending force on the lateral cortex of the femur. Among these factors, the genu varus alignment may, at least in part, be altered by aging. The progression of such age-related changes in the femur, which are frequently observed in Asian populations, shifts the area of maximal tensile stress to a more distal site in the femoral shaft. Indeed, the patients with atypical Ds were significantly older than those with atypical STs in our study (77.2 years vs. 54.8 years; $p < 0.01$).

On the other hand, the presence of a genu valgus alignment, which is frequently observed in Asian patients with collagen diseases, shifted the maximal loading site to a more proximal location in the femoral cortex (Fig. 6.13). The patients with a ST had a higher number of chronic diseases and were more frequently of Asian origin

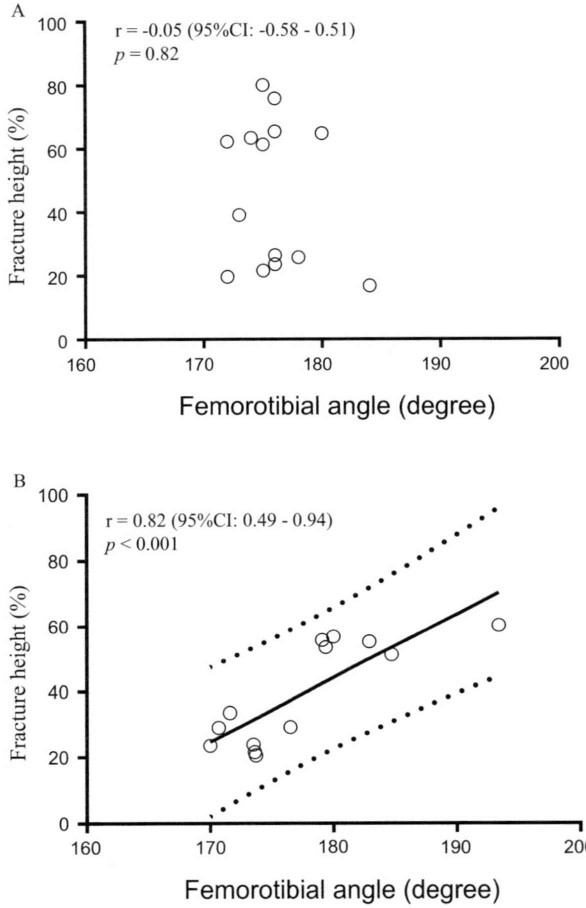

Fig. 6.14 Association between the fracture site and the lower limb alignment in patients with AFFs. Relationships between the standing femorotibial angle (FTA, as shown in Fig. 6.13) and the fracture site (the proportion of the fracture site per full length of the femur, as shown in Fig. 6.12) in patients with typical subtrochanteric and diaphyseal femoral fractures (typical femoral fractures) (**A**) and atypical subtrochanteric and diaphyseal femoral fractures (atypical femoral fractures) (**B**). *Solid lines*, approximate line; *dotted curves*, 95 % prediction intervals; *n.s.*, not significant (Reprinted with permission from the Elsevier [11])

compared to those with a femoral shaft fracture [75]. In our study, all of the patients with atypical ST suffered from collagen diseases, and the FTA of these patients was low (172.8° on average) in comparison with that of the Japanese general population (177.6° on average in women). In addition, in the patients with collagen disease, the joint motion of hip abduction is decreased and the hip abductor moment is low in the patients with collagen disease in comparison to healthy controls [76]. These biomechanical factors of the lower limb would be one of the reasons why atypical STs frequently occur in the patients with multiple chronic diseases and especially in the patients with collagen diseases in Japan.

These studies indicated that biomechanical factors, such as the femoral bone geometry and lower limb alignment, are related to the location at which the mechanical stresses are concentrated. Therefore, malalignment and/or age-related changes in the lower limbs would be one of the risk factors for the accumulation of microcracks in the lateral cortex and the progression of microcracks to AFFs.

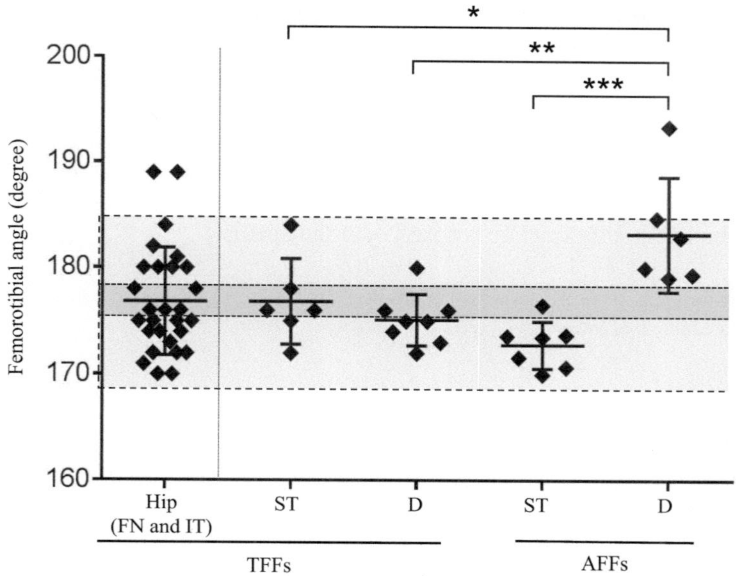

Fig. 6.15 Comparison of FTA in patients with TFFs and AFFs. The mean, standard deviation, and data plots of femorotibial angle (FTA) in the patients with femoral fractures [typical femoral fractures (TFFs) and atypical femoral fracture (AFFs)] were shown. *Gray zone* between *dotted lines* indicates the 95 % confidence interval of the mean value of the standing FTA of a Japanese general population over 40 years of age calculated from the population-based cohort study ($n = 5860$, 175.1 to 178.0°) [74]. *Gray zone* between *dashed line* indicates the 95 % prediction interval of standing FTA (168.6° to 184.6°) [74]. *, $p < 0.05$; **, $p < 0.01$; *FN*, femoral neck fractures; *IT*, intertrochanteric fractures; *ST*, subtrochanteric fractures; *D*, femoral diaphyseal fractures (Reprinted with permission from the Elsevier [11])

6.7 Conclusions

The management of osteoporosis is improving [77]. Recently, osteoporosis management is starting to follow risk-based strategies that have already been adopted in other disease areas, such as cardiovascular disease. The implementation of the concepts of "goal-directed therapy" and "treat-to-target therapy" into future osteoporosis management strategies is an ongoing challenge [78, 79]. Although further discussion is needed for such concepts to be accepted, the long-term treatment of osteoporosis cannot be avoided if we are to really achieve success in the prevention of fractures in patients with osteoporosis. The absolute incidence of AFFs in patients with osteoporosis is low (Fig. 6.1). However, there is an association between antiresorptive agents, such as BPs, and probably also denosumab, and the incidence of AFFs. Although the pathogenesis of AFFs has not been fully understood, a large number of factors may be involved in their occurrence. The long-term suppression of bone remodeling, as one of the factors related to AFFs, would contribute to the deterioration of the bone microarchitecture, reduce the bone repair process, and lead to the accumulation of microdamage, resulting in the progression of AFFs. Geometrical factors, such as the bowing of the femur, coxa vara, and lower limb alignment, which are factors that are related to AFFs, may alter both the mechanical properties of the femora and the concentration of mechanical force to the femora. Given the large number of problems that remain unresolved, further research into the role of the geometric factors is required to contribute not only the understanding of the occurrence of AFFs but also for the prevention of fragility fractures caused by osteoporosis.

Acknowledgments This work was not funded by any research or training grants. The authors declare no conflicts of interest.

References

1. Rachner TD, Khosla S, Hofbauer LC (2011) Osteoporosis: now and the future. Lancet 377 (9773):1276–1287. doi:10.1016/S0140-6736(10)62349-5
2. Harris ST, Watts NB, Genant HK, McKeever CD, Hangartner T, Keller M, Chesnut CH 3rd, Brown J, Eriksen EF, Hoseyni MS, Axelrod DW, Miller PD (1999) Effects of risedronate treatment on vertebral and nonvertebral fractures in women with postmenopausal osteoporosis: a randomized controlled trial. Vertebral Efficacy with Risedronate Therapy (VERT) Study Group. JAMA 282(14):1344–1352
3. Russell RG, Xia Z, Dunford JE, Oppermann U, Kwaasi A, Hulley PA, Kavanagh KL, Triffitt JT, Lundy MW, Phipps RJ, Barnett BL, Coxon FP, Rogers MJ, Watts NB, Ebetino FH (2007) Bisphosphonates: an update on mechanisms of action and how these relate to clinical efficacy. Ann N Y Acad Sci 1117:209–257
4. Donnelly E, Meredith DS, Nguyen JT, Gladnick BP, Rebolledo BJ, Shaffer AD, Lorich DG, Lane JM, Boskey AL (2012) Reduced cortical bone compositional heterogeneity with bisphosphonate treatment in postmenopausal women with intertrochanteric and subtrochanteric fractures. J Bone Miner Res 27(3):672–678
5. Saito M, Mori S, Mashiba T, Komatsubara S, Marumo K (2008) Collagen maturity, glycation induced-pentosidine, and mineralization are increased following 3-year treatment with incadronate in dogs. Osteoporos Int 19(9):1343–1354. doi:10.1007/s00198-008-0585-3
6. Shane E, Burr D, Ebeling PR, Abrahamsen B, Adler RA, Brown TD, Cheung AM, Cosman F, Curtis JR, Dell R, Dempster D, Einhorn TA, Genant HK, Geusens P, Klaushofer K, Koval K, Lane JM, McKiernan F, McKinney R, Ng A, Nieves J, O'Keefe R, Papapoulos S, Sen HT, van der Meulen MC, Weinstein RS, Whyte M (2010) Atypical subtrochanteric and diaphyseal femoral fractures: report of a task force of the American Society for Bone and Mineral Research. J Bone Miner Res 25(11):2267–2294. doi:10.1002/jbmr.253
7. Tan SC, Koh SB, Goh SK, Howe TS (2011) Atypical femoral stress fractures in bisphosphonate-free patients. Osteoporos Int 22(7):2211–2212
8. Sasaki S, Miyakoshi N, Hongo M, Kasukawa Y, Shimada Y (2012) Low-energy diaphyseal femoral fractures associated with bisphosphonate use and severe curved femur: a case series. J Bone Miner Metab 30(5):561–567
9. Oh Y, Wakabayashi Y, Kurosa Y, Ishizuki M, Okawa A (2014) Stress fracture of the bowed femoral shaft is another cause of atypical femoral fracture in elderly Japanese: a case series. J Orthop Sci 19(4):579–586
10. Saita Y, Ishijima M, Mogami A, Kubota M, Baba T, Kaketa T, Nagao M, Sakamoto Y, Sakai K, Homma Y, Kato R, Nagura N, Miyagawa K, Wada T, Liu L, Matsuoka J, Obayashi O, Shitoto K, Nozawa M, Kajihara H, Gen H, Kaneko K (2014) The incidence of and risk factors

for developing atypical femoral fractures in Japan. J Bone Miner Metab. doi:10.1007/s00774-014-0591-9
11. Saita Y, Ishijima M, Mogami A, Kubota M, Baba T, Kaketa T, Nagao M, Sakamoto Y, Sakai K, Kato R, Nagura N, Miyagawa K, Wada T, Liu L, Obayashi O, Shitoto K, Nozawa M, Kajihara H, Gen H, Kaneko K (2014) The fracture sites of atypical femoral fractures are associated with the weight-bearing lower limb alignment. Bone 66:105–110
12. Aspenberg P (2014) Denosumab and atypical femoral fractures. Acta Orthop 85(1):1. doi:10.3109/17453674.2013.859423
13. Schilcher J, Aspenberg P (2014) Atypical fracture of the femur in a patient using denosumab – a case report. Acta Orthop 85(1):6–7. doi:10.3109/17453674.2014.885355
14. Hagen JE, Miller AN, Ott SM, Gardner M, Morshed S, Jeray K, Alton TB, Ren D, Abblitt WP, Krieg JC (2014) Association of atypical femoral fractures with bisphosphonate use by patients with varus hip geometry. J Bone Joint Surg Am 96(22):1905–1909. doi:10.2106/JBJS.N.00075
15. Odvina CV, Zerwekh JE, Rao DS, Maalouf N, Gottschalk FA, Pak CY (2005) Severely suppressed bone turnover: a potential complication of alendronate therapy. J Clin Endocrinol Metab 90(3):1294–1301. doi:jc.2004-0952 [pii] 10.1210/jc.2004-0952
16. Khan AA, Rios LP, Sandor GK, Khan N, Peters E, Rahman MO, Clokie CM, Dore E, Dubois S (2011) Bisphosphonate-associated osteonecrosis of the jaw in Ontario: a survey of oral and maxillofacial surgeons. J Rheumatol 38(7):1396–1402. doi:10.3899/jrheum.100221
17. Brown JP, Morin S, Leslie W, Papaioannou A, Cheung AM, Davison KS, Goltzman D, Hanley DA, Hodsman A, Josse R, Jovaisas A, Juby A, Kaiser S, Karaplis A, Kendler D, Khan A, Ngui D, Olszynski W, Ste-Marie LG, Adachi J (2014) Bisphosphonates for treatment of osteoporosis: expected benefits, potential harms, and drug holidays. Can Fam Physician 60 (4):324–333. doi:60/4/324 [pii]
18. Shane E, Burr D, Abrahamsen B, Adler RA, Brown TD, Cheung AM, Cosman F, Curtis JR, Dell R, Dempster DW, Ebeling PR, Einhorn TA, Genant HK, Geusens P, Klaushofer K, Lane JM, McKiernan F, McKinney R, Ng A, Nieves J, O'Keefe R, Papapoulos S, Howe TS, van der Meulen MC, Weinstein RS, Whyte MP (2014) Atypical subtrochanteric and diaphyseal femoral fractures: second report of a task force of the American society for bone and mineral research. J Bone Miner Res 29(1):1–23. doi:10.1002/jbmr.1998
19. Abrahamsen B, Eiken P, Eastell R (2009) Subtrochanteric and diaphyseal femur fractures in patients treated with alendronate: a register-based national cohort study. J Bone Miner Res 24 (6):1095–1102. doi:10.1359/jbmr.081247
20. Abrahamsen B, Eiken P, Eastell R (2010) Cumulative alendronate dose and the long-term absolute risk of subtrochanteric and diaphyseal femur fractures: a register-based national cohort analysis. J Clin Endocrinol Metab 95(12):5258–5265
21. Hsiao FY, Huang WF, Chen YM, Wen YW, Kao YH, Chen LK, Tsai YW (2011) Hip and subtrochanteric or diaphyseal femoral fractures in alendronate users: a 10-year, nationwide retrospective cohort study in Taiwanese women. Clin Ther 33(11):1659–1667
22. Kim SY, Schneeweiss S, Katz JN, Levin R, Solomon DH (2011) Oral bisphosphonates and risk of subtrochanteric or diaphyseal femur fractures in a population-based cohort. J Bone Miner Res 26(5):993–1001
23. Wang Z, Bhattacharyya T (2011) Trends in incidence of subtrochanteric fragility fractures and bisphosphonate use among the US elderly, 1996–2007. J Bone Miner Res 26(3):553–560
24. Abrahamsen B (2012) Atypical femur fractures: refining the clinical picture. J Bone Miner Res 27(5):975–976. doi:10.1002/jbmr.1610
25. Capeci CM, Tejwani NC (2009) Bilateral low-energy simultaneous or sequential femoral fractures in patients on long-term alendronate therapy. J Bone Joint Surg Am 91 (11):2556–2561
26. Dell RM, Adams AL, Greene DF, Funahashi TT, Silverman SL, Eisemon EO, Zhou H, Burchette RJ, Ott SM (2012) Incidence of atypical nontraumatic diaphyseal fractures of the femur. J Bone Miner Res 27(12):2544–2550

27. Girgis CM, Sher D, Seibel MJ (2010) Atypical femoral fractures and bisphosphonate use. N Engl J Med 362(19):1848–1849, doi:362/19/1848 [pii]10.1056/NEJMc0910389
28. Giusti A, Hamdy NA, Dekkers OM, Ramautar SR, Dijkstra S, Papapoulos SE (2011) Atypical fractures and bisphosphonate therapy: a cohort study of patients with femoral fracture with radiographic adjudication of fracture site and features. Bone 48(5):966–971, doi:S8756-3282(10)02147-2 [pii]10.1016/j.bone.2010.12.033
29. Lenart BA, Neviaser AS, Lyman S, Chang CC, Edobor-Osula F, Steele B, van der Meulen MC, Lorich DG, Lane JM (2009) Association of low-energy femoral fractures with prolonged bisphosphonate use: a case control study. Osteoporos Int 20(8):1353–1362. doi:10.1007/s00198-008-0805-x
30. Lo JC, Huang SY, Lee GA, Khandelwal S, Provus J, Ettinger B, Gonzalez JR, Hui RL, Grimsrud CD (2012) Clinical correlates of atypical femoral fracture. Bone 51(1):181–184
31. Meier RP, Perneger TV, Stern R, Rizzoli R, Peter RE (2012) Increasing Occurrence of Atypical Femoral Fractures Associated With Bisphosphonate Use. Arch Intern Med 172(12):930–936, doi:1160667 [pii]10.1001/archinternmed.2012.1796
32. Schilcher J, Michaelsson K, Aspenberg P (2011) Bisphosphonate use and atypical fractures of the femoral shaft. N Engl J Med 364(18):1728–1737. doi:10.1056/NEJMoa1010650
33. Thompson RN, Phillips JR, McCauley SH, Elliott JR, Moran CG (2012) Atypical femoral fractures and bisphosphonate treatment: experience in two large United Kingdom teaching hospitals. J Bone Joint Surg (Br) 94(3):385–390, doi:94-B/3/385 [pii]10.1302/0301-620X.94B3.27999
34. Feldstein AC, Black D, Perrin N, Rosales AG, Friess D, Boardman D, Dell R, Santora A, Chandler JM, Rix MM, Orwoll E (2012) Incidence and demography of femur fractures with and without atypical features. J Bone Miner Res 27(5):977–986. doi:10.1002/jbmr.1550
35. Warren C, Gilchrist N, Coates M, Frampton C, Helmore J, McKie J, Hooper G (2012) Atypical subtrochanteric fractures, bisphosphonates, blinded radiological review. ANZ J Surg 82(12):908–912
36. Gedmintas L, Solomon DH, Kim SC (2013) Bisphosphonates and risk of subtrochanteric, femoral shaft, and atypical femur fracture: a systematic review and meta-analysis. J Bone Miner Res 28(8):1729–1737
37. Wang Z, Ward MM, Chan L, Bhattacharyya T (2014) Adherence to oral bisphosphonates and the risk of subtrochanteric and femoral shaft fractures among female medicare beneficiaries. Osteoporos Int 25(8):2109–2116
38. Nieves JW, Bilezikian JP, Lane JM, Einhorn TA, Wang Y, Steinbuch M, Cosman F (2010) Fragility fractures of the hip and femur: incidence and patient characteristics. Osteoporos Int 21(3):399–408. doi:10.1007/s00198-009-0962-6
39. Mashiba T, Hirano T, Turner CH, Forwood MR, Johnston CC, Burr DB (2000) Suppressed bone turnover by bisphosphonates increases microdamage accumulation and reduces some biomechanical properties in dog rib. J Bone Miner Res 15(4):613–620. doi:10.1359/jbmr.2000.15.4.613
40. Jamal SA, Dion N, Ste-Marie LG (2011) Atypical femoral fractures and bone turnover. N Engl J Med 365(13):1261–1262
41. Schilcher J, Sandberg O, Isaksson H, Aspenberg P (2014) Histology of 8 atypical femoral fractures: remodeling but no healing. Acta Orthop 85(3):280–286
42. Ettinger B, Burr DB, Ritchie RO (2013) Proposed pathogenesis for atypical femoral fractures: lessons from materials research. Bone 55(2):495–500. doi:10.1016/j.bone.2013.02.004
43. Wright AA, Hegedus EJ, Lenchik L, Kuhn KJ, Santiago L, Smoliga JM (2015) Diagnostic accuracy of various imaging modalities for suspected lower extremity stress fractures: a systematic review with evidence-based recommendations for clinical practice. Am J Sports Med. doi:10.1177/0363546515574066
44. Brukner P, Bradshaw C, Khan KM, White S, Crossley K (1996) Stress fractures: a review of 180 cases. Clin J Sport Med 6(2):85–89

45. Matheson GO, Clement DB, McKenzie DC, Taunton JE, Lloyd-Smith DR, MacIntyre JG (1987) Stress fractures in athletes. A study of 320 cases. Am J Sports Med 15(1):46–58
46. Orava S (1980) Stress fractures. Br J Sports Med 14(1):40–44
47. Bennell KL, Brukner PD (1997) Epidemiology and site specificity of stress fractures. Clin Sports Med 16(2):179–196
48. Blatz DJ (1981) Bilateral femoral and tibial shaft stress fractures in a runner. Am J Sports Med 9(5):322–325
49. Butler JE, Brown SL, McConnell BG (1982) Subtrochanteric stress fractures in runners. Am J Sports Med 10(4):228–232
50. Hershman EB, Lombardo J, Bergfeld JA (1990) Femoral shaft stress fractures in athletes. Clin Sports Med 9(1):111–119
51. Masters S, Fricker P, Purdam C (1986) Stress fractures of the femoral shaft – four case studies. Br J Sports Med 20(1):14–16
52. Kang L, Belcher D, Hulstyn MJ (2005) Stress fractures of the femoral shaft in women's college lacrosse: a report of seven cases and a review of the literature. Br J Sports Med 39 (12):902–906. doi:10.1136/bjsm.2004.016626
53. DeFranco MJ, Recht M, Schils J, Parker RD (2006) Stress fractures of the femur in athletes. Clin Sports Med 25 (1):89–103, ix. doi:10.1016/j.csm.2005.08.003
54. Gebhardt MC, Campbell CJ, Schiller AL, Mankin HJ (1985) Desmoplastic fibroma of bone. A report of eight cases and review of the literature. J Bone Joint Surg Am 67(5):732–747
55. Milgrom C, Giladi M, Stein M, Kashtan H, Margulies JY, Chisin R, Steinberg R, Aharonson Z (1985) Stress fractures in military recruits. A prospective study showing an unusually high incidence. J Bone Joint Surg (Br) 67(5):732–735
56. Mohan PC, Howe TS, Koh JS, Png MA (2013) Radiographic features of multifocal endosteal thickening of the femur in patients on long-term bisphosphonate therapy. Eur Radiol 23 (1):222–227. doi:10.1007/s00330-012-2587-y
57. Ivkovic A, Bojanic I, Pecina M (2006) Stress fractures of the femoral shaft in athletes: a new treatment algorithm. Br J Sports Med 40 (6):518–520; discussion 520. doi:10.1136/bjsm.2005.023655
58. Koh JS, Goh SK, Png MA, Ng AC, Howe TS (2011) Distribution of atypical fractures and cortical stress lesions in the femur: implications on pathophysiology. Singap Med J 52 (2):77–80
59. Martelli S, Pivonka P, Ebeling PR (2014) Femoral shaft strains during daily activities: implications for atypical femoral fractures. Clin Biomech 29(8):869–876, 10.1016/j.clinbiomech.2014.08.001S0268-0033(14)00191-0[pii]
60. Boonen S, Ferrari S, Miller PD, Eriksen EF, Sambrook PN, Compston J, Reid IR, Vanderschueren D, Cosman F (2012) Postmenopausal osteoporosis treatment with antiresorptives: effects of discontinuation or long-term continuation on bone turnover and fracture risk – a perspective. J Bone Miner Res 27(5):963–974. doi:10.1002/jbmr.1570
61. Kwek EB, Koh JS, Howe TS (2008) More on atypical fractures of the femoral diaphysis. N Engl J Med 359(3):316–317
62. Aamodt A, Lund-Larsen J, Eine J, Andersen E, Benum P, Husby OS (1997) In vivo measurements show tensile axial strain in the proximal lateral aspect of the human femur. J Orthop Res 15(6):927–931. doi:10.1002/jor.1100150620
63. Duda GN, Heller M, Albinger J, Schulz O, Schneider E, Claes L (1998) Influence of muscle forces on femoral strain distribution. J Biomech 31(9):841–846
64. Saleh A, Hegde VV, Potty AG, Schneider R, Cornell CN, Lane JM (2012) Management strategy for symptomatic bisphosphonate-associated incomplete atypical femoral fractures. HSS J 8(2):103–110, 10.1007/s11420-012-9275-y9275 [pii]
65. Oh Y, Wakabayashi Y, Kurosa Y, Fujita K, Okawa A (2014) Potential pathogenic mechanism for stress fractures of the bowed femoral shaft in the elderly: mechanical analysis by the CT-based finite element method. Injury 45(11):1764–1771

66. Antapur P, Prakash D (2006) Proximal femoral geometry: a radiological assessment. J Arthroplasty 21(6):897–898. doi:10.1016/j.arth.2005.11.003
67. Gong H, Zhang M, Fan Y, Kwok WL, Leung PC (2012) Relationships between femoral strength evaluated by nonlinear finite element analysis and BMD, material distribution and geometric morphology. Ann Biomed Eng 40(7):1575–1585. doi:10.1007/s10439-012-0514-7
68. Koch J (1917) The laws of bone architecture. Am J Anat 21:177–298
69. Taormina DP, Marcano AI, Karia R, Egol KA, Tejwani NC (2014) Symptomatic atypical femoral fractures are related to underlying hip geometry. Bone 63:1–6
70. Buckland-Wright JC, Macfarlane DG, Williams SA, Ward RJ (1995) Accuracy and precision of joint space width measurements in standard and macroradiographs of osteoarthritic knees. Ann Rheum Dis 54(11):872–880
71. Ravaud P, Auleley GR, Chastang C, Rousselin B, Paolozzi L, Amor B, Dougados M (1996) Knee joint space width measurement: an experimental study of the influence of radiographic procedure and joint positioning. Br J Rheumatol 35(8):761–766
72. Bauer GC, Insall J, Koshino T (1969) Tibial osteotomy in gonarthrosis (osteo-arthritis of the knee). J Bone Joint Surg Am 51(8):1545–1563
73. Moreland JR, Bassett LW, Hanker GJ (1987) Radiographic analysis of the axial alignment of the lower extremity. J Bone Joint Surg Am 69(5):745–749
74. Oka H, Muraki S, Akune T, Nakamura K, Kawaguchi H, Yoshimura N (2010) Normal and threshold values of radiographic parameters for knee osteoarthritis using a computer-assisted measuring system (KOACAD): the ROAD study. J Orthop Sci 15(6):781–789
75. Giusti A, Hamdy NA, Papapoulos SE (2010) Atypical fractures of the femur and bisphosphonate therapy: a systematic review of case/case series studies. Bone 47(2):169–180
76. Weiss RJ, Wretenberg P, Stark A, Palmblad K, Larsson P, Grondal L, Brostrom E (2008) Gait pattern in rheumatoid arthritis. Gait Posture 28(2):229–234
77. McCloskey E, Leslie WD (2013) Goal-directed therapy in osteoporosis. J Bone Miner Res 28 (3):439–441. doi:10.1002/jbmr.1859
78. Cummings SR, Cosman F, Eastell R, Reid IR, Mehta M, Lewiecki EM (2013) Goal-directed treatment of osteoporosis. J Bone Miner Res 28(3):433–438. doi:10.1002/jbmr.1854
79. Lewiecki EM, Cummings SR, Cosman F (2013) Treat-to-target for osteoporosis: is now the time? J Clin Endocrinol Metab 98(3):946–953, 10.1210/jc.2012-3680jc.2012-3680 [pii]

Chapter 7
Spondylosis and Osteoporotic Vertebral Fractures

Naohisa Miyakoshi, Hiroyuki Kodama, Yuji Kasukawa, Takashi Kobayashi, Tetsuya Suzuki, Toshiki Abe, Eiji Abe, and Yoichi Shimada

Abstract Osteoporosis and spondylosis are the most common age-related conditions affecting the spine. Some of the literature on osteoporosis and spondylosis has demonstrated an inverse relationship between them, though insufficient support for such a relationship has also been documented. Our previous study showed that osteophyte formation and intervertebral disc degeneration were positively correlated with bone mineral density (BMD) for all measurement sites of the lumbar spine and proximal femur. Our most recent study, presented here, showed that, in an early phase of alendronate and/or alfacalcidol therapy ($\leq$6 months), fewer osteophytes were one of the significant factors for incident vertebral fractures. The existence of spondylosis may thus have a protective effect against osteoporotic vertebral fractures. With the increased aging of society, the demand for spine surgery in elderly patients with osteoporosis and spondylosis is increasing. Our surgical strategies for such patients are based on their predominant spinal pathology. If the predominant pathology is in the vertebral bodies, we consider vertebral replacement, and, if it is in the intervertebral space, we consider multilevel posterior lumbar interbody fusion (PLIF).

N. Miyakoshi (✉) • Y. Kasukawa • Y. Shimada
Department of Orthopedic Surgery, Akita University Graduate School of Medicine, 1-1-1 Hondo, Akita 010-8543, Japan

Akita Spine Group (ASG), Akita, Japan
e-mail: miyakosh@doc.med.akita-u.ac.jp

H. Kodama
Minami-Akita Orthopedic Clinic, 96-2 Kaidoshita, Showa-Okubo, Katagami 018-1401, Japan

T. Kobayashi • T. Abe • E. Abe
Akita Spine Group (ASG), Akita, Japan

Akita Kosei Medical Center, 1-1-1 Nishibukuro, Iijima, Akita 010-0948, Japan

T. Suzuki
Akita Spine Group (ASG), Akita, Japan

Akita Red Cross Hospital, 222-1 Saruta-Nashirozawa, Kamikitate, Akita 010-1495, Japan

Y. Shimada, N. Miyakoshi (eds.), *Osteoporosis in Orthopedics*,
DOI 10.1007/978-4-431-55778-4_7

Keywords Alendronate • Osteophyte • Posterior lumbar interbody fusion • Vertebral fracture • Vitamin D

7.1 Relationship Between Osteoporosis and Spondylosis

7.1.1 Prevalence of Osteoporosis and Spondylosis

Both osteoporosis and spondylosis increase with age [67]. Osteoporosis is a skeletal disorder characterized by compromised bone strength predisposing a person to an increased risk of fracture [40]. From 30 to 50 % of women will suffer an osteoporosis-related fracture in their lifetime [49]. Among osteoporotic fractures, vertebral fractures are the most common. In Japan, it has been estimated that 6,400,000 people aged ≥40 years are affected by osteoporosis when evaluated by bone mineral density (BMD) of the lumbar spine, and 10,700,000 people aged ≥40 years are affected by osteoporosis when evaluated by BMD of the femoral neck [67].

Spondylosis is a degenerative spinal disease characterized by a series of degenerative changes at the intervertebral discs, spinal end plates, and vertebral bodies, with consequent formation of osteophytes and sclerosis, in combination with osteoarthritis (OA) of the facet (zygapophyseal) joints. Spondylosis is a common cause of back pain and spinal canal stenosis in the elderly. Osteophytosis of the lumbar spine is more common in men than in women [43, 66], whereas disc space narrowing is more prevalent in women [66]. Studies have reported associations between disc height narrowing and back pain [25, 64]. A recent study has shown that the presence and extent of severe facet joint OA on computed tomography (CT) imaging was associated with back pain in community-based older adults, independent of sociodemographics, health factors, and disc height narrowing [59].

As to the prevalence of spondylosis, Kilshaw et al. [20] reviewed 2718 abdominal and kidney-ureter-bladder (KUB) radiographs in a population of random patients over the age of 20 years (male 52.6 %), and the prevalence of spinal OA was determined by the presence of osteophytes. The prevalence of OA of the spine in the age groups of 20–29, 30–39, 40–49, 50–59, 60–69, 70–79, 80–89, and 90+ years was 0 %, 0 %, 25.3 %, 72.9 %, 84.2 %, 99.5 %, 100 %, and 100 %, respectively [20].

In Japan, with a large-scale population-based cohort, it has been estimated that 37,900,000 individuals aged ≥40 years are affected by radiographic lumbar spondylosis [67]. In this cohort study in Japan with a mean age of 69.8 years in men ($n = 758$) and 68.3 years in women ($n = 1524$) at baseline, given 3.3 years of follow-up, the incidence of Kellgren and Lawrence (KL) grade ≥ 2 radiographic lumbar spondylosis was 50.0 % and 34.4 % (15.3 % and 10.5 % per year), while that of KL grade ≥ 3 lumbar spondylosis was 20.5 % and 27.4 % (6.2 % and 8.3 % per year) in men and women, respectively [35]. The KL classification is a widely used radiographic scale for evaluating OA: KL grade 0, normal or no radiographic features of OA; KL grade 1, slight osteophytes; KL grade 2, definite osteophytes; KL grade 3, intervertebral space narrowing with large osteophytes; and KL grade 4, bone sclerosis, intervertebral space narrowing, and large osteophytes [19].

However, the actual prevalence of spondylosis remains unknown because there are no definitive diagnostic criteria. In previous studies, only rudimentary qualitative grading systems like the KL scale (e.g., grades 1–4) were used to evaluate the severity of spondylosis [15–17, 21, 27, 35, 46, 50, 67]. More quantitative scoring methods for spondylosis appear necessary to achieve more accurate and better determination of the correlation between bone mass and degeneration [32]. We have previously developed a semiquantitative scoring of osteophytes and intervertebral disc height to evaluate the severity of spondylosis, which is mentioned later in this chapter [32].

7.1.2 Studies Showing an Inverse Relationship Between Osteoporosis and Spondylosis

Although osteoporosis and spondylosis often occur simultaneously, many studies indicate that there is an inverse relationship between osteoporosis and spondylosis [11, 21, 32, 38, 41, 47, 57, 63]. Several researchers have examined the coexistence of osteoporosis and spondylosis in the spine, and they have reported an inverse relationship between decreased BMD and intervertebral disc degeneration [11, 41, 57, 63]. BMD is known to be higher in subjects with osteophyte formation or facet joint OA than in normal controls [21]. In these subjects, increased BMD is observed not only at the lumbar spine but also throughout the skeleton [9, 46].

Many studies on systemic OA (OA in both the spine and extremities) or OA in the extremities also support the view that osteoporosis and spondylosis are different diseases and are possibly due to different pathomechanisms. Studies have suggested that systemic OA is associated with a decreased incidence of low bone mass [1, 12, 32, 38, 47]. Several observational studies have reported an inverse association between OA and osteoporosis, and longitudinal studies suggested a protective effect of one disease on the other one [6, 63]. There have been studies inferring that patients with OA have a generally high BMD [5, 8, 26, 58]. More recent studies have also shown that men and women with idiopathic hip OA have a phenotype with higher BMD, higher body mass index, proportionally higher fat mass, and proportionally lower lean body mass [18].

In addition, although environmental factors may also promote osteoporosis or spondylosis, studies have revealed differences in biochemistry and in the involvement of genetic factors between these two diseases [7, 14, 39, 42]. Increased bone density in patients with OA may be associated with increased skeletal concentrations of insulin-like growth factor (IGF)-I, IGF-II, and transforming growth factor (TGF)-β [7]. Studies indicate that bone density is associated with genes for the vitamin D receptor, estrogen receptor, collagen Iα1, calcitonin receptor, peroxisome proliferator-activated receptor-γ, Heremans-Schmid glycoprotein, and TGF-β1 [39]. Evidence suggests that the Werner helicase (WRN) gene is involved in the genetic regulation of osteoporosis but not spondylosis [42]. Other findings indicate that OA is associated with mutations or polymorphisms in genes encoding type II procollagen, type XI collagen, the vitamin D receptor, IGF-I, and TGF-β [14].

7.1.3 Studies Showing No Inverse Relationship Between Osteoporosis and Spondylosis

However, several studies have failed to show an inverse relationship between osteoporosis and spondylosis [2, 4, 10, 15, 53, 55, 65]. One study showed that vertebral trabecular BMD measured by quantitative CT was not higher in men with osteophytes than in men without osteophytes [15]. Another study showed that BMD at the distal radius and midshaft in patients with generalized OA was not significantly different from normal controls when age, height, and weight were taken into account [48]. Hannan et al. [10] observed that radius BMD was not associated with knee OA in subjects of either sex. Furthermore, Bultink et al. [2] recently showed that increased subchondral bone loss is a characteristic feature of osteoporosis and the early stage of OA.

In addition, a recent histomorphometric study of femoral heads obtained from patients undergoing hip arthroplasty for severe OA with and without osteoporosis defined by WHO criteria and those undergoing hip arthroplasty for osteoporosis-related femoral neck fractures showed that the cancellous bone volume fraction (bone volume/tissue volume) was significantly lower ($p < 0.01$) in subjects with femoral neck fractures (20.77 % ± 4.34 %, mean ± standard deviation (SD)) than in subjects with nonosteopenic OA (36.49 % ± 7.73 %), whereas there was no difference between subjects with femoral neck fractures and those with combined OA and osteoporosis (20.71 % ± 5.23 %) [62]. This study also supports the view that OA and osteoporosis can coexist in some cases. However, the possibility of impaired bone volume fraction in OA patients may also likely be caused by their decreased mobility without loading. Although such bone atrophy caused by disuse or less weight-bearing may occur in bones in the lower extremities, whether a similar phenomenon occurs in the spinal bone remains unclear.

7.1.4 Authors' Investigations

We previously investigated the possible inverse relationship between osteoporosis and spondylosis by evaluating the association between BMD and osteophyte formation or intervertebral disc narrowing using a semiquantitative scoring system

[32]. In this study, a total of 104 postmenopausal women aged over 60 years underwent BMD measurement of the lumbar spine (anteroposterior, lateral, and mid-lateral) and proximal femur (femoral neck, trochanter, and Ward's triangle) using dual-energy X-ray absorptiometry (DXA). Raw data representing semiquantitative osteophyte scores and disc scores and the number of vertebral fractures were obtained using spinal X-rays, and correlations between BMD and radiographic variables were then analyzed [32].

In the study, we assessed osteophyte formation according to Nathan's classification (0–4 degrees) [36]. The degree of osteophyte formation of each vertebra was scored as 0 (0 or 1 degrees), 1 (2 degrees), or 2 (3 or 4 degrees), and the total score from T4–T5 to L4–L5 was defined as the semiquantitative "osteophyte score" [32]. For the counting and grading of osteophytes according to Nathan's criteria, each separate end plate at one intervertebral level was counted as a combined entity [32]. Lumbar intervertebral disc degeneration was assessed based on the narrowing of the intervertebral disc height as previously described [30, 31]. The degree of narrowing of the intervertebral disc was scored as 0 (0–20 % reduction in disc height compared to L1–L2 intervertebral discs), 1 (20–50 % reduction), or 2 (more than 50 % reduction), and the total score from the L1–L2 to L5–S intervertebral discs was defined as the semiquantitative "disc score" [32].

Consequently, marginal/moderate positive correlations were observed between the osteophyte score and all BMD data ($0.263 \leq r \leq 0.580$, $p < 0.05$) and between the disc score and all BMD data ($0.233 \leq r \leq 0.570$, $p < 0.05$) (Table 7.1) [32]. All BMD data showed significant decreases with increasing age and increasing number of vertebral fractures [32]. Based on these findings that spondylotic changes showed positive correlations with not only lumbar BMD but also remote site hip BMD, our study results support the view that osteoporosis has an inverse relationship with spondylosis.

The effects of spondylosis on increasing BMD in the lumbar spine have been emphasized [16, 46, 50]. However, the methodology of our study eliminated the substantial contribution of osteophyte formation and disc degeneration to the BMD measurement, because higher BMD in Ward's triangle, which is a subregion primarily consisting of the trabecular bone, and higher BMD in the proximal femur, which is a site remote from the lumbar spine, were observed in patients with higher osteophyte scores and disc scores.

7.2 Pharmacotherapy for Osteoporosis and the Effect of Coexistent Spondylosis

7.2.1 Anti-Vertebral Fracture Effect of Spondylosis

Since osteoporosis and spondylosis often occur simultaneously, treatment of osteoporosis with antiosteoporotic agents may be affected by the coexistence of

Table 7.1 Correlations between BMD in the lumbar spine and proximal femoral and radiological variables

	Age	AP-BMD	L-BMD	Mid-BMD	FN-BMD	TR-BMD	WD-BMD	Osteophyte score	Disc score	No. of vertebral fractures
Age		−0.218*	−0.306**	−0.254*	−0.327**	−0.328**	−0.291*	−0.027	0.016	0.295**
AP-BMD			0.727***	0.669***	0.740***	0.590***	0.656***	0.580***	0.570***	−0.395***
L-BMD				0.912***	0.526***	0.464***	0.523***	0.349***	0.480***	−0.390***
Mid-BMD					0.445***	0.400***	0.462***	0.344***	0.445***	−0.347***
FN-BMD						0.847***	0.806***	0.417***	0.340**	−0.524***
TR-BMD							0.765***	0.330**	0.233*	−0.406***
WD-BMD								0.263*	0.298*	−0.466***
Osteophyte score									0.741***	−0.152
Disc score										−0.266**
No. of vertebral fractures										

From Ref. [32]. Published, with permission, from Miyakoshi N et al. Inverse relation between osteoporosis and spondylosis in postmenopausal women as evaluated by bone mineral density and semiquantitative scoring of spinal degeneration. Spine (Phila Pa 1976) 2003; 28(5): 492–5

BMD bone mineral density, *AP* anteroposterior lumbar, *L* lateral lumbar, *Mid* mid-lumbar, *FN* femoral neck, *TR* trochanter, *WD* Ward's triangle

r, Pearson's correlation coefficient

$^*p < 0.05$, $^{**}p < 0.01$, or $^{***}p < 0.001$

spondylosis in many patients. The presence of spondylosis may have a preventive effect against vertebral fractures. However, there are few reports about the effects of osteoporosis medication on the incidence of vertebral fractures in people with spondylosis.

We previously conducted a retrospective investigation of the effects of alfacalcidol alone or in combination with elcatonin on the incidence of osteoporotic vertebral fractures in women with spondylosis [34]. The severity of spondylosis was evaluated with the aforementioned "osteophyte score" [32]. The study subjects were 101 postmenopausal women with osteoporosis aged >60 years, divided into three groups: the D group ($n = 45$), treated for >5 years with alfacalcidol; the D + ECT group ($n = 26$), treated for >5 years with alfacalcidol plus elcatonin; and the control group ($n = 30$), received no medications for >5 years. Over the 5-year treatment period, the number of incident vertebral fractures per patient was significantly higher in the control group (2.9) than in the D group (1.2) and D + ECT group (1.5) ($p < 0.01$) [34]. However, in all three groups, the number of incident vertebral fractures was positively correlated with the number of prevalent vertebral fractures ($0.303 \leq r \leq 0.434$), and it was negatively correlated with baseline BMD ($-0.703 \leq r \leq -0.329$) and the osteophyte score ($-0.769 \leq r \leq -0.365$) [34]. Further multiple regression analysis showed that pharmacotherapy (D or D + ECT, $p < 0.001$) and the osteophyte score ($p < 0.001$) were the most significant contributors to the number of incident vertebral fractures [34]. These results showed that the presence of spondylosis (indicated by a high osteophyte score) appears to have an effect on the prevention of vertebral fractures. Because this study was designed as a retrospective study, for this chapter, we further evaluated the anti-vertebral fracture efficacy of pharmacotherapy and spondylosis in a prospective, randomized study described below.

7.2.2 *Effect of Spondylosis on the Results of Early-Phase Osteoporosis Treatment with Alendronate and Alfacalcidol: A 6-Month, Prospective, Randomized Study*

7.2.2.1 Background

Bisphosphonates are the most popular antiosteoporotic agents and are used worldwide. However, because the effects on the bone are exerted in an indirect manner by reducing the remodeling space and prolonging the duration of mineralization, several months are required to increase bone mass and strength. Previous reports have shown that significant antifracture effects of alendronate can be expected after 6 months of treatment [24]. Alfacalcidol also shows preventive effects against osteoporotic fractures, despite a small effect on bone mass [45]. We thus conducted a 6-month, prospective, randomized trial of postmenopausal women with osteoporosis to evaluate the possibility of early-phase superiority using combined treatment with alendronate and alfacalcidol compared to either alone, with radiographically diagnosed vertebral fracture as the primary end point. The preliminary results related only to fracture incidence were reported in Japanese and showed that combination therapy with alendronate and alfacalcidol was superior in terms of preventing vertebral fractures over either treatment alone in early-phase treatment ($\leq$6 months) [33]. However, because many of the enrolled osteoporotic patients also had spondylosis, the antifracture efficacy of spondylosis might also have affected the results. In addition, several other risk factors, such as spinal hyperkyphosis, lower BMD, and higher bone turnover markers, were not included in the preliminary report. Because we have many unpublished data from this study, we reevaluated the anti-vertebral fracture efficacy of alendronate and alfacalcidol in the presence of spondylosis for this chapter.

7.2.2.2 Methods

A total of 441 Japanese women with postmenopausal osteoporosis aged 60 years and over who initially attended one of two institutions (Minamiakita Orthopedic Clinic, Katagami, Japan, and Igarashi Memorial Hospital, Akita, Japan) and showed interest in participating in this study was enrolled. Osteoporosis was diagnosed according to the year 2000 version of the *Diagnostic Criteria for Primary Osteoporosis* published by the Japanese Society for Bone and Mineral Research [44]. The exclusion criteria were as follows: (1) women with a history of metabolic bone disease except for postmenopausal osteoporosis, malignancy, or previous antiosteoporotic treatment, (2) chronic glucocorticoid usage, and (3) patients with documented vertebral and/or nonvertebral fractures within the last 6 months.

The patients were randomized to one of three groups: ALN group, treated with daily oral administration of 5 mg of alendronate (Bonalon; Teijin Pharma, Tokyo, Japan); D group, treated with daily oral administration of 1 μg of alfacalcidol (Alfarol; Chugai Pharmaceutical, Tokyo, Japan); and ALN + D group, treated with daily oral administration of 5 mg of alendronate plus 1 μg of alfacalcidol. This study was conducted with a prospective, randomized, open-label design, with a duration of 6 months. Spinal X-rays, BMD of the distal radius, and serum samples for bone turnover markers were obtained at baseline and final follow-up (at 6 months). This study was performed in accordance with the recommendations of the Declaration of Helsinki, and patients' informed consent was obtained before randomization.

Thoracic and lumbar spine X-rays with anteroposterior and lateral views in a neutral position were taken using a film-tube distance of 1.0 m [32]. The thoracic radiographs were centered at T8 and the lumbar radiographs at L3 [32]. Vertebral fracture was considered present if at least one of three height measurements (anterior, middle, and posterior) for one vertebra had decreased by >20 % compared with the height of the nearest uncompressed vertebral body [45]. Angles of kyphosis for the thoracic (T4–T12) and lumbar (L1–L5) spines were also measured from lateral radiography using the Cobb angle method. As an indicator of spondylosis, osteophyte formation was assessed at baseline using the semiquantitative osteophyte score as mentioned above [32]. All radiographic assessments were made by two expert spine surgeons (NM, YK) masked to the BMD values and treatment groups.

BMD was measured at the distal 1/3 radius by DXA (DTX-200; Toyo Medic, Tokyo, Japan). Serum samples were obtained before noon after at least a 3-h fast, and N-terminal telopeptide of type I collagen (NTX) and bone-specific alkaline phosphatase (BAP) were measured at baseline and 6 months after the beginning of the treatment. Serum NTX was measured by an enzyme-linked immunosorbent assay (Osteomark; Mochida Pharmaceutical, Tokyo, Japan; reference range 9.5–17.7 nmolBCE/L) as a marker of bone resorption. Serum BAP was measured with an enzyme immunoassay kit (Osteolinks-BAP; Sumitomo Pharmaceuticals, Tokyo, Japan; reference range 13.0–33.9 U/L) as a marker of bone formation.

Statistical analysis of differences among the three groups was performed using Fisher's protected least significant difference method (a post hoc test) for multiple comparisons in one-way analysis of variance (ANOVA). A paired or unpaired t-test was used for the comparison between two groups, as appropriate. The chi-square test was used for categorical variables. Logistic regression analysis was used for analyzing risk factors for the incidence of vertebral fractures. Probability values of <0.05 were considered significant.

7.2.2.3 Results

The flow chart of the disposition of the patients is shown in Fig. 7.1. Seventeen patients were excluded before randomization because fresh fractures were identified before randomization. Of the 424 randomized patients, 61 were excluded from the data analysis because of the withdrawal of consent or dropout before completion of this study. Thus, 363 patients were included in the analysis of vertebral fracture incidence. Furthermore, 21 patients were excluded from the assessment of changes in BMD and bone turnover markers because of missing data at follow-up.

Table 7.2 shows the baseline characteristics of the study subjects. There were no significant differences among the three groups in mean age, serum NTX and BAP levels, BMD, angles of thoracic and lumbar kyphosis, number of prevalent vertebral fractures per patient, or osteophyte scores.

During the 6-month treatment period, new vertebral fractures included 11 fractures in 9 ALN group patients (7.6 %), 9 fractures in 9 D group patients (7.4 %), and 3 fractures in 3 ALN + D group patients (2.5 %). No significant difference was observed among the groups in the incidence of new vertebral fractures per patient. However, the incidence of new vertebral fractures per total vertebral body examined from T4 to L5 was significantly lower in the ALN + D group (three fractures in 1708 vertebral bodies examined, 0.18 %) than in the ALN group (11 fractures in 1666 vertebral bodies examined, 0.66 %) ($p = 0.029$). The incidence of new

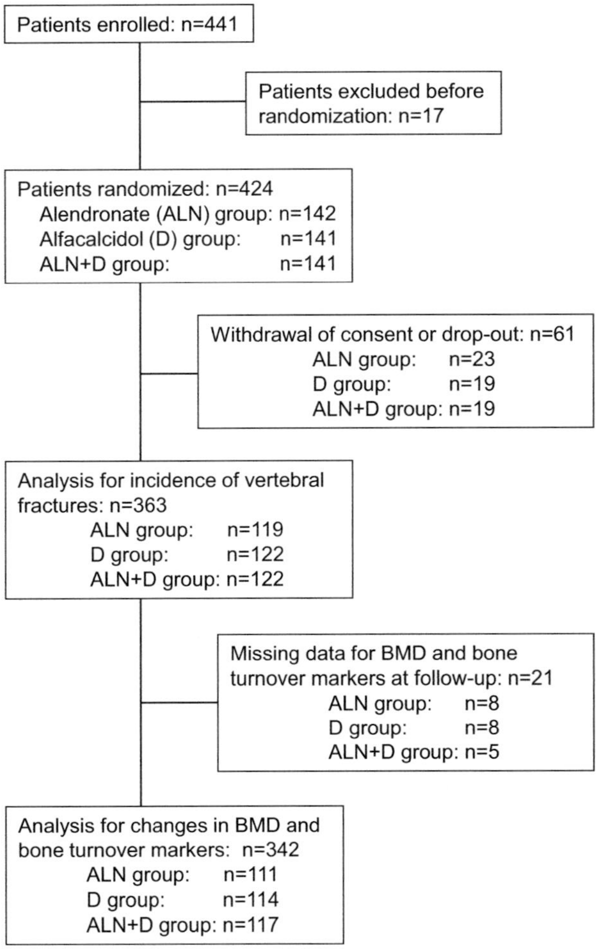

Fig. 7.1 Flow chart of patient disposition

vertebral fractures per total vertebral body examined was not significantly different in the D group (nine fractures in 1708 vertebral bodies examined, 0.52 %) compared with the ALN group or the ALN + D group.

The longitudinal changes in BMD of the distal radius and serum NTX and BAP levels over the 6 months are shown in Table 7.3. No significant changes of BMD from baseline were observed after treatment in any of the groups. No significant differences in BMD were observed among the groups 6 months after treatment. Serum NTX was significantly decreased compared to baseline in the ALN group and the ALN + D group ($p < 0.05$) but not in the D group. Serum BAP decreased significantly in all groups after treatment ($p < 0.05$). Serum NTX and BAP levels at 6 months after treatment were significantly lower in the ALN group and ALN + D group than in the D group ($p < 0.05$).

We then focused on the factors protecting against incident vertebral fractures. Patients were divided into groups with and without incident vertebral fractures

Table 7.2 Characteristics of the study subjects at baseline by treatment group

Variable	ALN ($n = 119$)	D ($n = 122$)	ALN + D ($n = 122$)	*P*-value[a]
Age (years)	74.1 ± 7.0	75.1 ± 7.0	74.0 ± 7.5	0.449
Serum NTX (nmolBCE/L)	16.6 ± 5.5	15.8 ± 5.5	16.7 ± 4.2	0.376
Serum BAP (U/L)	36.1 ± 13.5	33.8 ± 12.8	35.5 ± 12.6	0.359
Distal radius BMD (g/cm^2)	0.276 ± 0.056	0.279 ± 0.058	0.270 ± 0.053	0.474
Angle of thoracic kyphosis (°)	38.6 ± 10.4	38.6 ± 12.0	37.2 ± 9.8	0.490
Angle of lumbar kyphosis (°)	−22.6 ± 14.4	−20.4 ± 15.1	−20.6 ± 13.3	0.431
No. of prevalent thoracic vertebral fractures	1.0 ± 1.1	1.2 ± 1.1	1.1 ± 1.2	0.438
No. of prevalent lumbar vertebral fractures	0.6 ± 0.9	0.5 ± 0.9	0.6 ± 1.0	0.688
No. of prevalent vertebral fractures	1.6 ± 1.5	1.7 ± 1.7	1.7 ± 1.7	0.811
Thoracic osteophyte score	3.1 ± 2.4	2.8 ± 2.5	3.0 ± 2.0	0.581
Lumbar osteophyte score	3.6 ± 2.1	3.5 ± 2.3	3.6 ± 2.1	0.999
Osteophyte score	6.6 ± 3.8	6.3 ± 4.2	6.6 ± 3.7	0.817

Data are means ± SD
BMD bone mineral density, *ALN* alendronate, *D* alfacalcidol, *NTX* N-terminal telopeptide of type I collagen, *BAP* bone-specific alkaline phosphatase
[a]ANOVA

Table 7.3 BMD and bone turnover markers at follow-up and % changes from baseline

Variable	ALN ($n = 111$)	D ($n = 114$)	ALN + D ($n = 117$)	*P*-value[a]
Distal radius BMD at follow-up (g/cm^2)	0.276 ± 0.057	0.280 ± 0.060	0.272 ± 0.054	0.532
Serum NTX at follow-up (nmolBCE/L)	12.4 ± 3.3*	15.0 ± 4.3[b]	12.8 ± 3.7[c],*	<0.001
Serum BAP at follow-up (U/L)	24.1 ± 7.3*	28.0 ± 8.0[b],*	23.1 ± 8.2[c],*	<0.001
%Δ distal radius BMD (%)	+0.34 ± 0.38	−0.01 ± 0.37	+0.63 ± 0.37	0.470
%Δ serum NTX (%)	−22.3 ± 2.3	0.6 ± 2.3	−21.6 ± 2.2	<0.001
%Δ serum BAP (%)	−28.6 ± 2.2	−11.5 ± 2.2	−31.2 ± 2.1	<0.001

Data are means ± SD
BMD bone mineral density, *ALN* alendronate, *D* alfacalcidol, *NTX* N-terminal telopeptide of type I collagen, *BAP* bone-specific alkaline phosphatase
*Significantly different from baseline (paired *t*-test, $p < 0.05$)
[a]ANOVA
[b]$p < 0.05$ vs ALN group; [c]$p < 0.05$ vs D group

($n = 21$ and 342, each), and measured variables were compared between the groups. Compared with the patients without incident vertebral fractures, patients with incident vertebral fractures were significantly older and had higher baseline serum NTX levels, lower BMD, more prevalent vertebral fractures with increased thoracic kyphosis, and lower osteophyte scores (Table 7.4). Treatment regimen,

Table 7.4 Comparisons of variables with or without incident vertebral fractures (VFs)

Variable	Patients w/o incident VFs ($n = 342$)	Patients w/ incident VFs ($n = 21$)	P-value
Treatment	ALN:110, D:113, ALN +D:119	ALN:9, D:9, ALN +D:3	0.155[a]
Age (years)	74.1 ± 7.1	79.9 ± 6.8	<0.001[b]
Serum NTX (nmolBCE/L)	16.0 ± 4.6	22.2 ± 8.3	<0.001[b]
Serum BAP (U/L)	34.8 ± 12.8	39.7 ± 15.6	0.092[b]
Distal radius BMD (g/cm^2)	0.279 ± 0.053	0.216 ± 0.065	<0.001[b]
Angle of thoracic kyphosis (°)	37.4 ± 10.0	50.9 ± 14.4	<0.001[b]
Angle of lumbar kyphosis (°)	−21.2 ± 14.3	−21.0 ± 14.1	0.946[b]
No. of prevalent vertebral fractures	0:93, 1:104, 2:83, 3:24, 4:19, 5:19	0:0, 1:0, 2:4, 3:8, 4:4, 5:5	<0.001[a]
Osteophyte score	6.7 ± 3.9	3.6 ± 2.2	<0.001[b]
%Δ distal radius BMD	+0.41 ± 3.96	−0.99 ± 4.05	0.118[b]
%Δ serum NTX	−14.8 ± 25.7	−9.4 ± 33.9	0.364[b]
%Δ serum BAP	−24.2 ± 24.0	−17.0 ± 33.9	0.194[b]

Data are means ± SD or numbers
BMD bone mineral density, *ALN* alendronate, *D* alfacalcidol, *NTX* N-terminal telopeptide of type I collagen, *BAP* bone-specific alkaline phosphatase
[a]Chi-square test
[b]Unpaired *t*-test

baseline serum BAP, lumbar lordosis angle, percent change of BMD, percent change of NTX, and percent change of BAP showed no significant differences between the groups. Finally, multivariate logistic regression analysis showed that age, baseline serum NTX level, number of prevalent vertebral fractures, and osteophyte scores significantly affected incident vertebral fractures (Table 7.5).

7.2.2.4 Comments

It is known that increased bone turnover is significantly associated with an increased risk of osteoporotic fracture in postmenopausal women [52]. Postmenopausal women with previous or incident vertebral fractures are at higher risk of both vertebral and nonvertebral fractures than women without previous vertebral fractures, independent of bone density [3, 22, 37, 51]. The results of the present study indicated that, within the early phase of alendronate and/or alfacalcidol therapy, the presence of spondylosis has a protective effect on the incidence of vertebral

Table 7.5 Multivariate logistic regression analysis for binary data of new fractures

Variables	Unit	Odds ratio	95 % CI	*P*-value
Treatment group				
ALN (based on ALN + D)	–	3.04	0.56–16.44	0.197
D (based on ALN + D)	–	1.19	0.19–7.57	0.852
Age	1	1.12	1.01–1.25	0.031
NTX at baseline	1	1.20	1.09–1.32	<0.001
BAP at baseline	1	1.01	0.97–1.06	0.537
YAM at baseline	1	1.01	0.95–1.08	0.724
Angle of thoracic kyphosis (°)	1	1.07	0.99–1.15	0.074
Angle of lumbar kyphosis (°)	1	0.99	0.95–1.04	0.819
Prevalent vertebral fractures	1	1.73	1.15–2.61	0.008
Osteophyte score	1	0.57	0.41–0.79	<0.001

CI confidence interval
ALN alendronate, *D* alfacalcidol, *NTX* N-terminal telopeptide of type I collagen, *BAP* bone-specific alkaline phosphatase, *YAM* young adult mean of bone mineral density

fractures, even when analyzed simultaneously with other risk factors, such as increased bone turnover and prevalent vertebral fractures.

We hypothesize that the protective effect of spondylosis against vertebral fractures is not only due to the higher bone mass, but is also probably due to a process in which the osteophyte proliferation and endplate sclerosis form a strong cortical shell that increases the mechanical strength of the vertebral body. Osteophytes are defensive reactions of the bone to changes in the mechanical environment [13], and a biomechanical study indicated that overall stiffness of degenerated spinal columns increases with the severity of degeneration [23]. Thus, the protective effect of spondylosis (indicated by a high osteophyte score) against vertebral fracture appears to be caused not only by the increased BMD due to the spondylotic changes but also by increased mechanical strength due to the resulting morphology.

7.3 Our Surgical Strategies for Osteoporotic Vertebral Fractures and Spondylosis

7.3.1 PAVREC

Most elderly patients with osteoporotic vertebral fractures and/or painful spondylosis are usually treated conservatively with pharmacotherapy and braces, and these are sometimes combined with physiotherapy. However, with the increased aging of society, the demand for spine surgery in elderly patients is increasing, especially for progressive vertebral body collapse, severe kyphotic deformity, and late nerve palsy. Our surgical strategies for such patients are based on their predominant spinal pathology. If the pathology is in the vertebral bodies (i.e., vertebral fractures), we consider vertebral replacement, and, if it is in the intervertebral space (i.e., spondylosis), we consider intervertebral fusion using posterior lumbar interbody fusion (PLIF) technique.

For spinal reconstruction of vertebral collapse, we began performing posterior-approach vertebral replacement with a cylinder cage in 2004 [60]. The clinical results were satisfactory, but subsidence of the cage into the vertebrae was seen in several cases [60]. Thus, since 2005, we have been using a modified technique with large-sized rectangular parallelepiped cages (REC cages) to prevent subsidence. We named this novel technique PAVREC (posterior-approach vertebral replacement with REC cages) [61]. Basically, if a collapsed vertebra involved both upper and lower endplate fractures (i.e., Denis type A fracture), the collapsed vertebral body was totally excised with upper and lower intervertebral discs and replaced with two large REC cages with autologous bone grafting, and pedicle screwing for 1–3 levels above and below the lesion was applied, considering the affected vertebral level and the severity of osteoporosis. However, if the caudal end plate of the affected vertebra was intact (Denis type B fracture), the lower one-third to one-fourth of the pedicles was spared to connect with the lower half of the vertebra, and the upper surface of the vertebra was trimmed parallel to the lower disc [61] (Fig. 7.2). The details of the PAVREC surgical procedure with clinical and radiological outcomes have been described elsewhere [61].

7.3.2 Multilevel PLIF

Multilevel PLIF technique is indicated for patients with osteoporosis and spondylosis, if the pathology is mainly caused by the spondylosis resulting in spinal deformity. This technique can correct spinal deformity three dimensionally. Thus, lumbar kyphosis, scoliosis, and kyphoscoliosis due to degeneration are good indications for this procedure. However, because of the higher invasiveness of this surgery, in principle, we apply this procedure for healthy individuals without serious comorbidities.

Multilevel PLIF provides sufficient spinal correction regardless of age. In our hands, when multilevel PLIFs were performed within the lumbar spine levels, preoperative lumbar kyphosis angles of $10.1 \pm 19.9°$ (mean $\pm$ SD) in the non-old group (<65 years old; $n = 17$), $9.6 \pm 22.2°$ in the young-old group (≤ 65 years old and <75 years old; $n = 35$), and $14.4 \pm 17.8°$ in the old-old group (≥ 75 years old; $n = 18$) were all significantly and remarkably corrected, with postoperative lumbar lordosis angles of $26.8 \pm 10.6°$, $28.5 \pm 9.0°$, and $23.4 \pm 9.9°$, respectively ($p < 0.001$, $p < 0.001$, $p < 0.001$, respectively) [28]. The correction angles were comparable among the age groups. The operation time, the intraoperative blood loss, and the incidence of perioperative medical complications were also comparable among the age groups if multilevel PLIF was performed for healthy individuals [29].

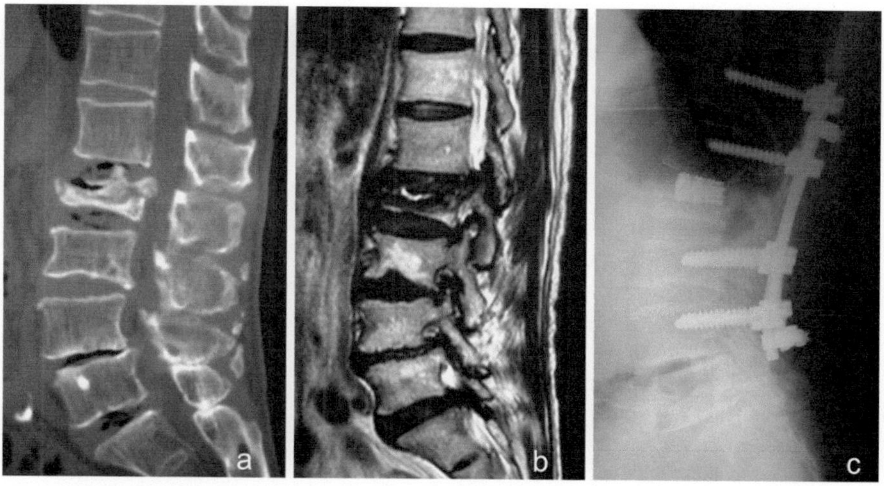

Fig. 7.2 An 88-year-old male with spondylosis and L2 osteoporotic vertebral collapse. Preoperative sagittal reconstructed computed tomogram (**a**) and sagittal T2-weighted magnetic resonance imaging (**b**) showing upper endplate destruction of the L2 vertebra. Lateral X-ray taken after PAVREC surgery showing good spinal alignment (**c**)

Recently, to obtain more significant correction and better global spinal balance, we have extended the fusion level from the lower thoracic spine to the ilium (Fig. 7.3). Our preliminary data of 16 female patients (mean age, 70 years) with lumbar kyphosis or kyphoscoliosis who underwent multilevel PLIF with extended fusion (lower thoracic to ilium) showed better spinal alignment correction compared with our previous series mentioned above. Their mean preoperative lumbar kyphosis angle ($10.0 \pm 20.4°$) was comparable with the previous series mentioned above, but the postoperative lumbar lordosis angle ($40.1 \pm 6.9°$) was significantly larger than the previous series at the mean follow-up of 1.1 years postoperatively ($p < 0.05$). The sagittal vertical axis (SVA), a parameter of sagittal plane alignment defined as the horizontal offset from the posterosuperior corner of S1 to the vertebral body of C7 [56], improved significantly after this surgery. Their preoperative SVA (148.1 ± 69.1 mm) was significantly decreased postoperatively (postoperative SVAs 16.1 ± 25.1 mm; $p < 0.001$).

7.3.3 *CBT-EP Technique*

Since patients with spondylosis frequently have lumbar spinal stenosis, once they sustain vertebral fractures, the canal compromise tends to be greater, and they frequently show neurological deficits requiring surgery. If such patients have comorbidities that affect peri- and postoperative general conditions, the aforementioned techniques are not indicated, and we should consider lesser invasive

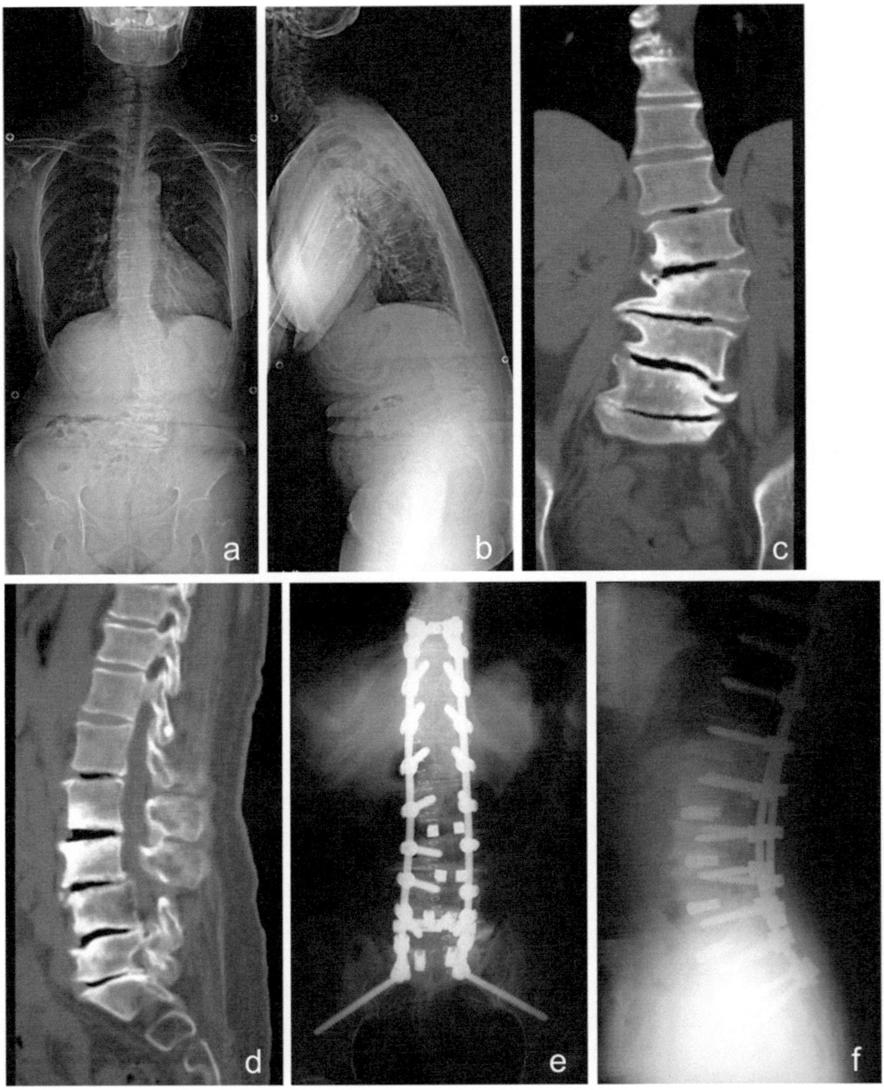

Fig. 7.3 A 62-year-old female with spondylotic lumbar kyphoscoliosis and osteoporosis. Preoperative standing anteroposterior and lateral X-rays showing lumbar scoliosis and a stooped trunk (**a** and **b**). Preoperative coronal and sagittal reconstructed computed tomograms showing severe spondylotic changes with narrowing of intervertebral discs and large osteophytes (**c** and **d**). Postoperative anteroposterior and lateral X-rays taken after multilevel PLIF with extended instrumented fusion (from lower thoracic to ilium) showing good spinal alignment (**e** and **f**)

surgeries. However, posterior decompression alone is usually insufficient, and stabilization with instrumentation is usually necessary. In such cases, posterior decompression and instrumented fusion with cortical bone trajectory (CBT) pedicle screwing are considered preferable as a lesser invasive form of instrumentation

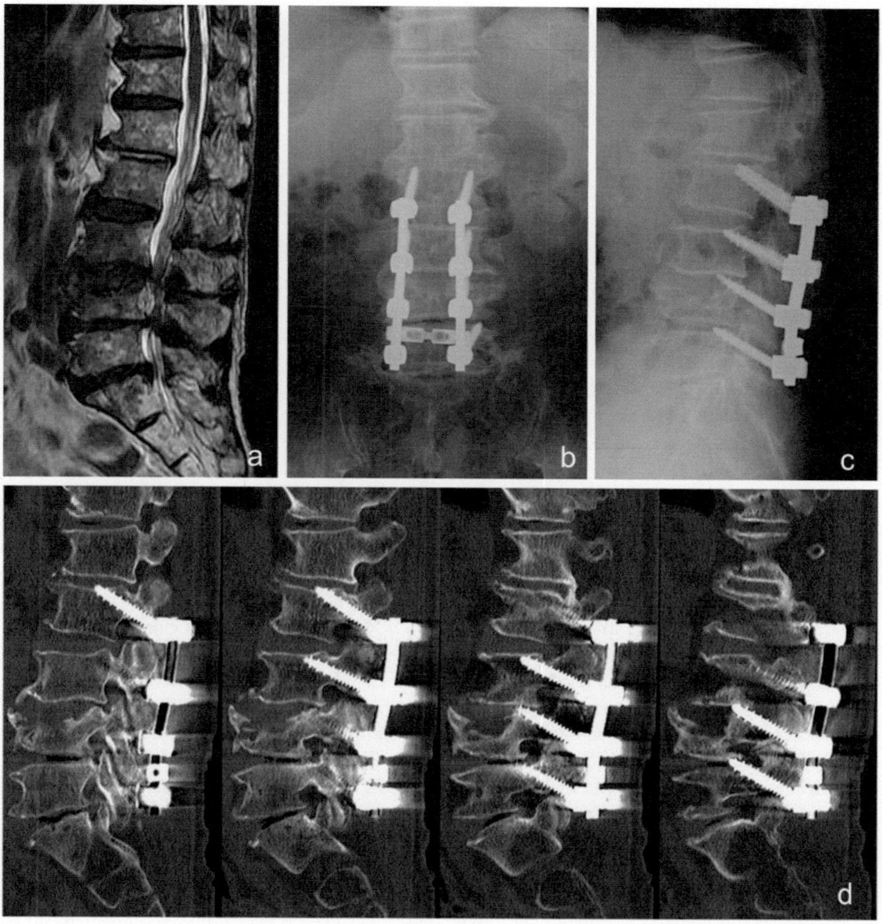

Fig. 7.4 A 79-year-old male with spondylosis and L4 osteoporotic vertebral collapse. Preoperative sagittal T2-weighted magnetic resonance imaging showing spinal canal stenosis at the level of vertebral collapse (**a**). Postoperative anteroposterior and lateral X-rays taken after posterior decompression and instrumented fusion showing placement of CBT pedicle screwing from L2–L5 (**b** and **c**). Postoperative sequential parasagittal reconstructed computed tomogram to check the placement of the screws on the right side showing that the L2, L4, and L5 vertebrae were fixed with CBT-EP technique (**d**)

surgery. CBT pedicle screwing directed medial-to-lateral/caudal-to-cephalad with an entry point on the lateral pars can obtain solid implant fixation to the osteoporotic bone [54]. For spondylotic patients with osteoporotic vertebral fractures, we use longer pedicle screws for CBT to penetrate the upper end plate to obtain more rigid stabilization. This modified technique was named the CBT-endplate penetrating technique (CBT-EP technique) (Fig. 7.4). Because spondylosis has hard bony end plates, bicortical screwing with the CBT-EP technique for lumbar pedicle screwing seems to be a more rigid and reliable technique than the conventional CBT technique for patients with osteoporosis and spondylosis.

References

1. Belmonte-Serrano MA, Bloch DA, Lane NE, Michel BE, Fries JF (1993) The relationship between spinal and peripheral osteoarthritis and bone density measurements. J Rheumatol 20:1005–1013
2. Bultink IE, Lems WF (2013) Osteoarthritis and osteoporosis: what is the overlap? Curr Rheumatol Rep 15:328. doi:10.1007/s11926-013-0328-0
3. Burger H, van Daele PL, Algra D, Hofman A, Grobbee DE, Schütte HE, Birkenhäger JC, Pols HA (1994) Vertebral deformities as predictors of non-vertebral fractures. BMJ 309:991–992
4. De Pedro JA, Martin AP, Blanco JF, Salvado M, Perez MA, Cardoso A, Collía F, Ellis SS, Domínguez J (2007) Histomorphometric study of femoral heads in hip osteoarthritis and osteoporosis. Histol Histopathol 22:1091–1097
5. Dequeker J, Aerssens J, Luyten FP (2003) Osteoarthritis and osteoporosis: clinical and research evidence of inverse relationship. Aging Clin Exp Res 15:426–439
6. Dequeker J, Johnell O (1993) Osteoarthritis protects against femoral neck fracture: the MEDOS study experience. Bone 14:S51–S56
7. Dequeker J, Mohan S, Finkelman RD, Aerssens J, Baylink DJ (1993) Generalized osteoarthritis associated with increased insulin-like growth factor types I and II and transforming growth factor beta in cortical bone from the iliac crest. Possible mechanism of increased bone density and protection against osteoporosis. Arthritis Rheum 36:1702–1708
8. Felson DT, Lawrence RC, Dieppe PA, Hirsch R, Helmick CG, Jordan JM, Kington RS, Lane NE, Nevitt MC, Zhang Y, Sowers M, McAlindon T, Spector TD, Poole AR, Yanovski SZ, Ateshian G, Sharma L, Buckwalter JA, Brandt KD, Fries JF (2000) Osteoarthritis: new insights. Part 1: the disease and its risk factors. Ann Intern Med 133:635–646
9. Gevers G, Dequeker J, Geusens P, Nyssen-Behets C, Dhem A (1989) Physical and histomorphological characteristics of iliac crest bone differ according to the grade of osteoarthritis at the hand. Bone 10:173–177
10. Hannan MT, Anderson JJ, Zhang Y, Levy D, Felson DT (1993) Bone mineral density and knee osteoarthritis in elderly men and women. The Framingham study. Arthritis Rheum 36:1671–1680
11. Harada A, Okuizumi H, Miyagi N, Genda E (1998) Correlation between bone mineral density and intervertebral disc degeneration. Spine (Phila Pa 1976) 23:857–862
12. Hart DJ, Mootoosamy I, Doyle DV, Spector TD (1994) The relationship between osteoarthritis and osteoporosis in the general population: the Chingford study. Ann Rheum Dis 53:158–162
13. He G, Xinghua Z (2006) The numerical simulation of osteophyte formation on the edge of the vertebral body using quantitative bone remodeling theory. Joint Bone Spine 73:95–101
14. Holderbaum D, Haqqi TM, Moskowitz RW (1999) Genetics and osteoarthritis: exposing the iceberg. Arthritis Rheum 42:397–405
15. Ito M, Hayashi K, Yamada M, Uetani M, Nakamura T (1993) Relationship of osteophytes to bone mineral density and spinal fracture in men. Radiology 189:497–502
16. Jones G, Nguyen T, Sambrook PN, Kelly PJ, Eisman JA (1995) A longitudinal study of the effect of spinal degenerative disease on bone density in the elderly. J Rheumatol 22:932–936
17. Jones G, White C, Nguyen T, Sambrook PN, Kelly PJ, Eisman JA (1996) Prevalent vertebral deformities: relationship to bone mineral density and spinal osteophytosis in elderly men and women. Osteoporos Int 6:233–239

18. Karlsson MK, Magnusson H, Cöster MC, Vonschewelov T, Karlsson C, Rosengren BE (2014) Patients with hip osteoarthritis have a phenotype with high bone mass and low lean body mass. Clin Orthop Relat Res 472:1224–1229. doi:10.1007/s11999-013-3395-7
19. Kellgren JH, Lawrence JS (1957) Radiological assessment of osteo-arthrosis. Ann Rheum Dis 16:494–502
20. Kilshaw M, Baker RP, Gardner R, Charosky S, Harding I (2011) Abnormalities of the lumbar spine in the coronal plane on plain abdominal radiographs. Eur Spine J 20:429–433. doi:10.1007/s00586-010-1610-8
21. Kinoshita H, Tamaki T, Hashimoto T, Kasagi F (1998) Factors influencing lumbar spine bone mineral density assessment by dual-energy X-ray absorptiometry: comparison with lumbar spinal radiogram. J Orthop Sci 3:3–9
22. Kotowicz MA, Melton LJ 3rd, Cooper C, Atkinson EJ, O'Fallon WM, Riggs BL (1994) Risk of hip fracture in women with vertebral fracture. J Bone Miner Res 9:599–605
23. Kumaresan S, Yoganandan N, Pintar FA, Maiman DJ, Goel VK (2001) Contribution of disc degeneration to osteophyte formation in the cervical spine: a biomechanical investigation. J Orthop Res 19:977–984
24. Kushida K, Shiraki M, Nakamura T, Kishimoto H, Morii H, Yamamoto K, Kaneda K, Fukunaga M, Inoue T, Nakashima M, Orimo H (2002) The efficacy of alendronate in reducing the risk for vertebral fracture in Japanese patients with osteoporosis: a randomized, double-blind, active-controlled, double-dummy trial. Curr Ther Res 63:606–620
25. Livshits G, Popham M, Malkin I, Sambrook PN, Macgregor AJ, Spector T, Williams FM (2011) Lumbar disc degeneration and genetic factors are the main risk factors for low back pain in women: the UK Twin Spine study. Ann Rheum Dis 70:1740–1745. doi:10.1136/ard.2010.137836
26. Marcelli C, Favier F, Kotzki PO, Ferrazzi V, Picot MC, Simon L (1995) The relationship between osteoarthritis of the hands, bone mineral density, and osteoporotic fractures in elderly women. Osteoporos Int 5:382–388
27. Masud T, Langley S, Wiltshire P, Doyle DV, Spector TD (1993) Effect of spinal osteophytosis on bone mineral density measurements in vertebral osteoporosis. BMJ 307:172–173
28. Miyakoshi N, Abe E, Kobayashi T, Abe T, Shimada Y (2012) Spinal corrective fusion using multilevel PLIF technique for lumbar spinal deformities: comparison of the surgical outcomes between the elderly and the non-elderly patients. J East Jpn Orthop Traumatol 24:62–65 (in Japanese)
29. Miyakoshi N, Abe E, Kobayashi T, Suzuki T, Abe T, Hongo M, Kasukawa Y, Murai H, Shimada Y (2011) Perioperative complications of instrumented corrective surgery for spinal deformity in the healthy elderly. J Spine Res 2:337–340
30. Miyakoshi N, Abe E, Shimada Y, Hongo M, Chiba M, Sato K (1999) Anterior decompression with single segmental spinal interbody fusion for lumbar burst fracture. Spine (Phila Pa 1976) 24:67–73
31. Miyakoshi N, Abe E, Shimada Y, Okuyama K, Suzuki T, Sato K (2000) Outcome of one-level posterior lumbar interbody fusion for spondylolisthesis and postoperative intervertebral disc degeneration adjacent to the fusion. Spine (Phila Pa 1976) 25:1837–1842
32. Miyakoshi N, Itoi E, Murai H, Wakabayashi I, Ito H, Minato T (2003) Inverse relation between osteoporosis and spondylosis in postmenopausal women as evaluated by bone mineral density and semiquantitative scoring of spinal degeneration. Spine (Phila Pa 1976) 28:492–495
33. Miyakoshi N, Kasukawa Y, Noguchi H, Sasaki H, Kamo K, Shimada Y, Kodama H (2008) Antifracture efficacy of combined treatment with alendronate and alfacalcidol for osteoporotic vertebrae in early-phase treatment: a preliminary report. Osteoporos Jpn 16:206–208 (in Japanese)
34. Miyakoshi N, Shimada Y, Ando S, Minato T, Itoi E (2006) Effects of alfacalcidol alone or in combination with elcatonin on incidence of osteoporotic vertebral fractures in postmenopausal women with spondylosis. J Bone Miner Metab 24:491–497

35. Muraki S, Akune T, Oka H, Ishimoto Y, Nagata K, Yoshida M, Tokimura F, Nakamura K, Kawaguchi H, Yoshimura N (2012) Incidence and risk factors for radiographic lumbar spondylosis and lower back pain in Japanese men and women: the ROAD study. Osteoarthr Cartil 20:712–718. doi:10.1016/j.joca.2012.03.009
36. Nathan H (1962) Osteophytes of the vertebral column. An anatomical study of their development according to age, race, and sex with considerations as to their etiology and significance. J Bone Joint Surg Am 44:243–268
37. Nevitt MC, Ettinger B, Black DM, Stone K, Jamal SA, Ensrud K, Segal M, Genant HK, Cummings SR (1998) The association of radiographically detected vertebral fractures with back pain and function: a prospective study. Ann Intern Med 128:793–800
38. Nevitt MC, Lane NE, Scott JC, Hochberg MC, Pressman AR, Genant HK, Cummings SR (1995) Radiographic osteoarthritis of the hip and bone mineral density. The Study of Osteoporotic Fractures Research Group. Arthritis Rheum 38:907–916
39. Nguyen TV, Blangero J, Eisman JA (2000) Genetic epidemiological approaches to the search for osteoporosis genes. J Bone Miner Res 15:392–401
40. NIH Consensus Development Panel on Osteoporosis Prevention, Diagnosis, and Therapy (2001) Osteoporosis prevention, diagnosis, and therapy. JAMA 285:785–795
41. Nuti R, Righi G, Martini G, Turchetti V, Lepore C, Doretti V (1988) Diagnostic approach to osteoporosis and spondyloarthrosis in post-menopausal women by total body dual-photon absorptiometry. Clin Exp Rheumatol 6:47–51
42. Ogata N, Shiraki M, Hosoi T, Koshizuka Y, Nakamura K, Kawaguchi H (2001) A polymorphic variant at the Werner helicase (WRN) gene is associated with bone density, but not spondylosis, in postmenopausal women. J Bone Miner Metab 19:296–301
43. O'Neill TW, McCloskey EV, Kanis JA, Bhalla AK, Reeve J, Reid DM, Todd C, Woolf AD, Silman AJ (1999) The distribution, determinants, and clinical correlates of vertebral osteophytosis: a population based survey. J Rheumatol 26:842–848
44. Orimo H, Hayashi Y, Fukunaga M, Sone T, Fujiwara S, Shiraki M, Kushida K, Miyamoto S, Soen S, Nishimura J, Oh-Hashi Y, Hosoi T, Gorai I, Tanaka H, Igai T, Kishimoto H (2001) Diagnostic criteria for primary osteoporosis: year 2000 revision. J Bone Miner Metab 19:331–337
45. Orimo H, Shiraki M, Hayashi Y, Hoshino T, Onaya T, Miyazaki S, Kurosawa H, Nakamura T, Ogawa N (1994) Effects of 1 alpha-hydroxyvitamin D3 on lumbar bone mineral density and vertebral fractures in patients with postmenopausal osteoporosis. Calcif Tissue Int 54:370–376
46. Orwoll ES, Oviatt SK, Mann T (1990) The impact of osteophytic and vascular calcifications on vertebral mineral density measurements in men. J Clin Endocrinol Metab 70:1202–1207
47. Peel NF, Barrington NA, Blumsohn A, Colwell A, Hannon R, Eastell R (1995) Bone mineral density and bone turnover in spinal osteoarthrosis. Ann Rheum Dis 54:867–871
48. Price T, Hesp R, Mitchell R (1987) Bone density in generalized osteoarthritis. J Rheumatol 14:560–562
49. Randell A, Sambrook PN, Nguyen TV, Lapsley H, Jones G, Kelly PJ, Eisman JA (1995) Direct clinical and welfare costs of osteoporotic fractures in elderly men and women. Osteoporos Int 5:427–432
50. Reid IR, Evans MC, Ames R, Wattie DJ (1991) The influence of osteophytes and aortic calcification on spinal mineral density in postmenopausal women. J Clin Endocrinol Metab 72:1372–1374
51. Ross PD, Davis JW, Epstein RS, Wasnich RD (1991) Pre-existing fractures and bone mass predict vertebral fracture incidence in women. Ann Intern Med 114:919–923
52. Ross PD, Kress BC, Parson RE, Wasnich RD, Armour KA, Mizrahi IA (2000) Serum bone alkaline phosphatase and calcaneus bone density predict fractures: a prospective study. Osteoporos Int 11:76–82
53. Roux C, Fechtenbaum J, Briot K, Cropet C, Liu-Léage S, Marcelli C (2008) Inverse relationship between vertebral fractures and spine osteoarthritis in postmenopausal women with osteoporosis. Ann Rheum Dis 67:224–228

54. Santoni BG, Hynes RA, McGilvray KC, Rodriguez-Canessa G, Lyons AS, Henson MA, Womack WJ, Puttlitz CM (2009) Cortical bone trajectory for lumbar pedicle screws. Spine J 9:366–373. doi:10.1016/j.spinee.2008.07.008
55. Schnitzler CM, Mesquita JM, Wane L (1992) Bone histomorphometry of the iliac crest, and spinal fracture prevalence in atrophic and hypertrophic osteoarthritis of the hip. Osteoporos Int 2:186–194
56. Schwab F, Lafage V, Patel A, Farcy JP (2009) Sagittal plane considerations and the pelvis in the adult patient. Spine (Phila Pa 1976) 34:1828–1833. doi:10.1097/BRS.0b013e3181a13c08
57. Silberberg R (1988) Histologic and morphometric observations on vertebral bone of aging sand rats. Spine (Phila Pa 1976) 13:202–208
58. Sowers M (2001) Epidemiology of risk factors for osteoarthritis: systemic factors. Curr Opin Rheumatol 13:447–451
59. Suri P, Hunter DJ, Rainville J, Guermazi A, Katz JN (2013) Presence and extent of severe facet joint osteoarthritis are associated with back pain in older adults. Osteoarthr Cartil 21:1199–1206. doi:10.1016/j.joca.2013.05.013
60. Suzuki T, Abe E, Miyakoshi N, Murai H, Kobayashi T, Abe T, Kikuchi K, Shimada Y (2012) Anterior decompression and shortening reconstruction with a titanium mesh cage through a posterior approach alone for the treatment of lumbar burst fractures. Asian Spine J 6:123–130. doi:10.4184/asj.2012.6.2.123
61. Suzuki T, Abe E, Miyakoshi N, Murai H, Kobayashi T, Abe T, Kikuchi K, Shimada Y (2013) Posterior-approach vertebral replacement with rectangular parallelepiped cages (PAVREC) for the treatment of osteoporotic vertebral collapse with neurological deficits. J Spinal Disord Tech 26:E170–E176. doi:10.1097/BSD.0b013e318286fc18
62. Tarantino U, Celi M, Rao C, Feola M, Cerocchi I, Gasbarra E, Ferlosio A, Orlandi A (2014) Hip osteoarthritis and osteoporosis: clinical and histomorphometric considerations. Int J Endocrinol 2014:372021. doi:10.1155/2014/372021
63. Verstraeten A, Van Ermen H, Haghebaert G, Nijs J, Geusens P, Dequeker J (1991) Osteoarthrosis retards the development of osteoporosis. Observation of the coexistence of osteoarthrosis and osteoporosis. Clin Orthop Relat Res 264:169–177
64. Videman T, Battié MC, Gibbons LE, Maravilla K, Manninen H, Kaprio J (2003) Associations between back pain history and lumbar MRI findings. Spine (Phila Pa 1976) 28:582–588
65. Wolf O, Ström H, Milbrink J, Larsson S, Mallmin H (2009) Differences in hip bone mineral density may explain the hip fracture pattern in osteoarthritic hips. Acta Orthop 80:308–313. doi:10.3109/17453670903039528
66. Yoshimura N, Dennison E, Wilman C, Hashimoto T, Cooper C (2000) Epidemiology of chronic disc degeneration and osteoarthritis of the lumbar spine in Britain and Japan: a comparative study. J Rheumatol 27:429–433
67. Yoshimura N, Muraki S, Oka H, Mabuchi A, En-Yo Y, Yoshida M, Saika A, Yoshida H, Suzuki T, Yamamoto S, Ishibashi H, Kawaguchi H, Nakamura K, Akune T (2009) Prevalence of knee osteoarthritis, lumbar spondylosis, and osteoporosis in Japanese men and women: the research on osteoarthritis/osteoporosis against disability study. J Bone Miner Metab 27:620–628. doi:10.1007/s00774-009-0080-8

Chapter 8
Sarcopenia and Osteoporosis

Atsushi Harada

Abstract In the patient group investigated in this study, there was a positive correlation between bone and muscle mass. This finding showed the possibility that a balance between these two tissue types is maintained by some mechanism. There is a similar correlation between osteoporosis and sarcopenia, and it is suggested that the concurrent occurrence of the two diseases in the same individual is not rare. Considering the fact that the concurrent occurrence of these diseases increases the risk of fall fractures, more attention should be paid to the concurrent occurrence of osteoporosis and sarcopenia. Our study showed that sarcopenia, independent of bone density, is related to the risk of hip fractures. This result supports the need for attention in this area. There is no reliable treatment for sarcopenia other than exercise. A new treatment that is effective for both osteoporosis and sarcopenia, if there is any, must be given high priority in the selection to treat. We look forward to further investigations in search of such treatments.

Keywords Osteoporosis • Sarcopenia • Fracture

8.1 Introduction

In Japan, which is on the forefront of an unprecedented super-aging society, the objective of medical care is rapidly shifting from the mere extension of life span to the extension of healthy life expectancy, the significance of which is further increasing. When an individual's healthy life expectancy is decreased, their risk of needing medical authorization for care or support increases. The National Livelihood Survey by the Ministry of Health, Labour and Welfare for 2013 shows that the proportion of persons who were authorized to receive care or support because of joint disease and fall/fracture was 23 %, which was larger than the proportion of persons who were authorized to receive the same for a cerebrovascular disorder (18 %) (Fig. 8.1) [1].

A. Harada, M.D., Ph.D. (✉)
National Center for Geriatrics and Gerontology, 7-430, Morioka-machi, Obu, Aichi, Japan, 474-8511
e-mail: aharada@ncgg.go.jp

Y. Shimada, N. Miyakoshi (eds.), *Osteoporosis in Orthopedics*,
DOI 10.1007/978-4-431-55778-4_8

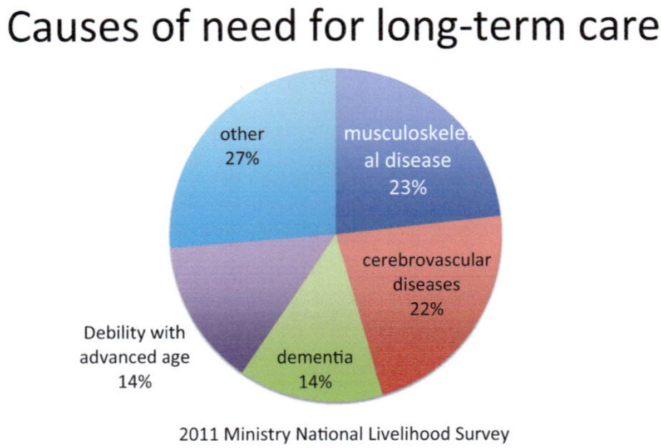

Fig. 8.1 Causes of need for long-term care. The proportions of the top four causes in the Ministry National Livelihood Survey for 2011. The proportion of persons for whom care became necessary because of locomotorium-related causes including fall/fracture, joint disease, and spinal cord injury ranked first at 23 %

Such circumstances are the background for the unique proposal in 2007 by the Japanese Orthopaedic Association of the concept of locomotive syndrome (hereafter referred to as "locomo"), which is based on the idea that locomotorium disorders inhibit healthy longevity [2]. The definition of this concept was revised in 2014 as a condition of decreased locomotive function due to locomotorium disorder [3]. The literature describes that osteoporosis, sarcopenia, fracture, osteoarthritis, spinal osteoarthritis, and neuropathy are the main diseases underlying locomo (Fig. 8.2). These locomotorium disorders are obviously the main factors that inhibit healthy longevity. Of them, sarcopenia is a relatively new disease concept [4].

Among the above-described causes of need for support or care, fall/fracture accounted for 12 % and is thought to result from sarcopenia (factor of fall) and concurrent osteoporosis (factor of fracture). The main reason that osteoporosis and sarcopenia are addressed in this chapter seems to be the serious condition that the concurrent occurrence of these two diseases leads to.

The science of osteoporosis, including definition, diagnosis, prophylaxis, and treatment, has dramatically advanced over the past 20 years and boasts of drug treatment with strong evidence. It is considered a skeletal disease that is characterized by decreased bone strength and likely to increase the risk of fractures [5]. A cohort study of community residents aged ≥ 40 years showed that the prevalence of osteoporosis by transcervical bone density was 12 % in men and 27 % in women and that the estimated number of patients is 10.7 million [6, 7]. Decreased bone strength alone does not produce any symptoms, nor does it directly decrease locomotive function. In the Japanese diagnostic criteria, osteoporosis is diagnosed when the patient has a history of fragility fracture due to a slight external force. In the absence of a history of fracture, osteoporosis is diagnosed when bone density is <70 % of the young adult mean (YAM) [8].

On the other hand, in the science of sarcopenia, the definition and diagnostic criteria have just been established and there is little evidence for prophylaxis and treatment other than exercise and nutrition. Sarcopenia is thought to lead to health problems such as movement disorder, increased risk for fall/fracture, decreased

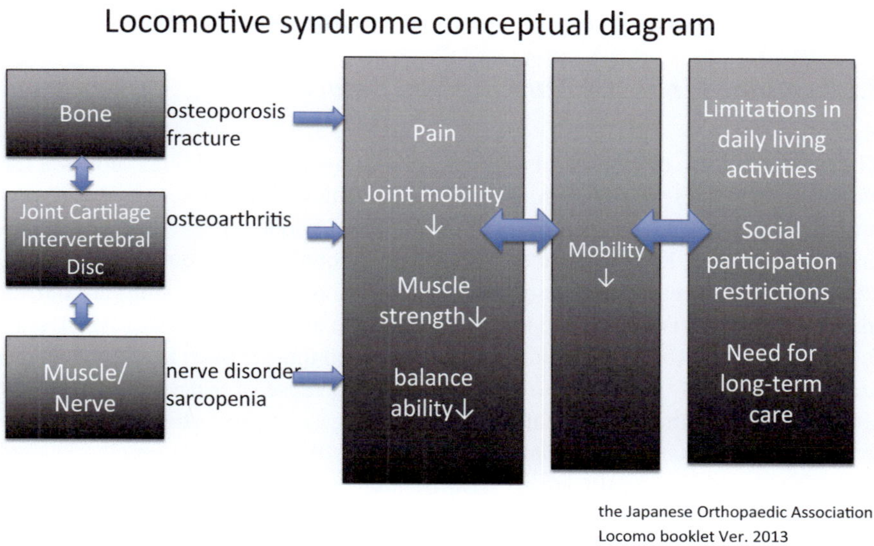

Fig. 8.2 Locomotive syndrome conceptual diagram. According to a brochure on locomotive syndrome prepared in 2013 by the Japanese Orthopaedic Association. This diagram shows the underlying disease to which bone, articular cartilage/intervertebral disc, and muscle/nerve tissues are related, the symptoms that are caused by the disease, and their effects on mobility and correlation with activity

ability to perform activities of daily living, increased disability, loss of independence, and an increased risk of death [9–12].

A consensus report published in 2010 by the European Geriatric Medicine Society and related organizations (European Working Group on Sarcopenia in Older People [hereafter referred to as "EWGSOP"]) [13] defines sarcopenia as "a syndrome characterised by progressive and generalised loss of skeletal muscle mass and strength with a risk of adverse outcomes such as physical disability, poor quality of life, and death."[14] Sarcopenia was initially diagnosed by muscle mass alone [15] and changes in diagnostic procedures occurred subsequently. EWGSOP and the Asian Working Group for Sarcopenia [16] proposed a diagnostic algorithm using gait speed and grip strength for screening and muscle mass for diagnosis. In addition, the International Sarcopenia Consensus Conference Working Group [17] proposed a diagnostic algorithm that uses gait speed alone for screening and muscle mass for diagnosis. As is seen from the above description, although the diagnostic procedure has not yet been internationally standardized, muscle mass is the criterion used for the final diagnosis of sarcopenia and the most important factor in any procedure. In our study of sarcopenia as described below, it was diagnosed using muscle mass.

Only a limited number of studies have examined the correlation between osteoporosis and sarcopenia; [18] thus, this article addresses the question.

8.2 Relationship Between Bone Mass and Muscle Mass

8.2.1 Bone Mass and Muscle Mass Database

The human body is composed of oxygen, carbon, hydrogen, and other atoms at the atomic level; water, fat, protein, and other molecules at the molecular level; and muscle, fat, bones, blood, and other tissues at the tissue level. The body composition at the tissue level continues to change gradually even during adulthood, although not as greatly as during the growth period [19]. Bone, muscle, and fat mass all decrease in old age, and these decreases are expected to increase the risk of fall/fracture in the following manner: the decrease in muscle mass is likely to cause falls, which in turn are likely to cause fractures because of a decrease in impact absorption due to the reduced fat mass and a decrease in bone strength due to the reduced bone mass. However, only a small number of studies have been conducted on these changes and most were cross sectional. Hence, much of the details remain unknown. Thus, we used the database of bone mass and muscle mass in our hospital to study the correlation between the two parameters.

Bone density measurements have long been taken using dual energy X-ray absorptiometry (DXA) to diagnose osteoporosis. The typical sites at which bone density is measured by DXA are the lumbar spine, proximal femur, and distal radius. The actual principle of measurement by DXA is that the accurate calculation of fat and lean masses is always performed internally and automatically for the purpose of obtaining an accurate bone mass from body composition. However, DXA devices that are used to measure bone mass at these sites do not show the lean mass value since it is unnecessary for the diagnosis of osteoporosis.

On the other hand, DXA devices that are used to measure the whole-body bone mass show both the whole-body bone mass and the regional fat and lean masses as the body composition. In other words, in this measurement mode, muscle mass, which can be calculated from lean mass, can be obtained in addition to bone mass.

To measure bone density, we have been using the entire body in addition to the lumbar spine and proximal femur since the 1990s in routine examinations of outpatients and inpatients of the departments of orthopedic surgery, internal medicine, rehabilitation, and gerontology of our hospital who are suspected to have osteoporosis. This patient database contains the bone mass values at the lumbar spine and proximal femur and of the whole body, and the muscle mass values calculated from lean mass as described later, and it can be used as a bone and muscle mass database.

The data used in this investigation represented that obtained from 2800 patients (655 men, 2118 women; age range, 20–102 years) who underwent body composition measurements by DXA between June 2002 and January 2009. The mean values for age, body height, body weight, bone mass, muscle mass (appendicular lean mass and the corresponding skeletal muscle index [SMI], a value corrected for body height), and fat mass for this database are shown in Table 8.1. Appendicular lean mass is the sum of arm lean mass and leg lean mass. SMI is a value obtained by

Table 8.1 Values for the parameters in the bone and muscle mass database

Sex		Age (year)	Height (cm)	Body weight (kg)	SMI (kg/m^2)	Total bone mineral content (g)	Total fat mass (g)	Appendicular lean mass (g)	Arm lean mass (g)	Leg lean mass (g)
Men: 655 patients	Average	71.1	152.4	51.7	6.081	1746	14,196	14,068	3487	10,759
Women: 2118 patients	SD	12.1	9.1	11.5	0.976	531	7428	3609	1027	2413
	Range	20–102	125–186	24–136	1.608–10.586	469–4531	876–59,991	3280–30,353	769–8998	2512–25,637

SD standard deviation
SMI skeletal muscle index

Table 8.2 Mean bone, muscle, and fat mass values by age bracket

Age (year)	n	Total bone mineral content (g)	Total fat mass (g)	Appendicular lean mass (g)
20–30	5	2510	14,499	19,901
30–40	31	2628	20,356	19,548
40–45	29	2457	17,393	17,008
45–50	123	2399	19,034	16,601
55–60	212	2044	16,857	15,546
60–65	356	1930	15,678	15,150
65–70	379	1829	15,465	14,872
70–75	482	1758	15,418	14,213
75–80	422	1642	13,110	13,668
85–90	202	1319	10,367	12,384
90–95	105	1262	8967	11,917
95–	30	1283	9279	12,148

correcting appendicular lean mass for body size as described later and is considered an international standard parameter of muscle mass.

Furthermore, Table 8.2 and Fig. 8.3 show variations in mean values for bone, muscle, and fat mass by age group. The data shown seem to show a tendency of these three tissue mass types to decrease with age in the investigated patient group. However, SMI, which is obtained by correcting for body height and considered to reflect muscle mass more accurately, did not necessarily show a tendency to decrease linearly with age (Fig. 8.4).

8.2.2 *Measurement of Bone Mass and Diagnosis of Osteoporosis*

Bone mass was measured by DXA (DPX-NT; GE Medical Systems Lunar, Madison, WI, USA) at three sites, i.e., with the anteroposterior views of the lumbar spine and the proximal femur and as the whole-body bone mass. In all three sites, two-dimensional bone density is calculated in grams per squared centimeters. In patients with a hip fracture, the measurement was performed at the unaffected proximal femur as soon as the patient was admitted to the hospital (within 3 days). Of the three sites, the lumbar spine and the proximal femur are most commonly used for the diagnosis of osteoporosis. However, as a patient ages, bone growth and sclerosis occur more often in the lumbar spine because of spinal osteoarthritis, making the lumbar spine less likely to reflect the accurate bone density of the vertebral body. Thus, the proximal femur was selected as the osteoporosis diagnostic site in this study. In the current diagnosis of osteoporosis, a history of fragility fractures is considered in addition to bone density as described above. There are also two proposals for the normal value of bone density: “less than the

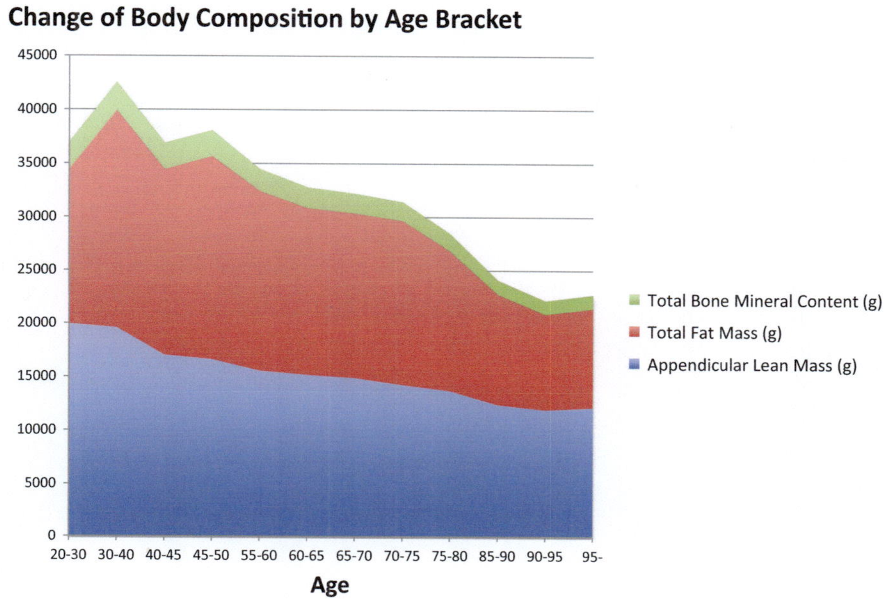

Fig. 8.3 Change of body composition by age bracket. Data of 2800 patients including outpatients and inpatients in the bone and muscle mass database in whom bone and muscle mass were measured by dosimetry X-ray absorptiometry for suspected osteoporosis. This figure shows the distribution of body composition (bone, fat, and fat-free mass) by age bracket in this patient group

YAM – 2.5 SD" by the World Health Organization and "less than the YAM – 30 %" by the Japanese Society for Bone and Mineral Research and the Japan Osteoporosis Society. The latter was selected in this study. In summary, osteoporosis is diagnosed when the transcervical bone density is <30 % of the YAM, osteopenia is diagnosed when the density is ≥70 % and <80 % of the YAM, and osteoporosis is diagnosed when both osteopenia and a fragility fracture are present [8].

8.2.3 Measurement of Muscle Mass and Diagnosis of Sarcopenia

In the measurement of muscle mass, body composition and bone mass are measured using the same DXA device. Body composition, including bone mineral content, fat mass, and lean mass, was measured separately for each part of the body. Muscle mass was calculated from lean mass according to the method by Baumgartner et al. The lean masses of the arms and legs were nearly equal to the skeletal muscle mass and are known as the appendicular lean mass. Since appendicular lean mass is affected by body size and ethnicity, SMI as described below is often used to correct the effect.

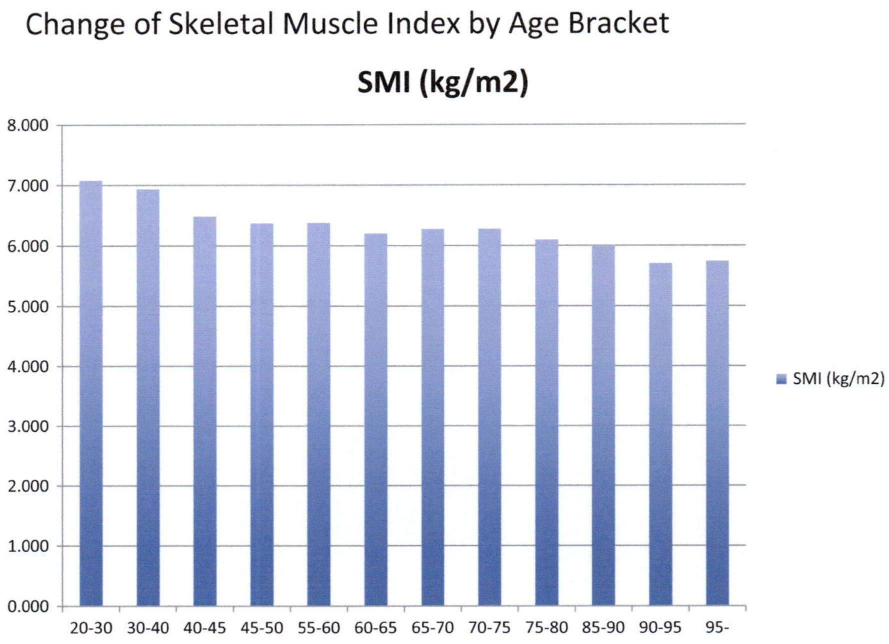

Fig. 8.4 Change of skeletal muscle index by age bracket. This figure shows the distribution of skeletal muscle index (SMI) by age bracket in 2800 patients in the bone and muscle mass database. *SMI* is an international standard indicator used to assess muscle mass and is calculated by the following formula: SMI = appendicular lean mass (kg)/height (m^2). Appendicular lean mass is the sum of arm lean mass and leg lean mass

SMI was calculated by the following formula:

$$\text{SMI} = \text{appendicular lean mass}\ (\text{kg})/\text{height}^2\left(\text{m}^2\right).$$

Sarcopenia was defined according to only the skeletal muscle mass index (SMI) in this database, using the criteria for the Japanese based on the report by Sanada et al. [20]. The value of Japanese criterion was an SMI below 5.46 kg/m^2 in women and below 6.87 kg/m^2 in men.

As mentioned above, EWGSOP' paper suggested an algorithm for sarcopenia case finding in older individuals based on measurements of gait speed, grip strength, and muscle mass [13].

However, as is obvious from their algorithm, muscle mass has the largest effect on the diagnosis. Thus, the diagnosis of sarcopenia by muscle mass alone is thought to be the most basic approach with the greatest significance.

8.2.4 *Relationship Between Bone Mass and Muscle Mass: Proximal Femur Bone Density and SMI*

The abovementioned investigation of bone and muscle mass based on our database showed a strong positive correlation between total bone mineral content and appendicular lean mass, which are uncorrected bone and muscle mass, respectively (Table 8.3 and Fig. 8.5). In other words, bone and muscle mass seem to be nearly in direct proportion from a cross-sectional aspect.

A similar investigation was conducted of the correlation between bone and muscle mass, except that SMI, which is a standard indicator of muscle mass that is obtained by correction for body height, was used as the parameter of muscle mass. The investigation showed a moderate but similar positive correlation between them (Table 8.3 and Fig. 8.6). Another similar investigation was conducted of the correlation between bone and muscle mass except that proximal femur bone density, a representative indicator of bone mass, and SMI were used. The investigation showed a little weaker but similar significant positive correlation between them ($R = 0.349$, $p = 0.000$) (Table 8.3 and Fig. 8.7). On the basis of these combined results, a positive correlation is considered to exist between bone and muscle mass in the patient group investigated in this study.

Multiple linear regression analysis using appendicular lean mass and SMI as the dependent variables as well as age, body height, body weight, total bone

Table 8.3 Pearson's correlation coefficient

		Age	Height	Body weight	SMI	Total bone mineral content	Total fat mass	Appendicular lean mass
Age	*r*		−0.459	−0.429	−0.236	−0.55	−0.33	−0.422
	p		.000	.000	.000	.000	.000	.000
Height	*r*			0.633	0.233	0.733	0.25	0.712
	p			.000	.000	.000	.000	.000
Body weight	*r*				0.538	0.768	0.789	0.737
	p				.000	.000	.000	.000
SMI	*r*					0.507	0.218	0.842
	p					.000	.000	.000
Total bone mineral content	*r*						0.466	0.77
	p						.000	.000
Total fat mass	*r*							0.29
	p							.000
Appendicular lean mass	*r*							
	p							

SMI skeletal muscle index
r Pearson's correlation coefficient

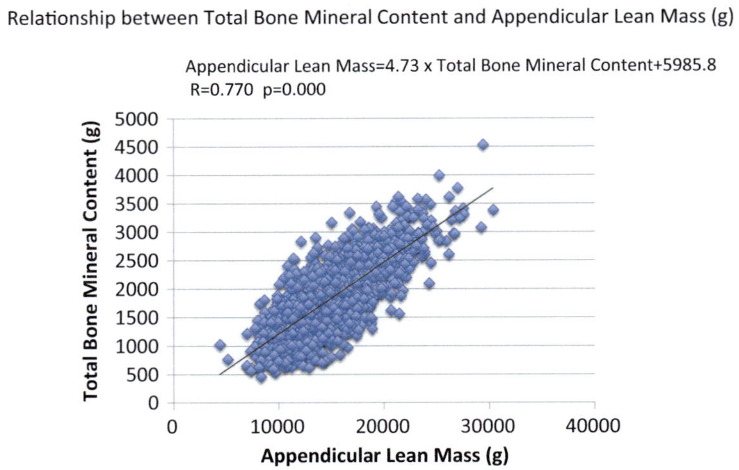

Fig. 8.5 Relationship between total bone mineral content and appendicular lean mass. This figure shows the regression of total bone mineral content to appendicular lean mass in 2800 patients in the bone and muscle mass database. The following significant positive regression line was obtained from the two parameters. Appendicular lean mass = 4.73 × total bone mineral content + 5985.8 $R = 0.770$ $p = 0.000$

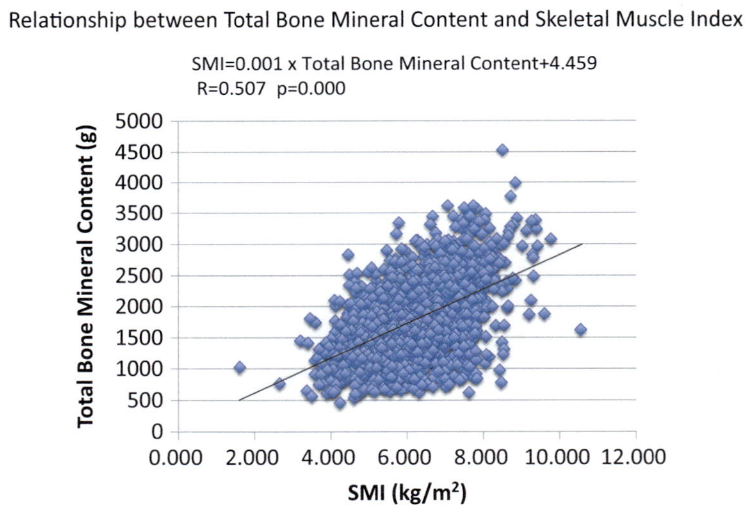

Fig. 8.6 Relationship between total bone mineral content and skeletal muscle index. This figure shows the regression of total bone mineral content to skeletal muscle index in 2800 patients in the bone and muscle mass database. The following significant positive regression line was obtained from the two parameters. SMI = 0.001 × total bone mineral content + 4.459 $R = 0.507$ $p = 0.000$

mineral content, and total fat mass as the independent variables showed that, for the prediction of SMI, all independent variables including body height are useful and that, for the prediction of appendicular lean mass, body height does

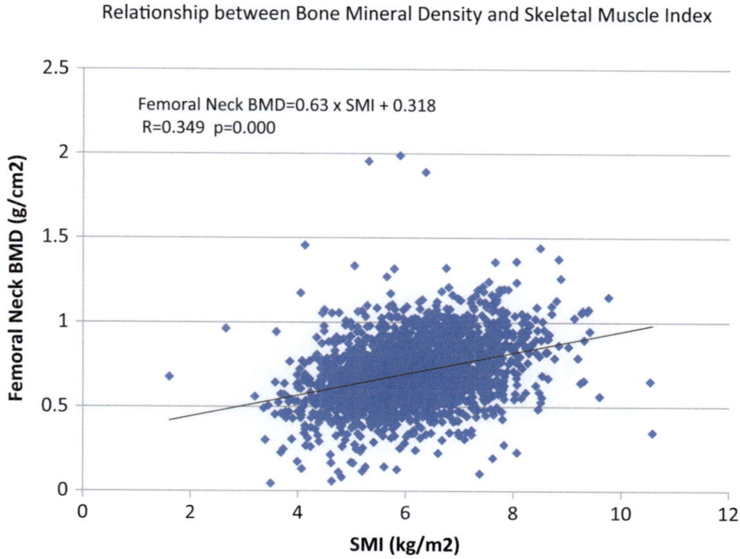

Fig. 8.7 Relationship between bone mineral density and skeletal muscle index. This figure shows the regression of femoral neck bone mineral density (BMD) to skeletal muscle index in 2800 patients in the bone and muscle mass database. The following significant positive regression line was obtained from the two parameters. Femoral neck $\text{BMD} = 0.63 \times \text{SMI} + 0.318$ $R = 0.349$ $p = 0.000$

Table 8.4 Results of multiple linear regression analysis using appendicular lean mass and skeletal muscle index (SMI) as the dependent variables

Dependent variable	Appendicular lean mass		SMI	
Independent variable	Standardized regression coefficient	Significance probability	Standardized regression coefficient	Significance probability
Intercept	749.584	.290	12.438	.000
Age	−16.612	.000	−.007	.000
Height	5.193	.304	−.075	.000
Body weight	306.905	.000	.123	.000
Total bone mineral content	1.324	.000	.001	.000
Total fat mass	−.302	.000	.000	.000

not produce significant results and all other independent variables are useful (Table 8.4).

One report shows that bone size or strength was not obviously correlated with gait speed but was strongly related with muscle size and strength in both men and women even after the adjustment for influential factors [21]. Many other reports [22–27] have argued that a positive correlation also exists between bone and muscle mass.

A study by Miyakoshi et al. showed a significant positive correlation between the bone densities of the lumbar spine and the proximal femur and SMI and reported that multivariate analysis using factors such as age and BMI showed a weak but significant correlation between proximal femur bone density and SMI but no significant correlation between lumbar spine bone density and SMI [18]. In our analysis in this study, there was also a positive correlation between the two parameters as described above as shown on multivariate analysis. This result is consistent with those of past reports.

8.3 Concurrent Occurrence of Osteoporosis and Sarcopenia: Status of Concurrent Occurrence of Osteoporosis and Sarcopenia as Diagnosed Using the Japanese Criteria

8.3.1 Prevalence of Osteoporosis

With respect to the prevalence of osteoporosis as determined by the criterion, transcervical bone density is <70 % of the YAM, 977 (35 %) of the patients in this database had osteoporosis, 689 (25 %) had osteopenia, and 1107 (40 %) had normal bone mass. With respect to the proportion of patients diagnosed with osteoporosis by sex, 145 men (22 %) had osteoporosis and 510 men (78 %) had decreased or normal bone mass, while 832 women (39 %) had osteoporosis and 1286 women (61 %) had decreased or normal bone mass. There was a significant difference between the sexes in the prevalence of osteoporosis (Pearson's chi-square test, $p = 0.000$) (Table 8.5).

8.3.2 Prevalence of Sarcopenia

With respect to the prevalence of sarcopenia, on the other hand, as determined by the criterion YAM of SMI – 2SD, 976 patients (35 %) had sarcopenia, while 1797 (65 %) were normal (Fig. 8.8). With respect to the proportion of patients diagnosed with sarcopenia by sex, 359 men (55 %) had sarcopenia and 296 men (45 %) were

Table 8.5 Percentages of persons diagnosed with osteoporosis and sarcopenia by sex

	Diagnosis of sarcopenia by SMI		Diagnosis of osteoporosis by BMD	
	Normal	Sarcopenia	Normal + decreased bone mass	Osteoporosis
Women	1501	617	1286	832
Men	296	359	510	145

Pearson's chi-square test: $p = 0.000$

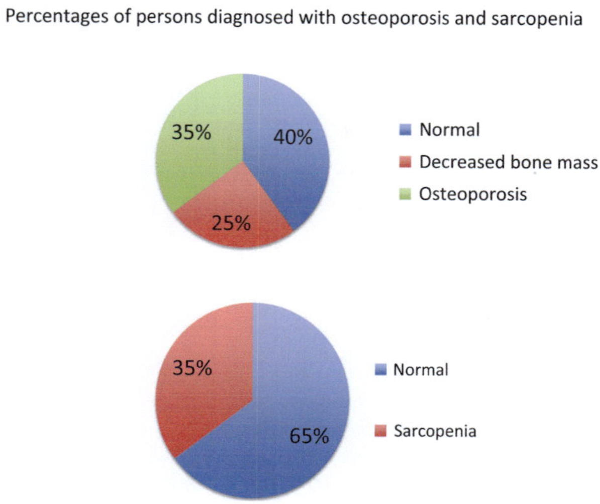

Fig. 8.8 Percentages of persons diagnosed with osteoporosis and sarcopenia. This figure shows the percentages of persons diagnosed with osteoporosis and osteopenia on the basis of femoral neck bone mineral density and the percentages of persons diagnosed with sarcopenia on the basis of skeletal muscle index in 2800 patients in the bone and muscle mass database

Table 8.6 Correlation between sarcopenia and osteoporosis

		Femoral neck BMD	
	Normal + decreased bone mass	Osteoporosis	
SMI	Normal	1260	537
	Sarcopenia	536	440

Pearson's chi-square test, $p = 0.000$
SMI skeletal muscle index
BMD bone mineral density

normal, while 617 women (29 %) had sarcopenia and 1501 women (71 %) were normal. There was a significant difference between the sexes in the prevalence of sarcopenia (Pearson's chi-square test, $p = 0.000$) (Table 8.5).

A cross-sectional survey was performed of 2419 subjects from the general population in their 40s and older who were living in the Obu-Higashiura district of Aichi-ken, which is substantially the same health care region as the district from which the patient group of the database of bone and muscle mass that was investigated in this study. The results show that the proportion of persons who were diagnosed with sarcopenia according to the muscle mass criterion was 25.0 % in men and 24.2 % in women. The results also show a difference between the sexes in the change in muscle mass with age. The number of persons diagnosed with sarcopenia by the muscle mass criterion significantly increased with age in men, whereas there was no significant difference between age groups in women [28]. These findings show that the prevalence of sarcopenia is obviously higher in the patient group than in the general population.

Moreover, the proportions of patients who were diagnosed with sarcopenia and osteoporosis by the SMI criterion in the patient group of the bone and muscle mass are shown in Table 8.6.

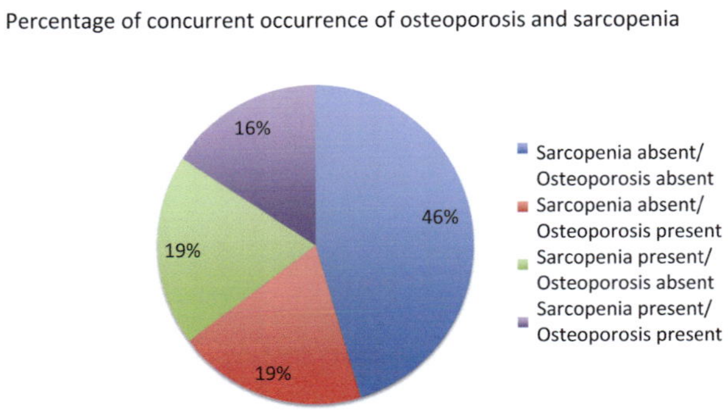

Fig. 8.9 Percentage of concurrent occurrence of osteoporosis and sarcopenia. This figure shows the proportions of patients who were not diagnosed with osteoporosis or sarcopenia, patients who were diagnosed with osteoporosis but not sarcopenia, patients who were not diagnosed with osteoporosis but were diagnosed with sarcopenia, and patients who were diagnosed with both diseases on the basis of the diagnosis of osteoporosis by transcervical bone mineral density and the diagnosis of sarcopenia by skeletal muscle index in 2800 patients in the bone and muscle mass database

8.3.3 Status of Concurrent Osteoporosis and Sarcopenia

It is well known that muscle and bone mass decrease with age. Pathological decreases in muscle and bone mass are referred to as sarcopenia and osteoporosis, respectively. To date, these two diseases have been studied separately. The correlation between them in patients in clinical settings has been studied by Miyawaki et al. [18] and other researchers but has not been fully elucidated. A survey of the concurrent occurrence of the two diseases showed that 1260 patients (45.4 %) had no sarcopenia and no osteoporosis, 537 patients (19.4 %) had no sarcopenia but osteoporosis, 536 patients (19.3 %) had sarcopenia but no osteoporosis, and 440 patients (15.9 %) had sarcopenia and osteoporosis (Fig. 8.9). In other words, of the 976 patients who were diagnosed with sarcopenia, 440 (45.1 %) had osteoporosis, and of 977 patients who were diagnosed with osteoporosis, 440 (45.0 %) had sarcopenia. The proportion of patients with one disease complicated by the other disease was shown to be substantially the same between the two diseases.

Table 8.7 shows the values of age, body-size factors, bone mass, and muscle mass in the groups according to complication status of the two diseases. A chi-square test showed a significant difference between the presence and absence of osteoporosis and between the presence and absence of sarcopenia (Table 8.6).

According to the Women's Health and Aging Study (WHAS) II, the presence of osteopenia was almost three times higher in the sarcopenic group, when compared to non-sarcopenics; moreover, the likelihood of being frail was substantially higher in the presence of both of osteoporosis and sarcopenia [29].

The concurrent occurrence of osteoporosis and sarcopenia is a dangerous duet for elderly patients because sarcopenia is likely to cause falls, and once a fall

Table 8.7 Age, body-size factors, and body composition values according to the presence or absence of the concurrent occurrence of osteoporosis and sarcopenia

			Age (year)	Height (cm)	Body weight (kg)	SMI (kg/m^2)	Total bone mineral content (g)	Total fat mass (g)	Appendicular lean mass (g)	Arm lean mass (g)	Leg lean mass (g)
Sarcopenia absent/ osteoporosis absent	$n = 1260$	Average	66.2	154.0	57.1	6.565	1990	17,371	15,709	3838	11,871
		SD	10.6	8.4	11.1	0.818	488	7145	3274	1043	2393
Sarcopenia absent/ osteoporosis present	$n = 537$	Average	78.2	146.0	45.9	6.364	1346	10,882	13,606	3360	10,245
		SD	9.7	7.6	8.5	0.742	322	6109	2208	875	1646
Sarcopenia present/ osteoporosis absent	$n = 536$	Average	69.1	157.0	52.3	5.481	1928	14,476	13,628	3357	10,272
		SD	12.5	8.4	9.2	0.768	449	6468	2859	917	2109
Sarcopenia present/ osteoporosis present	$n = 440$	Average	79.0	150.3	42.5	5.081	1312	8803	11,588	2794	8794
		SD	9.7	8.8	8.9	0.700	362	5814	2543	835	1890

SD standard deviation
SMI skeletal muscle index

occurs, the patient has an increased risk of fracture due to osteoporosis. Most of the fractures of the hip, distal radius, and proximal humerus and about half of vertebral compression fractures, which are representative fractures in the elderly, are caused by falls. Even in patients with osteoporosis, the likelihood of incurring bad outcomes, i.e., fractures, is likely to remain low if patients do not fall.

In this context, we should pay more attention to the concurrent occurrence of osteoporosis and sarcopenia.

8.4 Concurrent Occurrence of Osteoporosis and Sarcopenia in Hip Fractures

8.4.1 Status of Concurrent Occurrence of Osteoporosis and Sarcopenia in Patients with Hip Fractures

A total of 635 patients with hip fractures were treated in our hospital between June 2002 and January 2009. The patients were an average of 81.4 years and consisted of 535 women and 100 men. The types of fracture consisted of trochanteric fracture (326 patients) and femoral neck fracture (309 patients). Of them, 422 patients with hip fractures underwent bone density and body composition measurements using DXA. The measurements are included in the abovementioned database of bone and muscle mass.

As is well known, after such fractures, patients become nearly bedridden; thus, they are forced to submit to complete bed rest until treatment progresses and training in a standing position is started. Bone and muscle mass is markedly reduced during the period when patients are forced to take complete bed rest. Thus, the bone and muscle masses of patients with hip fractures need to be assessed as early as possible to obtain accurate values before injury. Of the 422 patients with hip fractures in the database of bone and muscle mass, 357 were assessed by DXA within 48 h after hospitalization.

Thus, these 357 patients, who are considered to maintain bone and muscle mass at near pre-injury levels before injury, were selected as subjects. The subjects consisted of 304 women with a mean age, body height, body weight, and body mass index (BMI) of 82.7 (SD, 9.3) years, 146.2 (SD, 7.2) cm, 43.1 (SD, 9) kg, and 20.1 (SD, 3.6) kg/m^2, respectively, as well as 53 men with a mean age, body height, and body weight of 80.3 (SD, 9.4) years, 160 (SD, 8.7) cm, 51.4 (SD, 10.6) kg, and 20.0 (SD, 3.3) kg/m^2, respectively [30].

The percentage of the concurrent occurrence of hip fractures and osteoporosis was determined by diagnosing osteoporosis at the unaffected proximal femur of these subjects with hip fractures. The proportion of subjects diagnosed with osteoporosis by transcervical bone mineral density (BMD) alone was 89.4 %, that of patients with a decreased BMD was 7.1 %, and that of subjects with a normal BMD was 3.5 %. Persons with bone density corresponding to "osteopenia" and a history

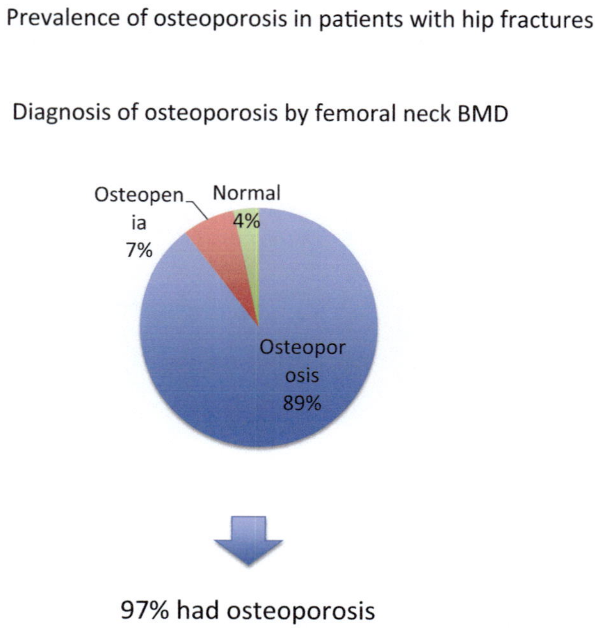

Fig. 8.10 Prevalence of osteoporosis in patients with hip fractures. Osteoporosis, osteopenia, and normal bone mass were diagnosed on the basis of transcervical bone mineral density in 357 patients with hip fractures. A total of 97 % were diagnosed with osteoporosis

of fragility fracture are diagnosed with osteoporosis; therefore, the prevalence of osteoporosis was 97 % (Fig. 8.10). The extremely high prevalence of osteoporosis in patients with hip fractures is thought to be natural.

On the other hand, with respect to the percentage of the concurrent occurrence of hip fractures and sarcopenia, SMI was 5.93 (SD, 0.0020) kg/m^2, while the prevalence of sarcopenia was 47.3 % in patients with hip fractures (Fig. 8.11) [30]. The evaluation of the prevalence of sarcopenia obtained in this investigation in patients with hip fractures requires comparison with a control group without fractures.

Thus, 2511 outpatients with osteoporosis who did not have fractures were extracted from the bone and muscle mass database and used as the control group for comparison with patients with hip fractures using the general linear model with correction for age and sex. The results showed that the SMI in the control group was 6.13 (SD, 0.0050) kg/m^2, demonstrating a significant decrease in muscle mass in patients with hip fractures ($p < 0.001$). Comparison of SMI at the upper and lower extremities separately showed that in patients with hip fractures, there was no significant difference in upper extremity SMI ($p > 0.95$), while lower extremity SMI was significantly decreased ($p < 0.001$). The prevalence of sarcopenia as diagnosed by the SMI criterion in Japanese was 31.8 % in the control group and 47.3 % in patients with hip fractures, showing a significant difference (Fig. 8.11). These findings have elucidated the actual serious condition of the concurrent occurrence of sarcopenia in patients with hip fractures [30].

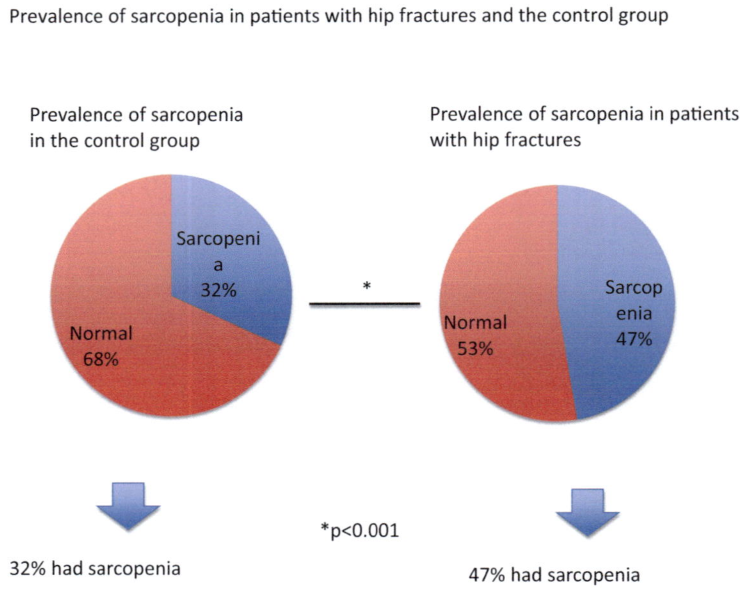

Fig. 8.11 Prevalence of sarcopenia in patients with hip fractures and the control group. Sarcopenia and normal muscle mass were diagnosed on the basis of the skeletal muscle index in 357 patients with hip fractures. A total of 47 % were diagnosed with sarcopenia. In addition, 2511 outpatients with osteoporosis who did not have fractures were extracted from the bone and muscle mass database and diagnosed as the control group for comparison. A total of 32 % were diagnosed with sarcopenia. The prevalence of sarcopenia was significantly higher in patients with hip fractures than in the control group

8.4.2 Correlation Between Sarcopenia and the Risk of Hip Fractures

Stepwise logistic regression analysis by age, sex, bone density, body weight, and body height showed that sarcopenia ($p = 0.002$), older age ($p < 0.001$), and low bone density ($p < 0.001$) were independently related to hip fractures. In other words, the analysis showed the possibility that sarcopenia is a potential independent risk factor for hip fractures [30].

A similar study by Di Monaco et al. reported that, of 313 women with hip fractures, 180 (58 %) had sarcopenia [31]. This is the first report of the prevalence of sarcopenia in patients with hip fractures. In this study, the effect of long-term immobility and malnutrition after fractures on muscle mass is undeniable because muscle mass was measured an average of 21 days after fracture injury. Our investigation is limited to patients in whom muscle mass was measured shortly after injury and is thought to show values that are closer to the actual condition.

It is needless to say that a further investigation is necessary because these analyses are cross sectional and not prospective by design.

References

1. National Livelihood Survey by the Ministry of Health, Labour and Welfare for 2001, 2004, 2007, 2010, and 2013 on the website of the Ministry of Health, Labour and Welfare: http://www.mhlw.go.jp/toukei/list/20-21.html
2. Nakamura K (2011) The concept and treatment of locomotive syndrome: its acceptance and spread in Japan. J Orthop Sci 16:489–491. doi:10.1007/s00776-011-0108-5
3. https://locomo-joa.jp/locomo/01.html
4. Rosenberg IH (1997) Sarcopenia: origins and clinical relevance. J Nutr 127:90S–991S
5. Klibanski A, Lucile, A-C, Bassford T, et al (2001) NIH consensus development panel on osteoporosis. JAMA 285:785–795
6. Yoshimura N, Muraki S, Oka H et al (2010) Cohort profile: research on osteoarthritis/osteoporosis against disability study. Int J Epidemiol 39:988–995
7. Yoshimura N, Muraki S, Oka H et al (2009) Prevalence of knee osteoarthritis, lumbar spondylosis and osteoporosis in Japanese men and women: the research on osteoarthritis/osteoporosis against disability study. J Bone Miner Metab 27:620–628
8. Orimo H, Hayashi Y, Fukunaga H et al (2001) Diagnostic criteria for primary osteoporosis (2001 edition). Jpn J Bone Metab 18:76–82
9. Cawthon PM, Marshall LM, Michael Y et al (2007) Frailty in older men: prevalence, progression, and relationship with mortality. J Am Geriatr Soc 55:1216–1223
10. Laurentani F, Russo C, Bandinelli S et al (2003) Age-associated changes in skeletal muscles and their effect on mobility: an operational diagnosis of sarcopenia. J Appl Physiol 95:1851–1860
11. Rolland Y, Czerwinski S, Abellan Van Kan G et al (2008) Sarcopenia: its assessment, etiology, pathogenesis, consequences and future perspectives. J Nutr Health Aging 12:433–450
12. Topinkova E (2008) Aging, disability and frailty. Ann Nutr Metab 52(Suppl 1):6–11
13. Cruz-Jentoft AJ, Baeyens JP, Bauer JM et al (2010) Sarcopenia: European consensus on definition and diagnosis: Report of the European Working Group on Sarcopenia in Older People. Age Ageing 39:412–423
14. Delmonico MJ, Harris TB, Lee JS et al (2007) Alternative definitions of sarcopenia, lower extremity performance, and functional impairment with aging in older men and women. J Am Geriatr Soc 55:769–774
15. Baumgartner RN, Koehler KM, Gallagher D et al (1998) Epidemiology of sarcopenia among the elderly in New Mexico. Am J Epidemiol 147:755–763
16. Chen LK, Liu LK, Woo J et al (2014) Sarcopenia in Asia: consensus report of the Asian Working Group for Sarcopenia. J Am Med Dir Assoc 15:95–101. doi:10.1016/j.jamda.2013.11.025
17. Fielding RA, Vellas B, Evans WJ et al (2011) Sarcopenia: an undiagnosed condition in older adults. Current consensus definition: prevalence, etiology, and consequences. International working group on sarcopenia. J Am Med Dir Assoc 12:249–56. doi:10.1016/j.jamda.2011.01.003
18. Miyakoshi N, Hongo M, Mizutani Y et al (2013) Prevalence of sarcopenia in Japanese women with osteopenia and osteoporosis. J Bone Miner Metab 31:556–561. doi:10.1007/s00774-013-0443-z
19. Van Loan MD (1996) Total body composition: birth to old age. In: Roche AF, Heymsfield SB, Lohman TG (eds) Human body composition. Human Kinetics, Champaign, pp 205–216. http://www.humankinetics.com
20. Sanada K, Miyachi M, Tanimoto M et al (2010) A cross-sectional study of sarcopenia in Japanese men and women: reference values and association with cardiovascular risk factors. Eur J Appl Physiol 110:57–65
21. Edwards MH, Gregson CL, Patel HP et al (1972) Muscle size, strength, and physical performance and their associations with bone structure in the Hertfordshire Cohort study. J Bone Miner Res 28:2295–2304. doi:10.1002/jbmr

22. Visser M, Deeg DJ, Lips P (2003) Low vitamin D and high parathyroid hormone levels as determinants of loss of muscle strength and muscle mass (sarcopenia): the Longitudinal Aging Study Amsterdam. J Clin Endocrinol Metab 88:5766–5772
23. Blain H, Vuillemin A, Teissier A et al (2001) Influence of muscle strength and body weight and composition on regional bone mineral density in healthy women aged 60 years and over. Gerontology 47:207–212
24. Pluijm SMF, Visser M, Smit JH et al (2001) Determinants of bone mineral density in older men and women: body composition as mediator. J Bone Miner Res 16:2142–2151
25. Moro M, van der Meulen MCH, Kiratli BJ et al (1996) Body mass is the primary determinant of midfemoral bone acquisition during adolescent growth. Bone 19:519–526
26. Barondess DA, Nelson DA, Schlaen SE (1997) Whole body bone, fat, and lean mass in black and white men. J Bone Miner Res 12:967–971
27. Walsh MC, Hunter GR, Livingstone MB (2006) Sarcopenia in premenopausal and postmenopausal women with osteopenia, osteoporosis and normal bone mineral density. Osteoporos Int 17:61–67
28. Shimokata H, Ando F, Yuki A et al (2014) Age-related changes in skeletal muscle mass among community-dwelling Japanese: a 12-year longitudinal study. Geriatr Gerontol Int 14(Suppl 1):85–92. doi:10.1111/ggi.12219
29. Frisoli A Jr, Chaves PH, Ingham SJM et al (2010) Severe osteopenia and osteoporosis, sarcopenia, and frailty status in community-dwelling older women: results from the Women's Health and Aging Study (WHAS) II. Bone 48:952–957. doi:10.1016/j.bone.2010.12.025
30. Hida T, Ishiguro N, Shimokata H et al (2013) High prevalence of sarcopenia and reduced leg muscle mass in Japanese patients immediately after a hip fracture. Geriatr Gerontol Int 13:413–420
31. Di Monaco M, Vallero F, Di Monaco R et al (2011) Prevalence of sarcopenia and its association with osteoporosis in 313 older women following a hip fracture. Arch Gerontol Geriatr 52:71–74

Part III
Clinical Applications of Antiosteoporotic Agents

Chapter 9
Effects of Vitamin D on Bone and Skeletal Muscle

Yuji Kasukawa, Naohisa Miyakoshi, and Yoichi Shimada

Abstract The native and active forms of vitamin D exert various effects on both bone and skeletal muscle. Vitamin D prevents osteoclastogenesis, reduces bone resorption in osteoporotic patients, and stimulates bone formation by acting on osteoblasts. A new active vitamin D analog, eldecalcitol, has unique effects on bone formation known as mini-modeling, which are independent of bone resorption. Vitamin D also has positive effects on skeletal muscle by increasing muscle strength and improving physical functions in older people, particularly in those who are vitamin D deficient. The mechanisms of vitamin D effects on skeletal muscle are both indirect via calcium and phosphate and direct via $1\alpha,25(OH)_2D_3$ activation of the vitamin D receptor on muscle cells. Based on these effects of vitamin D on both bone and skeletal muscle, many meta-analyses have shown that vitamin D decreases the risk of falls as well as osteoporotic vertebral and non-vertebral fractures. The interrelationships between muscle and bone related to vitamin D actions and the molecular mechanisms by which vitamin D affects both bone and skeletal muscle are still incongruent in the different backgrounds of subjects.

Keywords Vitamin D • Bone • Skeletal muscle • Falls • Osteoporotic fractures

9.1 Background of the Effects of Native and Active Forms of Vitamin D on the Bone and Skeletal Muscle

In an advanced aged society, maintenance of quality of life and reducing morbidity and mortality are very important goals. Osteoporosis is a systemic skeletal disease associated with low bone mass and microarchitectural deterioration of bone with a consequential increase in bone fragility and fractures. In addition to osteoporosis, sarcopenia, which is characterized by a decline in skeletal muscle volume, causes impairment of activity in older people.

Y. Kasukawa, M.D., Ph.D. (✉) • N. Miyakoshi • Y. Shimada
Department of Orthopedic Surgery, Akita University Graduate School of Medicine, 1-1-1 Hondo, Akita 010-8543, Japan
e-mail: kasukawa@doc.med.akita-u.ac.jp

Y. Shimada, N. Miyakoshi (eds.), *Osteoporosis in Orthopedics*,
DOI 10.1007/978-4-431-55778-4_9

To treat osteoporosis and sarcopenia is a reasonable target in older people by orthopedic surgeons. Among several types of medicine for osteoporosis, the native and active forms of vitamin D reduce the risk of falls and fractures [1, 2]. Vitamin D is a lipid-soluble hormone produced in the skin through ultraviolet irradiation and obtained from animal- (vitamin D_3) and plant-based (vitamin D_2) foods [3, 4] as the native form. In the human body, vitamin D is hydroxylated in the liver to 25-hydroxyvitamin D [25(OH)D] and subsequently in the kidney to its biologically active form, 1,25-dihydroxyvitamin D [calcitriol, $1\alpha,25(OH)_2D_3$]. Alfacalcidol, a synthetic calcitriol analog (1α-hydroxycholecalciferol), is hydroxylated to calcitriol in the liver [5]. Eldecalcitol [1α, 25-dihydroxy-2β-(3-hydroxypropyloxy) vitamin D_3, ED-71], which is a new analog of the active form of vitamin D, has a hydroxypropyloxy group at the 2β position of $1\alpha,25(OH)_2D_3$ [6, 7]. The binding activity of eldecalcitol to serum vitamin D-binding protein (DBP) is greater than that of $1\alpha,25(OH)_2D_3$, resulting in a longer half-life in circulation [8]. These native or active forms of vitamin D have been considered to exert their preventive effects on falls and fractures by acting on both bone and skeletal muscle. In this chapter, we describe the effects and mechanisms of vitamin D in bone metabolism, bone mineral density (BMD), and skeletal muscle and then review the preventive effects of vitamin D on falls and finally on osteoporotic fractures.

9.2 Effects on Bone Metabolism

9.2.1 Osteoclasts and Bone Resorption

The effects of active vitamin D on bone resorption in vitro and in vivo are opposing. Based on the results from in vitro studies, active vitamin D, $1\alpha,25(OH)_2D_3$, stimulates osteoclastic bone resorption by inducing expression of receptor activator of nuclear factor (NF)-κB ligand (RANKL) [9]. RANKL in osteoblasts is responsible for the activation and differentiation of osteoclasts [10, 11]. Using receptor activator of NF-κB (RANK)-deficient mice, a previous study showed that vitamin D directly acts on osteoclasts to stimulate bone resorption and maintain serum calcium levels [12]. This catabolic effect promotes bone resorption in both experimental animals and in vitro cultures of calvaria [11].

However, vitamin D is used to treat osteoporosis by suppressing bone resorption and increasing BMD. Vitamin D deficiency causes significant bone loss with increased bone resorption by RANKL-mediated osteoclastogenesis in rats [13]. Vitamin D exerts its effects on bone and skeletal muscle via binding to the vitamin D receptor (VDR) on osteoclasts, osteoblasts, and osteocytes in bone tissue. $1\alpha,25(OH)_2D_3$ inhibits osteoclastogenesis induced by RANKL following induction of c-Fos protein in a dose-dependent manner via binding to the VDR [14]. Previous studies have shown that active vitamin D suppresses bone resorption in parathyroidectomized rats [15] as well as inhibits bone resorption and stimulates bone formation in ovariectomized (OVX) rats [16, 17]. A recent study showed that eldecalcitol does not affect the number of osteoclast precursors and suppresses RANKL mRNA expression but not macrophage colony-stimulating factor (M-CSF) or RANK mRNA expression [18]. Furthermore, eldecalcitol has a greater effect on bone resorption than alfacalcidol in OVX rats [19].

Daily administration of vitamin D may alter the microenvironment of the bone, which supports osteoclastogenesis, as another mechanism by which vitamin D affects bone resorption. Vitamin D enhances intestinal calcium absorption, leading to an increase in serum calcium levels and suppression of bone resorption by suppressing RANKL expression in osteoblasts [20–24]. Moreover, autocrine/paracrine activities of vitamin D are detected in each of the three bone cell types [25]. Vitamin D has an autocrine action in the form of 1α,25$(OH)_2D_3$ synthesized within these bone cell types, and/or a paracrine action by synthesis of 1α,25$(OH)_2D_3$ in one cell type, which acts on adjacent cells [25]. The synthesis of adequate 1α,25$(OH)_2D_3$ by bone tissue is dependent on the level of the enzyme 25-hydroxyvitamin D-1α-hydroxylase (CYP27B1), which catalyzes the conversion of 25(OH)D to 1α,25$(OH)_2D_3$, and the level of the 25(OH)D [25]. Kogawa et al. demonstrated that 25(OH)D metabolism is an important intrinsic mechanism in optimization of osteoclast differentiation as well as osteoclast activity and might promote the coupling of bone resorption with formation [26, 27].

The details of vitamin D effects on bone resorption are still unclear. Thus, further studies will need to elucidate these important points.

9.2.2 Osteoblasts and Bone Formation

1α,25$(OH)_2D_3$ has been demonstrated to play a significant role in osteoblast differentiation and mineralization [28–31]. In addition to the indirect actions of 1α,25$(OH)_2D_3$ for mineralization in bone via control of calcium absorption in the intestine and reabsorption in the kidney, it exerts direct effects on bone via binding to the VDR on osteoblasts. 1α,25$(OH)_2D_3$ increases Runx2 expression, which stimulates osteoblast differentiation via the bone morphogenetic protein (BMP) pathway that cooperates with the Wnt signaling pathway in human osteoblasts [32, 33], but inhibits its expression in murine osteoblasts [33, 34]. Osteopontin is induced by 1α,25$(OH)_2D_3$ in osteoblasts, increasing cell survival and triggering ossification of the skeleton [35]. 1α,25$(OH)_2D_3$ also significantly increases the expression of LRP5 that stimulates osteoblast proliferation via enhanced canonical Wnt signaling and acts on bone as an anabolic factor [36, 37]. 1α,25$(OH)_2D_3$ also stimulates production of bone-specific proteins such as osteocalcin, osteopontin, and type I collagen [38]. However, the magnitude or results of these direct effects of 1α,25$(OH)_2D_3$ on osteoblasts are subject to the presence of many other factors, and there are different responses between murine and human/rat osteoblasts [39]. The reason for these discrepancies in 1α,25$(OH)_2D_3$ effects on osteoblasts between humans and mice is still unknown.

Recent studies have demonstrated increases in the bone mass, osteoid volume, and osteoblast numbers not only in VDR knockout mice but also in osteoblast-specific VDR knockout mice [40, 41]. As another mechanism of vitamin D in osteoblasts, autocrine $1\alpha,25(OH)_2D_3$ synthesis and activity are a common feature of human osteoblastic cells at different stages of development with critical roles in osteoblast development, differentiation, and mineralization [42]. Anderson and colleagues reported that $1\alpha,25(OH)_2D_3$ synthesis and expression of osteocalcin, RANKL, and CYP24 mRNA in response to 25(OH)D are dependent on osteoblastic expression of CYP27B1 [28]. $1\alpha,25(OH)_2D_3$ production in osteoblasts is modulated by factors that are synthesized locally in cells of the bone and/or marrow [42]. These effects of $1\alpha,25(OH)_2D_3$ are exerted in an autocrine/paracrine manner on osteoblasts.

Eldecalcitol shows stimulating effects on bone formation. Several animal studies have demonstrated that eldecalcitol maintains bone formation [43–45]. Such effects on bone formation are known as mini-modeling that is independent of bone resorption [18, 23]. The ability of eldecalcitol to induce bone mini-modeling is approximately tenfold higher than that of $1\alpha,25(OH)_2D_3$ [46].

9.2.3 Vitamin D Effects on Osteocytes

$1\alpha,25(OH)_2D_3$ binds to the VDR and regulates the expression of numerous genes in bone cells. Osteocytes are known to not only act in bone remodeling with other bone cell types but also exert endocrine functions as part of the regulatory network for calcium and phosphate homeostasis. Osteocyte-like cells convert physiological levels of 25(OH)D to $1\alpha,25(OH)_2D_3$ with changes in gene expression that is consistent with an increase in osteocyte maturation [47]. Furthermore, $1\alpha,25(OH)_2D_3$ induces the release of fibroblast growth factor 23 (FGF23) from osteocytes of the osteoblastic lineage [48]. Osteocytes are the major source of FGF23 under pathological conditions such as rickets and chronic kidney failure [49, 50]. FGF is a phosphate regulator and the second phosphaturic hormone following parathyroid hormone (PTH) [48]. Based on these findings, osteocytes exert a local effect on both mineralization and bone remodeling via FGF23. Thus, $1\alpha,25(OH)_2D_3$ is a major contributor to the regulation of FGF23 in osteocytes and osteoblasts, and active vitamin D_3 regulates some osteocyte functions via control of FGF23. However, the details of vitamin D effects on osteocytes are still under investigation.

9.3 Effects on BMD and Bone Quality

9.3.1 BMD

The 2011 Institute of Medicine reported that several studies found no association between a baseline or attenuated 25(OH)D status and changes in the BMD of healthy adults [51]. Reid et al. performed a systematic review and meta-analysis of the effects of vitamin D supplements on BMD [52]. The meta-analysis showed a small effect on the femoral neck BMD [95 % confidence interval (CI), 0.2–1.4] but not the total hip or lumbar spine [52]. Vitamin D supplementation significantly increased 25(OH)D levels in individuals at 53–92 nmol/L in all studies [52]. The effects of vitamin D supplementation on BMD might be different depending on age, calcium intake, and baseline 25(OH)D levels.

In a 2-year double-blind study, Shiraki et al. reported that alfacalcidol increased BMD of the lumbar spine by 2.32 % in osteoporotic women [53]. In addition to the effects of active vitamin D on BMD, several studies have demonstrated the beneficial effects of combined therapy with active vitamin D_3 such as alfacalcidol or calcitriol and antiresorptive agents. A large 3-year randomized double-blind, placebo-controlled study of 489 postmenopausal women compared placebo, hormone replacement therapy (HRT), calcitriol, and HRT + calcitriol that showed the strongest effect on BMD [54]. Another study of 120 postmenopausal osteoporotic women revealed that the combination of 1-μg alfacalcidol with 60 mg per day of raloxifene resulted in a greater decrease in bone turnover and increased BMD compared with the respective monotherapies [55]. Combinatorial therapy with alfacalcidol or calcitriol and alendronate is superior to monotherapy in terms of BMD in postmenopausal osteoporosis [56]. However, in our retrospective investigation, elcatonin showed no additive effects on BMDs of the lumbar spine (Fig. 9.1a) and proximal femur (Fig. 9.1b) or prevention of vertebral fractures in postmenopausal women receiving alfacalcidol therapy for a mean of 5 years [57].

Eldecalcitol suppresses bone resorption to a greater extent than alfacalcidol and has a similar effect on bone formation and calcium metabolism, resulting in a greater increase in the BMD of OVX rats [19]. Combined therapy with eldecalcitol and alendronate improves the mechanical properties of the lumbar spine and mid-shaft femur by additive suppression of bone resorption and maintenance of bone formation in OVX rats [58, 59]. Co-treatment with eldecalcitol and raloxifene improves mechanical strength by increasing BMD in OVX rats [60]. In a clinical study, 0.75 μg eldecalcitol significantly increased lumbar and hip BMD [61]. The enhancing effects of eldecalcitol on BMD are not dependent on the baseline level of 25(OH)D [62]. A recent review of eldecalcitol showed an increase in BMD with inhibitory effects on bone resorption [63].

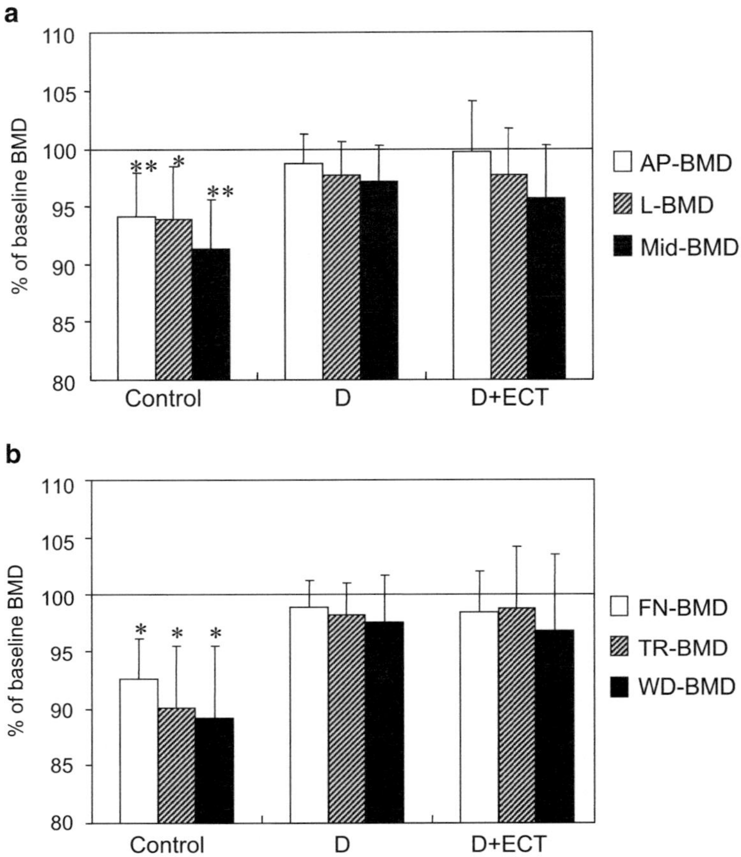

Fig. 9.1 (**a**) Changes in BMD of the lumbar spine after 5 years of treatment with alfacalcidol alone (D) or alfacalcidol and elcatonin (D + ECT). Data are presented as the mean + standard error the mean (SEM). *AP* anteroposterior, *L* lateral, *Mid* midlateral. $*P < 0.05$ and $**P < 0.001$ compared with the baseline BMD in each group (Reprint with permission from Springer). (**b**) Changes in proximal femoral BMD after 5 years of treatment with alfacalcidol alone (D) or alfacalcidol and elcatonin (D + ECT). Data are presented as the mean + SEM. *FN* femoral neck, *TR* trochanter, *WD* Ward's triangle. $*P < 0.001$ compared with the baseline BMD in each group (Reprint with permission from Springer)

9.3.2 Bone Quality and Mechanical Properties

In addition to the effects of vitamin D on BMD, there have been several studies of active vitamin D effects on bone quality including mechanical properties, collagen, and collagen cross-linking. Microcomputed tomography has shown that combined therapy with etidronate and alfacalcidol increased the mechanical properties of the trabecular and cortical bone without impairment of mineralization or connectivity, resulting in bone strengthening in OVX rats [64]. In the fracture repair rat model, alfacalcidol induced lamellar bone formation coinciding with an increase in enzymatic cross-linking and normalization of the cross-linking pattern in callus to a native bone pattern [65]. Alfacalcidol also improved the amount and cross-linking pattern of collagen in steroid-treated rats [66]. A recent study has shown that alfacalcidol not only increased the amount of collagen but also enhanced the maturation of collagen in OVX rats [67]. Eldecalcitol improved the biomechanical properties of the femoral cortical bone by inhibiting endocortical bone resorption and stimulating periosteal bone formation in SAM/P6 mice [68]. In a clinical study, eldecalcitol increased the cortical cross-sectional area and maintained the cortical thickness of the proximal femur better than alfacalcidol in osteoporotic patients as evaluated by clinical computed tomography [69]. This study showed that the biomechanical properties of the femoral neck, including cross-sectional moment of inertia and the section modulus, were improved more by eldecalcitol than alfacalcidol [69]. These studies indicate that active vitamin D improves both the quality and mechanical properties of bone.

9.4 Effects on Skeletal Muscle

9.4.1 Effects of Vitamin D Deficiency on Muscle

Many studies have shown that serum levels of 25(OH)D, but not $1\alpha,25(OH)_2D_3$, are related to bone variables and muscle functions. Some recent studies have reported that the incidence of 25(OH)D deficiency has increased in older people [70–72]. A lower serum 25(OH)D level predicted a decrease in grip strength and appendicular muscle mass in older men and women [73]. This study indicated that the 3-year risk of sarcopenia was twofold higher in older subjects with baseline 25(OH)D levels of less than 25 nmol/L [73]. Prospective studies have also reported an association between baseline 25(OH)D levels and declines in muscle function. Wicherts et al. reported that low baseline 25(OH)D levels (<50 nmol/L) were significantly correlated with a greater 3-year decline in physical performance including a walking test, chair standing, and tandem standing in people over 65 years of age [74].

Vitamin D deficiency also causes atrophy of type II muscle fibers [75, 76] and myopathy with muscle pain, fatigue, muscle weakness, and gait disturbance in older people [77]. These studies indicate that vitamin D has obvious effects on skeletal muscle.

9.4.2 Effects of Vitamin D on Muscle Strength and Fatigue

In an animal study, vitamin D deficiency induced by dietary restriction and housing under incandescent lighting caused a significant reduction in muscle strength of the soleus in rats as assessed by a force transducer to detect isometric contraction [78]. We performed several animal studies to clarify the effects of alfacalcidol on muscle strength and fatigue, and the histomorphometric changes in muscle tissues of normal and OVX rats as a model for aged osteoporotic women [79, 80]. Alfacalcidol administration significantly increased the maximum contraction tension of the calf muscle in the sham-operated group (5–7 % increase, $p < 0.01$) and OVX group (4–7 % increase, $p < 0.001$) compared with their respective controls. However, alfacalcidol administration did not significantly affect muscle fatigue in these groups as evaluated by the percentage strength at each cycle of the initial contraction strength [80]. Furthermore, we evaluated the effects of alfacalcidol on skeletal muscle strength and fatigue in prednisolone-administered rats and found steroid myopathy with muscle weakness and atrophy. Alfacalcidol significantly increased the maximum contractile muscle strength (Fig. 9.2a) and decreased muscle fatigue (Fig. 9.2b) as evaluated by the strength decrement index (SDI) of the calf muscle in prednisolone-administered rats [81]. These results indicate that the active form of vitamin D, alfacalcidol, increases muscle strength and decreases muscle fatigue, resulting in prevention of falls.

In a clinical situation, supplementation of more than 700 IU/day vitamin D led to an improvement in muscle strength and preserved bone in older people with vitamin D insufficiency (serum 25(OH)D, <50 nmol/L) [82]. Other studies also showed that vitamin D supplementation improved lower limb strength in institutionalized [83] and community-dwelling older individuals [84]. Stockton et al. reported that muscle fatigue was related to physical function but not vitamin D levels or maximal isometric strength in vitamin D-depleted patients with systemic lupus erythematosus (SLE) [85].

Treatment with 1 μg alfacalcidol increases muscle mass, muscle power, and balance and reduces fear of falling in older people [86]. Alfacalcidol (0.5 μg) has been shown to significantly improve muscle strength (isometric knee extension strength) and functional ability (walking distance over 2 min) after 6 months of treatment in older 25(OH)D-deficient women [87]. Another study demonstrated that alfacalcidol together with calcium and alendronate enhanced the beneficial effects of back extensor exercise in patients younger than those in their late 60s [88]. In addition, long-term treatment with alfacalcidol improved body sway in older women [89]. A recent study revealed that alfacalcidol maintains muscle mass and increases the skeletal muscle index in patients with low muscle mass [90].

However, a single high dose of vitamin D (300,000 IU) did not improve physical performance even in older patients with a low baseline 25(OH)D level (<12 nmol/L) [91]. A meta-analysis showed no effect on grip strength or proximal lower limb strength by vitamin D supplementation in adults with 25(OH)D levels of more than 25 nmol/L in 17 randomized controlled trials (RCTs) involving 5072 subjects

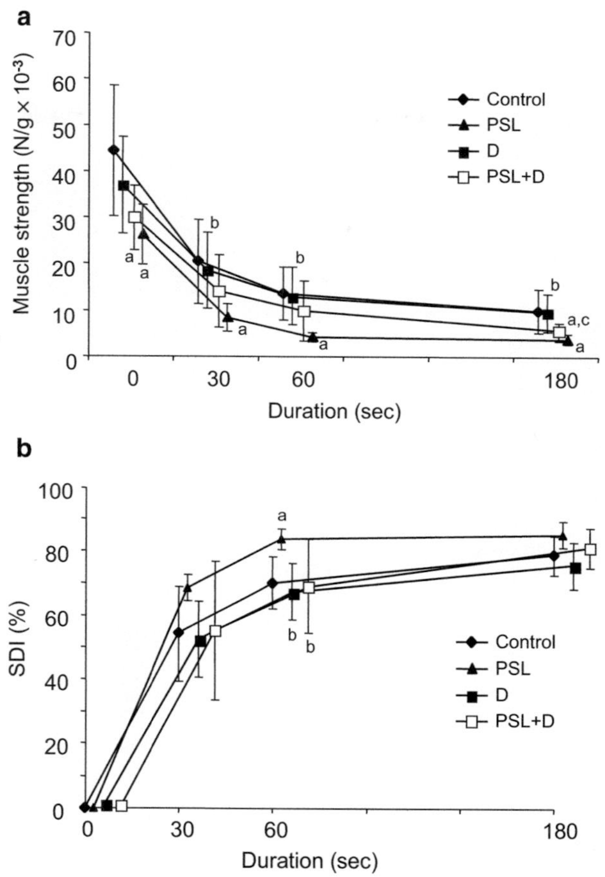

Fig. 9.2 (**a**) Changes in muscle strength during stimulation. Each data point for the Control (♦), PSL (▲), D (■), and PSL + D (□) groups is expressed as mean ± standard deviation (SD). [a,b,c] Significant differences ($P < 0.05$) between [a]Control, [b]PSL, and [c]D groups at each time point (Reprint with permission from Biomedical Research Press). (**b**) Changes in SDI during stimulation. Each data point for the Control (♦), PSL (▲), D (■), and PSL + D(□) groups is expressed as mean ± SD. [a,b] Significant differences ($P < 0.05$) between [a]Control and [b]PSL groups at each time point (Reprint with permission from Biomedical Research Press)

[92]. Annweiler et al. also performed a systematic review to examine the effects of low serum vitamin D and vitamin D supplementation on muscles, balance, and gait performance among people aged 65 years and older [93]. They concluded that the association between vitamin D and physical performance remains controversial [93].

9.4.3 *Effects of Vitamin D on Muscle Fiber Phenotypes*

Vitamin D supplementation may change the muscle fiber composition. Muscle fibers are divided into type I (slow twitch) and type II (fast twitch) with further subdivision into IIA, IIX, and IIB depending on the expression of different myosin heavy chain isoforms [70]. We have recently reevaluated the effects of vitamin D on the percentages of muscle fiber phenotypes in OVX rats. After 4 weeks of oral administration of alfacalcidol (0.1 μg/kg/day) to OVX rats, their calf muscle fibers

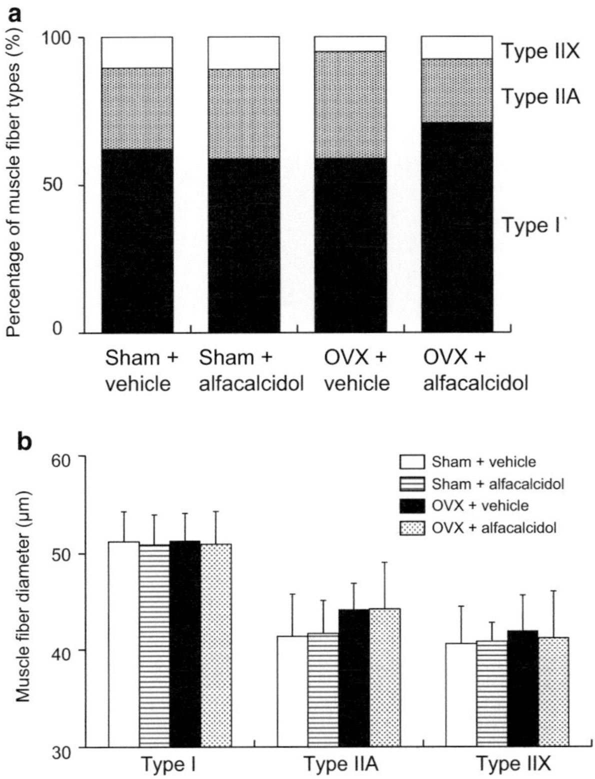

Fig. 9.3 (**a**) Effects of ovariectomy and/or alfacalcidol on the composition of muscle fiber types including type I (■), type IIA (▨), and type IIX (□). There was no significant difference in the composition of muscle fiber types induced by ovariectomy or alfacalcidol treatment. (**b**) Differences in the diameters of muscle fibers of each phenotype induced by ovariectomy (OVX) and alfacalcidol treatment. OVX or alfacalcidol administration did not affect the diameter of muscle fibers in any of the four groups

had a smaller diameter. Moreover, type I fibers increased from 83.6 to 88.3 % in OVX and control rats treated with or without alfacalcidol (Fig. 9.3a) [80]. Ovariectomy or alfacalcidol administration did not affect the smaller diameter of muscle fibers (Fig. 9.3b) [80]. Conversely, Sorenson et al. showed an increase in the relative fiber composition and size of type IIA fibers after treatment with alfacalcidol and calcium in muscle biopsies from older women [94]. A randomized controlled study found that daily treatment of older stroke patients with 1000 IU vitamin D_2 increased the type II muscle fiber diameter and percentage of type II fibers over 2 years [95]. Treatment with alfacalcidol and calcium for 3–6 months increased the proportion and cross-sectional area of type IIA fibers in the vastus lateralis of aged osteoporotic patients [94].

9.4.4 Effects of Eldecalcitol on Muscle

Eldecalcitol increases the expression of several factors related to muscle function in C2C12 cells in vitro, such as MyoD and myogenin [96]. To evaluate in vivo effects of eldecalcitol on skeletal muscle morphology and function, we treated glucocorticoid-induced myopathic and osteopenic rats with eldecalcitol. Four weeks of treatment with eldecalcitol prevented muscle atrophy of the tibialis anterior and loss of femoral BMD and increased calf muscle strength. However, there was no significant preventive effect on muscle fatigue induced by eldecalcitol [97]. A recent study has demonstrated that eldecalcitol enhances the expression of insulin-like growth factor-1 (IGF-1), myelin basic protein, and VDR in rat primary Schwann cells, and VDR signaling induced by eldecalcitol regulates neuromuscular maintenance and enhances locomotive ability following physical exercise [98].

In a clinical situation, eldecalcitol improved muscle power as evaluated by chair-rising time in postmenopausal women with osteoporosis treated with alendronate or risedronate [99]. We have also performed a prospective study to evaluate the effects of eldecalcitol on static and dynamic body balance in older osteoporotic women. Eldecalcitol and alendronate co-treatment improved muscle strength measured at the back extensor and dynamic body balance as evaluated by dynamic sitting balance and a timed up and go test [100]. These results indicate that eldecalcitol also exerts significant effects on muscle strength, body balance, and physical functions.

9.4.5 Genomic and Non-Genomic Effects on Muscle

As a genomic effect on muscle, it has been reported that $1\alpha,25(OH)_2D_3$ regulates muscle calcium uptake [101], affects the synthesis of muscle cytoskeletal proteins [102], and regulates phosphate metabolism in myoblasts [102]. Recently, it was found that $1\alpha,25(OH)_2D_3$ also affects muscle function through a transcription-enhancing effect on proteins such as IGF-1 and its binding proteins as well as proteins involved directly in calcium metabolism, revealing an anabolic effect on muscle tissue [103]. Eldecalcitol induces expression of MyoD and myogenin through induction of osteoglycin, which is secreted from myoblast and stimulates osteoblastic differentiation, in C2C12 cells when combined with $1\alpha,25(OH)_2D_3$ [96]. However, as a non-genomic effect on muscle, $1\alpha,25(OH)_2D_3$ activates protein kinase C (PKC) to release calcium into the cytosol [104]. These studies suggest that alfacalcidol also has positive effects on muscle strength via genomic and non-genomic effects on muscle functions.

9.5 Effects on Falling

9.5.1 Vitamin D Deficiency and Falls

Approximately 30 % of community-dwelling people over the age of 65 years fall each year [105]. Falls are a major risk factor for fracture and other injuries and worsen quality of life [106]. Several studies have demonstrated that low baseline 25 (OH)D levels are increased in older people at risk of subsequent falls [107, 108]. Older people in nursing homes and hostel residents who fall have lower serum 25(OH)D levels and higher serum PTH levels than other residents [109]. These studies indicate that low serum 25(OH)D levels are related to falling, especially in older people.

9.5.2 Prevention of Falls by Vitamin D Treatment

Although native vitamin D exerts small effects on BMD, many studies have demonstrated a beneficial effect of native vitamin D on fractures by prevention of falls [110–112]. In 2004, Bischoff et al. performed a meta-analysis based on five RCTs including people of more than 60 years of age (total number of subjects, 1237) to evaluate the effects of native vitamin D on falls [110]. They found that native vitamin D significantly reduced falls by 22 % (95 % CI, 0.64–0.92). The study also reported that treatment of 15 subjects with native vitamin D would prevent one fall [110]. Another meta-analysis with eight RCTs also demonstrated that native vitamin D treatment at more than 700 IU/day significantly reduced falls with a relative risk (RR) of 0.81 and 95 % CI of 0.77–0.92 [2]. The most recent meta-analysis included 26 RCTs with 45,782 participants, revealing that native vitamin D significantly reduced the risk of falls [odds ratio (OR) for suffering at least one fall, 0.86; 95 % CI, 0.77–0.96] [112].

Conversely, there have been several negative randomized studies between vitamin D supplementation and falls. Vitamin D (400 IU/day) treatment had no significant effect on falls among 354 older persons in the Netherlands [113]. Although a high dose of vitamin D (800 IU/day) showed positive effects on the risk of falls in nursing home residents, lower doses of vitamin D (200, 400, and 600 IU/day) did not demonstrate significant effects on the risk of falls [114]. Another two studies with larger numbers of subjects did not find a beneficial effect of 800 IU/day vitamin D on falls in people over 70 years of age or in older women living in nursing homes [115, 116]. However, a subgroup analysis of a recent meta-analysis demonstrated that the effect of vitamin D on prevention of falls was more significant in subjects with vitamin D deficiency (OR, 0.53; 95 % CI, 0.39–0.72) than in those with sufficient vitamin D (OR, 0.90; 95 % CI, 0.81–0.99). A high dose ($>$800 IU/day) of vitamin D (OR, 0.82; 95 % CI, 0.73–0.93) was more effective than a lower dose ($<$800 IU/day) of vitamin D (OR, 1.00; 95 % CI, 0.72–1.37). Furthermore, combined therapy with vitamin D and calcium (OR, 0.83; 95 % CI, 0.72–0.93) was more beneficial than monotherapy with vitamin D (OR, 0.97; 95 % CI, 0.84–1.11) [112].

Active vitamin D_3 also inhibits osteoporotic fractures by acting on bone tissue and improves muscle strength and sense of balance, thus helping to prevent falls [2, 117]. Alfacalcidol has been shown to decrease postural sway in older people during 12 months of treatment [118]; improve muscle power and balance, as evaluated by a timed up and go test; and reduce the incidence of falls [119]. Studies have also demonstrated the positive effects of eldecalcitol on physical functions [99] and body balance [100]. These effects of eldecalcitol on muscle and physical functions might contribute to reducing the risk of falls. In 1054 osteoporotic patients, the incidence of wrist fractures caused by falls was significantly lower in the eldecalcitol-treated group compared with that in the alfacalcidol-treated group after 36 months [120].

Based on these results, vitamin D supplementation and active vitamin D, including eldecalcitol, are probably effective in conjunction with calcium to prevent falls among older individuals. The effects appear to be optimal in those who are vitamin D deficient at baseline.

9.6 Preventive Effects on Osteoporotic Fractures

9.6.1 Vitamin D Deficiency and Fractures

Serum 25(OH)D level is related to the muscle strength [73, 74] and the incidence of falls [107–110]. Furthermore, serum 25(OH)D levels influence the risk of osteoporotic fractures. Serum 25(OH)D concentrations of 40 nmol/L or less result in a marked increase in the risk of hip fractures in older people, which is unrelated to their serum 1α,25$(OH)_2D_3$ levels [121, 122]. Meta-analyses of case-control studies have clearly demonstrated that a decrease in the serum 25(OH)D level is significantly associated with an increased risk of hip fractures among older people [123]. Conversely, this relationship is not obvious between the serum 1α,25 $(OH)_2D_3$ level and hip fractures [124].

9.6.2 Prevention of Fractures by Vitamin D Treatment

The most important goal of osteoporosis treatment is prevention of fractures including vertebral and non-vertebral fractures in older people. Vitamin D has obvious positive effects on both bone and skeletal muscle as shown by previous studies. There have been several RCTs that evaluated the effects of vitamin D supplementation and active vitamin D on prevention of osteoporotic fractures.

Papadimitropoulos et al. performed a meta-analysis of the preventive effects of vitamin D supplementation and active vitamin D on osteoporotic vertebral fractures. Their study demonstrated that vitamin D significantly reduced the risk of vertebral fractures (RR, 0.63; 95 % CI, 0.45–0.88) [1]. In terms of the preventive effects of vitamin D supplementation on non-vertebral fractures, Bischoff-Ferrari et al. reported a meta-analysis including 12 double-blind RCTs. Their study showed that vitamin D supplementation significantly decreased the risk of non-vertebral

Table 9.1 Fracture incidence among 31,022 participants, according to the vitamin D treatment dose and actual intake

Analysis	No. of participants	Hip fracture			Any nonvertebral fracture		
		No. of fractures	Relative risk (95% CI)	P value	No. of fractures	Relative risk (95% CI)	P value
Intention-to-treat analysis							
Control	15,495	586	1.00		1948	1.00	
Treatment	15,527	525	0.90 (0.80–1.01)	0.07	1822	0.93 (0.87–0.99)	0.03
Treatment-dose analysis							
Control	15,495	586	1.00		1948	1.00	
≤400 IU/day	10,111	255	0.89 (0.74–1.07)	0.20	1225	0.96 (0.89–1.05)	0.40
>400 IU/day[a]	5,416	270	0.91 (0.78–1.06)	0.22	597	0.89 (0.80–0.98)	0.02
Actual-intake analysis[b]							
Control	15,495	586	1.00		1948	1.00	
0–360 IU/day	3,935	100	1.00 (0.79–1.26)	0.99	425	0.96 (0.86–1.07)	0.44
361–637 IU/day	3,836	110	1.03 (0.83–1.29)	0.78	520	1.01 (0.91–1.12)	0.85
638–791 IU/day	3,790	164	1.01 (0.83–1.23)	0.92	419	0.90 (0.80–1.01)	0.08
792–2000 IU/day	3,966	151	0.70 (0.58–0.86)	<0.001	458	0.86 (0.76–0.96)	0.007
Sensitivity analysis							
Control	15,495	586	1.00		1948	1.00	
0–337 IU/day	3,353	84	1.01 (0.79–1.30)	0.91	465	1.06 (0.95–1.17)	0.32
338–360 IU/day	5,652	114	0.83 (0.66–1.05)	0.11	619	0.89 (0.80–0.98)[c]	0.02
361–699 IU/day	2,640	180	1.14 (0.93–1.41)	0.21	326	1.05 (0.91–1.22)	0.52
700–2000 IU/day	3,882	147	0.71 (0.58–0.87)	0.001	412	0.81 (0.72–0.91)	<0.001
Internal validation							
0–360 IU/day	18,153	639	1.00		2193	1.00	
361–637 IU/day	4,976	150	1.03 (0.84–1.26)	0.80	681	1.04 (0.95–1.15)	0.37
638–791 IU/day	3,865	168	1.02 (0.84–1.24)	0.83	431	0.92 (0.82–1.03)	0.16
792–2000 IU/day	4,028	154	0.70 (0.58–0.86)	<0.001	465	0.86 (0.77–0.97)	0.01

*All analyses were adjusted for study, age group, sex, and type of dwelling. To limit false positive results and correct for multiplicity, we used a *P* value of 0.0125 to indicate significance

[a]All trials included doses between 700 and 2000 IU per day

[b]Among 21,241 participants from the eight trials that used vitamin D combined with any dose of calcium supplementation, a benefit was present only at the highest actual-intake level of vitamin D

[c]In the sensitivity analysis for adherence-adjusted dose without supplements outside the study protocol, 511 participants in the Women's Health Initiative trial[17] shifted from the highest actual-intake level (792–2000 IU per day), and 1356 shifted from the second-highest actual-intake level (683–791 IU per day) to the second-lowest adherence-adjusted intake level (338–360 IU per day). See the Supplementary Appendix for additional information (Reprint with permission from the Massachusetts Medical Society)

fractures (RR, 0.86; 95 % CI, 0.77–0.96) and hip fractures (RR, 0.91; 95 % CI, 0.78–1.05) [111]. A recent analysis including 11 double-blind RCTs of 31,022 people (65 years of age or older) with 1111 incident hip fractures and 3770 non-vertebral fractures demonstrated that the highest doses (800–2000 IU/day) of vitamin D supplements reduced the risk of hip fractures by 30 % and any non-vertebral fracture by 14 % in older people [125] (Table 9.1). Another study showed that supplementation with both vitamin D and calcium improved hip BMD but had no effect on the risk of fracture [126]. It has been speculated that the effects of vitamin D supplementation on the risk of osteoporotic fractures may depend on the background of the subjects, such as age, baseline serum 25(OH)D level, and past history of osteoporotic fractures. A recent meta-analysis also reported no significant interactions between the highest actual intake of vitamin D and subgroups defined by age, type of dwelling, baseline 25(OH)D level, and additional calcium intake [125]. Instead of 25(OH)D, $1\alpha,25(OH)_2D_3$ administration showed no reduction in fracture risk in a meta-analysis [127].

Similar to native vitamin D, active vitamin D, calcitriol, also significantly reduced the incidence of osteoporotic vertebral fractures in older people [128, 129]. A 2-year double-blind study by Shiraki M et al. demonstrated that alfacalcidol decreased new osteoporotic fractures in one third of the control group [53]. A meta-analysis demonstrated that active vitamin D reduced the risk of vertebral fractures with an RR of 0.53 and non-vertebral fractures with an RR of 0.34 [130]. Furthermore, the effects of active vitamin D on the reduction of fracture risks are better than native vitamin D [131].

A new analog of the active form of vitamin D, eldecalcitol, has been approved for the treatment of osteoporosis in Japan since 2011. A phase III clinical trial of eldecalcitol for osteoporosis showed a significant reduction in the incidence of new vertebral fractures over 3 years (hazard ratio (HR), 0.74; 90 % CI, 0.56–0.97) compared with alfacalcidol [120]. The incidence of new severe vertebral fractures (grade III by semiquantitative classification) in the eldecalcitol treatment group was significantly lower than that in the alfacalcidol treatment group (HR, 0.53; 95 % CI, 0.29–0.96) [132]. Compared with alfacalcidol, the risk of non-vertebral osteoporotic fractures was significantly reduced by eldecalcitol (HR, 0.59; 95 % CI, 0.37–0.94) [133]. It has been also reported that eldecalcitol significantly reduces the risk of forearm fractures compared with alfacalcidol [120].

Based on these results, vitamin D supplementation and active vitamin D have significant preventive effects on osteoporotic vertebral and non-vertebral fractures.

9.7 Conclusion

Vitamin D increases BMD and mechanical properties and improves muscle strength and physical functions. Native and active forms of vitamin D are useful to prevent falls as well as osteoporotic vertebral and non-vertebral fractures by acting on both bone and skeletal muscle in older people. A new analog of the active form of vitamin D, eldecalcitol, also increases BMD and improves physical functions. Eldecalcitol reduces the incidence of vertebral and wrist fractures more than the conventional active form of vitamin D. These effects of vitamin D result in a decrease in falls and osteoporotic fractures.

References

1. Papadimitropoulos E, Well G, Shea B et al (2002) Osteoporosis Methodology Group and The Osteoporosis Research Advisory Group. Meta-analyses of therapies for postmenopausal osteoporosis. VIII: meta-analysis of the efficacy of vitamin D treatment in preventing osteoporosis in postmenopausal women. Endocr Rev 23:560–569
2. Bischoff-Ferrari HA, Dawson-Hughes B, Staehelin HB et al (2009) Fall prevention with supplement and active forms of vitamin D: a meta-analysis of randomized controlled trials. Br Med J 339:b3692. doi:10.1136/bmj.b3692
3. Lips P (2006) Vitamin D physiology. Prog Biophys Mol Biol 92:4–8
4. DeLuca HF (2004) Overview of general physiologic features and functions of vitamin D. Am J Clin Nutr 80:1689S–1696S
5. Menczel J, Foldes J, Steinberg R et al (1994) Alfacalcidol (alpha D3) and calcium in osteoporosis. Clin Orthop 300:241–247
6. Sanford M, McCormack PL (2011) Eldecalcitol: a review of its use in the treatment of osteoporosis. Drugs 71:1755–1770
7. Matsumoto T, Endo I (2012) Eldecalcitol for the treatment of osteoporosis. Drugs Today (Barc) 48:189–196
8. Okano T, Tsugawa S, Masuda A et al (1989) Regulatory activities of 2β-(3-hydroxypropoxy)-1α25-dihydroxy-vitamin D3, a novel vitamin D3 derivative, on calcium metabolism. Biochem Biophys Res Commun 163:1444–1449
9. Yasuda H, Shima N, Nakagawa N et al (1998) Osteoclast differentiation factor is a ligand for osteoprotegerin/osteoclastogenesis-inhibitory factor and is identical to TRANCE/RANKL. Proc Natl Acad Sci U S A 95:3597–3602
10. Goltzman D (2002) Discoveries, drugs and skeletal disorders. Nat Rev Drug Discov 1:784–796
11. Haussler MR, Hasussler CA, Whitfield GK et al (2010) The nuclear vitamin D receptor controls the expression of genes encoding factors with feed the "Fountain of Youth" to mediate healthful aging. J Steroid Biochem Mol Biol 121:88–97
12. Li J, Sarosi I, Yan XQ et al (2000) RANK is the intrinsic hematopoietic cell surface receptor that controls osteoclastogenesis and regulation of bone mass and calcium metabolism. Proc Natl Acad Sci U S A 97:1566–1571
13. Anderson PH, Sawyer RK, Moore AJ et al (2008) Vitamin D depletion induces RANKL-mediated osteoclastogenesis and bone loss in a rodent model. J Bone Miner Res 23:1789–1797
14. Takasu H, Sugita A, Uchiyama Y et al (2006) c-Fos protein as a target of anti-osteoclastogenic action of vitamin D and synthesis of new analogs. J Clin Invest 116:528–535
15. Endo K, Katsumata K, Hirata M et al (2000) 1,25-dihydroxy-vitamin D3 as well as its analogue OCT lower blood calcium through inhibition of bone resorption in hypercalcemic rats with continuous parathyroid hormone-related peptide infusion. J Bone Miner Res 15:175–181
16. Shiraishi A, Takeda S, Masaki T et al (2000) Alfacalcidol inhibits bone resorption and stimulates formation in an ovariectomized rat model of osteoporosis: distinct actions from estrogen. J Bone Miner Res 15:770–779

17. Shibata T, Shiraishi A, Sato T et al (2002) Vitamin D hormone inhibits osteoclastogenesis in vivo by decreasing the pool of osteoclast precursors in bone marrow. J Bone Miner Res 17:622–629
18. Harada S, Mizoguchi T, Kobayashi Y et al (2012) Daily administration of eldecalcitol (ED-71), an active vitamin D analog, increase bone mineral density by suppressing RANKL expression in mouse trabecular bone. J Bone Miner Res 27:461–473
19. Uchiyama Y, Higuchi Y, Takeda S et al (2002) ED-71, a vitamin D analog, is a more potent inhibitor of bone resorption than alfacalcidol in an estrogen-deficient rat model of osteoporosis. Bone 30:582–588
20. Gardiner EM, Baldock PA, Thomas GP et al (2000) Increased formation and decreased resorption of bone in mice with elevated vitamin D receptor in mature cells of the osteoblastic lineage. FASEB J 14:1908–1916
21. Atkins GJ, Kostakis P, Pan B et al (2003) RANKL expression is related to the differentiation state of human osteoblasts. J Bone Miner Res 18:1088–1098
22. Nakashima T, Hayashi M, Fukunaga T et al (2011) Evidence for osteocyte regulation of bone homeostasis through RANKL expression. Nat Med 17:1231–1234
23. De Freitas PHL, Hasegawa T, Takeda S et al (2011) Eldecalcitol, a second-generation vitamin D analog, drives bone minimodeling and reduces osteoclastic number in trabecular bone of ovariectomized rats. Bone 49:335–342
24. Lieben L, Masuyama R, Torrekens S et al (2012) Normocalcemia is maintained in mice under conditions of calcium malabsorption by vitamin D-induced inhibition of bone mineralization. J Clin Invest 122:1803–1815
25. Morris HA, Anderson PH (2010) Autocrine and paracrine actions of vitamin D. Clin Biochem Rev 31:129–138
26. Kogawa M, Anderson PH, Findlay DM et al (2010) The metabolism of 25(OH)-vitamin D3 by osteoclasts and their precursors regulates the differentiation of osteoclasts. J Steroid Biochem Mol Biol 121:277–280
27. Kogawa M, Findlay DM, Anderson PH et al (2010) Osteoclastic metabolism of 25(OH)-vitamin D3: a potential mechanism for optimization of bone resorption. Endocrinology 151:4613–4625
28. Atkins GJ, Anderson PH, Findlay DM et al (2007) Metabolism of vitamin D3 in human osteoblasts: evidence for autocrine and paracrine activities of 1 alpha,25-dihydroxyvitamin D3. Bone 40:1517–1528
29. Geng S, Zhou S, Glowacki J (2010) Effects of 25-hydroxyvitamin D3 on proliferation and osteoblast differentiation of human marrow stromal cells require CYP27B1/1alphoa-hydroxylase. J Bone Miner Res 26:1145–1153
30. van Driel M, Pols HA, van Leeuwen JP (2004) Osteoblast differentiation and control by vitamin D and vitamin D metabolites. Curr Pharm Des 10:253–255
31. van Driel M, Koedam M, Buurman CJ et al (2006) Evidence for auto/paracrine actions of vitamin D in bone: 1 alpha-hydroxylase expression and activity in human bone cells. FASEB J 20:2417–2419
32. Prince M, Banerjee C, Javed A et al (2001) Expression and regulation of Runx2/Cbfa1 and osteoblast phenotypic markers during the growth and differentiation of human osteoblasts. J Cell Biochem 80:424–440
33. Viereck V, Siggelkow H, Tauber S et al (2002) Differential regulation of Cbfa1/Runx2 and osteocalcin gene expression by vitamin-D3, dexamethasone, and local growth factors in primary human osteoblasts. J Cell Biochem 86:348–356
34. Drissi H, Pouliot A, Koolloos C et al (2002) 1,25-(OH)2-vitamin D3 suppresses the bone-related Runx2/Cbfa1 gene promoter. Exp Cell Res 274:323–333
35. Weissen-Plenz G, Nitschke Y, Rutsch F (2008) Mechanisms of arterial calcification: spotlight on the inhibitors. Adv Clin Chem 46:263–293

36. Fretz JA, Zella LA, Kim S et al (2006) 1,25-dihydroxyvitamin D3 regulates the expression of low-density lipoprotein receptor-related protein 5 via deoxyribonucleic acid sequence elements located downstream of the start site of transcription. Mol Endocrinol 20:2215–2230
37. Barthel TK, Mathern DR, Whitfield GK et al (2007) 1,25-dihydroxyvitamin D3/VDR-mediated induction of FGF23 as well as transcriptional control of other bone anabolic and catabolic genes that orchestrate the regulation of phosphate and calcium mineral metabolism. J Steroid Biochem Mol Biol 103:381–388
38. van de Peppel J, van Leeuwen JP (2014) Vitamin D and gene networks in human osteoblasts. Front Physiol 5:137. doi:10.3389/fphys.2014.00137. eCollection 2014
39. van Driel M, van Leeuwen JP (2014) Vitamin D endocrine system and osteoblasts. Bonekey Rep. doi:10.1038/bonekey.2013.227
40. Amling M, Priemel M, Holzmann T et al (1999) Rescue of the skeletal phenotype of vitamin D receptor-ablated mice in the setting of normal mineral ion homeostasis: formal histomorphometric and biomechanical analyses. Endocrinology 140:4982–4987
41. Yamamoto Y, Yoshizawa T, Fukuda T et al (2013) Vitamin D receptor in osteoblasts is a negative regulator of bone mass control. Endocrinology 154:1008–1020
42. Anderson PH, Atkins GJ, Turner AG et al (2011) Vitamin D metabolism within bone cells: effects on bone structure and strength. Mol Cell Endocrinol 347:42–47
43. Okuda N, Takeda S, Shinomiya K et al (2007) ED-71, a novel vitamin D analog, promotes bone formation and angiogenesis and inhibits bone resorption after bone marrow ablation. Bone 40:281–292
44. Tanaka Y, Nakamura T, Nishida S et al (1996) Effects of a synthetic vitamin D analog, ED-71, one bone dynamics and strength in cancellous and cortical bone in prednisolone-treated rats. J Bone Miner Res 11:325–336
45. Tsurukami H, Nakamura T, Suzuki K et al (1994) A novel synthetic vitamin D analogue, 2 beta-(3-hydroxyropoxy)1 alpha, 25-dihydroxyvitamin D3 (ED-71), increases bone mass by stimulating the bone formation in normal and ovariectomized rats. Calcif Tissue Int 54:142–149
46. Saito H, Takeda S, Amizuka N (2013) Eldecalcitol and calcitriol stimulates bone minimodeling focal bone formation without prior bone resorption, in rat trabecular bone. J Steroid Biochem Mol Biol 136:178–182
47. Turner AG, Hanrath MA, Morris HA et al (2014) The local production of 1,25(OH)2D3 promotes osteoblast and osteocyte maturation. J Steroid Biochem Mol Biol 144:114–118
48. Kolek OI, Hines ER, Jones MD et al (2005) 1α25-dihydroxyvitamin D3 upregulates FGF23 gene expression in bone: the final link in a renal-gastrointestinal-skeletal axis that controls phosphate transport. Am J Physiol Gastrointest Liver Physiol 289:G1036–G1042
49. Pereira RC, Juppner H, Azucena-Serrano CE et al (2009) Patterns of FGF-23, DMP1, and MEPE expression in patients with chronic kidney disease. Bone 45:1161–1168
50. Lanske B, Densmore MJ, Erben RG (2014) Vitamin D endocrine system and osteocytes. Bonekey Rep 3:494. doi:10.1038/bonekey.2013.228. eCollection 2014
51. Ross AC, Manson JE, Abrams SA et al (2011) The 2011 report on dietary reference intakes for calcium and vitamin D from the institute of medicine: what clinicians need to know. J Clin Endocrinol Metab 96:53–58
52. Reid IR, Bolland MJ, Grey A (2014) Effects of vitamin D supplements on bone mineral density: systematic review and meta-analysis. Lancet 383:146–155
53. Shiraki M, Kushida K, Yamazaki K et al (1996) Effects of 2 year's treatment of osteoporosis with 1α-hydroxy vitamin D3 on bone mineral density and incidence of fracture: a placebo-controlled, double-blind prospective study. Endocr J 43:211–220
54. Gallagher JC, Fowler SE, Detter JR et al (2001) Combination treatment with estrogen and calcitriol in prevention of age-related bone loss. J Clin Endocrinol Metab 86:3618–3628
55. Gorai I, Tanaka Y, Imacki Y (2006) Raloxifene when combined with 1a(OH) vitamin D more greatly suppresses bone turnover and increases bone density than when used alone in postmenopausal Japanese women with osteoporosis or osteopenia. J Bone Miner Res 21:S186

56. Frediani B, Allegri A, Bisohno S et al (1998) Effects of combined treatment with calcitriol plus alendronate on bone mass and bone turnover in postmenopausal osteoporosis. Two years of continuous treatment. Clin Drug Invest 14:235–244
57. Miyakoshi N, Shimada Y, Ando S et al (2006) Effects of alfacalcidol alone or in combination with elcatonin on incidence of osteoporotic vertebral fractures in postmenopausal women with spondylosis. J Bone Miner Metab 24:491–497
58. Sakai S, Endo K, Takeda S et al (2012) Combination therapy with eldecalcitol and alendronate has therapeutic advantages over monotherapy by improving bone strength. Bone 50:1054–1063
59. Sugimoto M, Futaki N, Harada M et al (2013) Effects of combined treatment with eldecalcitol and alendronate on bone mass, mechanical properties, and bone histomorphometry in ovariectomized rat: a comparison with alfacalcidol and alendronate. Bone 52:181–188
60. Takeda S, Sakai S, Shiraishi A et al (2013) Combination treatment with eldecalcitol (ED-71) and raloxifene improves bone mechanical strength by suppressing bone turnover and increasing bone mineral density in ovariectomized rats. Bone 53:167–173
61. Matsumoto T, Miki T, Hagino H et al (2005) A new active vitamin D. ED-71, increases bone mass in osteoporotic patients under vitamin D supplementation: a randomized, double-blind, placebo-controlled clinical trial. J Clin Endocrinol Metab 90:5031–5036
62. Matsumoto T, Kubodera N (2007) ED-71 Study Group. ED-71, a new active vitamin D3, increases bone mineral density regardless of serum 25(OH)D levels in osteoporotic subjects. J Steroid Biochem Mol Biol 103:584–586
63. Noguchi Y, Kawate H, Nomura M et al (2013) Eldecalcitol for the treatment of osteoporosis. Clin Interv Aging 8:1313–1321
64. Nishikawa T, Ogawa S, Kogita K et al (2000) Additive effects of combined treatment with etidronate and alfacalcidol on bone mass and mechanical properties in ovariectomized rats. Bone 27:647–654
65. Saito M, Shiraishi A, Ito M et al (2010) Comparison of effects of alfacalcidol and alendronate on mechanical properties and bone collagen cross-links of callus in the fracture repair rat model. Bone 46:1170–1179
66. Saito M, Marumo K, Ushiku C et al (2011) Effects of alfacalcidol on mechanical properties and collagen cross-links of the femoral diaphysis in glucocorticoid-treated rats. Calcif Tissue Int 88:314–324
67. Nagaoka H, Terajima M, Yamada S et al (2014) Alfacalcidol enhances collagen quality in ovariectomized rat bones. J Orthop Res 32:1030–1036
68. Shiraishi A, Sakai S, Saito H et al (2014) Eldecalcitol improves mechanical strength of cortical bones by stimulating the periosteal formation in the senescence-accelerated SAM/P6 mice- a comparison with alfacalcidol. J Steroid Biochem Mol Biol 144:119–123
69. Ito M, Nakamura T, Fukunaga M et al (2011) Effect of eldecalcitol, an active vitamin D analog, on hip structure and biomechanical properties: 3D assessment by clinical CT. Bone 49:328–334
70. Girgis CM, Clifton-Bligh RJ, Hamrick MW et al (2013) The roles of vitamin D in skeletal muscle: form, function, and metabolism. Endocr Rev 34:33–83
71. Daly RM, Gagnon C, Lu ZX et al (2012) Prevalence of vitamin D deficiency and its determinants in Australian adults aged 25 years and older: a national, population-based study. Clin Endocrinol (Oxf) 77:26–35
72. Forrest KY, Stuhldreher WL (2011) Prevalence and correlates of vitamin D deficiency in US adults. Nutr Res 31:48–54
73. Visser M, Deeg DJ, Lips P (2003) Longitudinal Aging Study Amsterdam. Low vitamin D and high parathyroid hormone levels as determinants of loss of muscle strength and muscle mass (sarcopenia): the Longitudinal Aging Study Amsterdam. J Clin Endocrinol Metab 88:5766–5772

74. Wicherts LS, van Schoor NM, Boeke AJ et al (2007) Vitamin D status predicts physical performance and its decline in older persons. J Clin Endocrinol Metab 92:2058–2065
75. Pfeifer M, Minne HW (1999) Vitamin D and hip fracture. Trends Endocrinol Metab 10:417–420
76. Sato Y, Inose M, Higuchi I et al (2002) Changes in the supporting muscles of the fractured hip in elderly women. Bone 30:325–330
77. Eriksen EF, Glerup H (2002) Vitamin D deficiency and aging: implications for general health and osteoporosis. Biogerontology 3:73–77
78. Schubert L, DeLuca HF (2010) Hypophosphatemia is responsible for skeletal muscle weakness of vitamin D deficiency. Arch Biochem Biophys 500:157–161
79. Maekawa S, Miyakoshi N, Kasukawa Y et al (2008) Effects of alfacalcidol on muscle strength, fatigue, and bone mineral density in aged rats. Akita J Med 35:53–58
80. Kasukawa Y, Miyakoshi N, Maekawa S et al (2010) Effects of alfacalcidol on muscle strength, muscle fatigue, and bone mineral density in normal and ovariectomized rats. Biomed Res 31:273–279
81. Miyakoshi N, Sasaki H, Kasukawa Y et al (2010) Effects of a vitamin D analog, alfacalcidol, on bone and skeletal muscle in glucocorticoid-treated rats. Biomed Res 31:329–336
82. Bischoff-Ferrari HA, Dawson-Hughes B et al (2011) Relevance of vitamin D deficiency in adult fracture and fall prevention. In: Vitamin D, vol 2. Elsevier, London, pp 114–1154
83. Moreira-Pfrimer LD, Pedrosa MA, Teixeira L et al (2009) Treatment of vitamin D deficiency increases lower limb muscle strength in institutionalized older people independently of regular physical activity: a randomized double-blind controlled trial. Ann Nutr Metab 54:291–300
84. Zhu K, Austin N, Devine A et al (2010) A randomized controlled trial of the effects of vitamin D on muscle strength and mobility in older women with vitamin D insufficiency. J Am Geriatr Soc 58:2063–2068
85. Stockton KA, Kandiah DA, Paratz JD et al (2012) Fatigue, muscle strength and vitamin D status in women with systemic lupus erythematosus compared with healthy controls. Lupus 21:271–278
86. Schacht E, Ringe JD (2012) Alfacalcidol improves muscle power, muscle function and balance in elderly patients with reduced bone mass. Rheumatol Int 32:207–215
87. Verhaar HJJ, Samson MM, Jansen PAF et al (2000) Muscle strength, functional mobility and vitamin D in older women. Aging Clin Exp Res 12:455–460
88. Hara S, Kishimoto KN, Okuno H et al (2013) Effects of alfacalcidol on back extensor strength gained through back extensor exercise in postmenopausal women with osteoporosis. Am J Phys Med Rehabil 92:101–110
89. Koike T, Okawa T, Wada M et al (2003) Effects of a long-term alfacalcidol or calcitonin administration on body sway in Japanese elderly women. J Bone Miner Res 18:S168
90. Ito S, Harada A, Kasai T et al (2014) Use of alfacalcidol in osteoporotic patients with low muscle mass might increase muscle mass: an investigation using a patient database. Geriatr Gerontol Int 14:122–128
91. Latham NK, Anderson CS, Lee A et al (2003) A randomized, controlled trial of quadriceps resistance exercise and vitamin D in frail older people: the frailty interventions trial in elderly subjects (FITNESS). J Am Geriatr Soc 51:291–299
92. Stockton KA, Mengersen K, Paratz JD et al (2012) Effect of vitamin D supplementation on muscle strength: a systematic review and meta-analysis. Osteoporos Int 22:859–871
93. Annweiler C, Schott AM, Berrut G et al (2009) Vitamin D-related changes in physical performance: a systematic review. J Nutr Health Aging 13:893–898
94. Sorensen OH, Lund B, Saltin B et al (1979) Myopathy in bone loss of ageing: improvement by treatment with 1 alpha-hydroxycholecalciferol and calcium. Clin Sci (Lond) 56:157–161
95. Sato Y, Iwamoto J, Kanoko T et al (2005) Low-dose vitamin D prevents muscular atrophy and reduces falls and hip fractures in women after stroke: a randomized controlled trial. Cerebrovasc Dis 20:187–192

96. Tanaka K, Kanazawa I, Yamaguchi T et al (2014) Active vitamin D possesses beneficial effects on the interaction between muscle and bone. Biochem Biophys Res Commun 450:482–487
97. Kinoshita H, Miyakoshi N, Hongo M et al (2014) Effects of eldecalcitol on body weight, bone mineral density and skeletal muscle in glucocorticoid-treated rats. http://www.asbmr.org/education/AbstractDetail?aid=288c5019-54bd-4dc4-88e4-24d77b687691. Accessed 5 Dec 2014
98. Sakai S, Suzuki M, Tashiro Y et al (2014) Vitamin D receptor signaling enhances locomotive ability in mice. J Bone Miner Res. doi:10.1002/jbmr.2317
99. Iwamoto J, Sato Y (2014) Eldecalcitol improves chair-rising time in postmenopausal osteoporotic women treated with bisphosphonate. Ther Clin Risk Manag 16:51–59
100. Saito K, Miyakoshi N, Hongo M et al (2013) Active vitamin D3 analog (eldecalcitol) improves muscle strength and dynamic balance in postmenopausal osteoporotic women. J Bone Miner Res 28. http://www.asbmr.org/education/AbstractDetail?aid=908e77b4-cca8-44f8-93d6-c72aa61d6d62. Accessed 5 Dec 2014
101. Boland R (1986) Role of vitamin D in skeletal muscle function. Endocrinol Rev 7:434–448
102. Boland R, de Boland AR, Marinissen MJ et al (1995) Avian muscle cells as targets for the secosteroid hormone 1,25-dihydroxy-vitamin D3. Mol Cell Endocrinol 114:1–8
103. Hamilton B (2009) Vitamin D and human skeletal muscle. Scand J Med Sci Sports 20:182–190
104. de Boland AR, Boland RL (1993) 1,25-dihydroxyvitamin D-3 induces arachidonate mobilization in embryonic chick myoblasts. Biochim Biophys Acta 1179:98–104
105. Gillespie LD, Gillespie WJ, Robertson MC et al (2003) Interventions for preventing falls in elderly people. Cochrane Database Syst Rev 4:CD000340
106. Vellas BJ, Wayne SJ, Romero LJ et al (1997) Fear of falling and restriction of mobility in elderly fallers. Age Ageing 26:189–193
107. Flicker L, Mead K, Maclnnis RJ et al (2003) Serum vitamin D and falls in older women in residential care in Australia. J Am Geriatr Soc 51:1533–1538
108. Snijder MB, van Schoor NM, Pluijm SM et al (2006) Vitamin D status in relation to one-year risk of recurrent falling in older men and women. J Clin Endocrinol Metab 91:2980–2985
109. Stein MS, Wark JD, Scherer SC et al (1999) Falls relate to vitamin D and parathyroid hormone in an Australian nursing home and hostel. J Am Geriatr Soc 47:1195–1201
110. Bischoff-Ferrari HA, Dawson-Hughes B, Willett WC, Staehelin HB, Bazemore MG, Zee RY, Wong JB (2004) Effect of Vitamin D on falls: a meta-analysis. JAMA 291:1999–2006
111. Bischoff-Ferrari HA, Willette WC, Wong JB et al (2009) Prevention of nonvertebral fractures with oral vitamin D and dose dependence: a meta-analysis of randomized controlled trials. Arch Int Med 169:551
112. Murad MH, Elamin KB, Abu Elnour NO et al (2011) The effect of vitamin D on falls: a systematic review and meta-analysis. J Clin Endocrinol Metab 96:2997–3006
113. Graafmans WC, Ooms ME, Hofstee HM et al (1996) Falls in the elderly: a prospective study of risk factors and risk profiles. Am J Epidemiol 143:1129–1136
114. Broe KE, Chen TC, Weinberg J et al (2007) A higher dose of vitamin D reduces the risk of falls in nursing home residents: a randomized, multiple-dose study. J Am Geriatr Soc 55:234–239
115. Grant AM, Avenell A, Campbell MK et al (2005) Oral vitamin D3 and calcium for secondary prevention of low-trauma fractures in elderly people (Randomised evaluation of calcium or vitamin D, RECORD): a randomised placebo-controlled trial. Lancet 365:1621–1628
116. Porthouse J, Cockayne S, King C et al (2005) Randomised controlled trial of calcium and supplementation with cholecalciferol (vitamin D3) for prevention of fractures in primary care. BMJ 330:1003
117. Dukas L, Bischoff HA, Lindpaintner LS et al (2004) Alfacalcidol reduces the number of fallers in a community-dwelling elderly population with a minimum calcium intake of more than 500 mg daily. J Am Geriatr Soc 52:230–236

118. Fujita T, Nakamura S, Ohue M et al (2007) Postural stabilizing effect of alfacalcidol and active absorbable algal calcium (AAA Ca) compared with calcium carbonate assessed by computerized posturography. J Bone Miner Metab 25:68–73
119. Dukas L, Schacht E, Runge M et al (2010) Effect of a six-month therapy with alfacalcidol on muscle power and balance and the number of fallers and falls. Arzneimittelforschung 60:519–525
120. Matsumoto T, Ito M, Hayashi Y et al (2011) A new active vitamin D3 analog, eldecalcitol, prevents the risk of osteoporotic fractures – a randomized, active comparator, double-blind study. Bone 49:605–612
121. Morris HA, Morrison GW, Burr M et al (1984) Vitamin D and femoral neck fractures in elderly South Australian women. Med J Aust 140:519–521
122. Lidor C, Sagiv P, Amdur B et al (1993) Decrease in bone levels of 1,25-dihydroxyvitamin D in women with subcapital fracture of the femur. Calcif Tissue Int 52:146–148
123. Lai JK, Lucas RM, Clements MS et al (2010) Hip fracture risk in relation to vitamin D supplementation and serum 25-hydroxyvitamin D levels: a systematic review and meta-analysis of randomized controlled trials and observational studies. BMC Public Health 10:331
124. Lips P, van Ginkel FC, Jongen MJ et al (1987) Determinants of vitamin D status in patients with hip fracture and in elderly control subjects. Am J Clin Nutr 46:1005–1010
125. Bischoff-Ferrari HA, Willett WC, Orav EJ et al (2012) A pooled analysis of vitamin D dose requirements for fracture prevention. N Engl J Med 367:40–49
126. Jackson RD, LaCroix AZ, Gass M et al (2006) Calcium plus vitamin D supplementation and the risk of fractures. N Engl J Med 354:669–683
127. Avenell A, Gillespie WJ, Gillespie LD et al (2009) Vitamin D and vitamin D analogues for preventing fractures associated with involutional and post-menopausal osteoporosis. Cochrane Database Syst Rev 15:CD000227. doi:10.1002/14651858.CD000227.pub3
128. Gallagher JC, Riggs BL, Recker RR et al (1989) The effect of calcitriol on patients with postmenopausal osteoporosis with special reference to fracture frequency. Proc Soc Exp Biol Med 191:287–292
129. Tilyard MW, Spears GF, Thomson J et al (1992) Treatment of postmenopausal osteoporosis with calcitriol or calcium. N Engl J Med 326:357–362
130. Richy F, Ethgen O, Bruyere O et al (2004) Efficacy of alphacalcidol and calcitriol in primary and corticosteroid-induced osteoporosis: a meta-analysis of their effects on bone mineral density and fracture rate. Osteoporos Int 15:301–310
131. Richy F, Schacht E, Bryere O et al (2005) Vitamin D analogs versus native vitamin D in preventing bone loss and osteoporosis-related fractures: a comparative meta-analysis. Calcif Tissue Int 76:176–186
132. Hagino H, Takano T, Fukunaga M et al (2013) Eldecalcitol reduces the risk of severe vertebral fractures and improves the health-related quality of life in patients with osteoporosis. J Bone Miner Metab 31:183–189
133. Nakamura T, Takano T, Fukunaga M et al (2013) Eldecalcitol is more effective for the prevention of osteoporotic fractures than alfacalcidol. J Bone Miner Metab 31:417–422

Chapter 10
Applications of Teriparatide for Fracture Repair and Osteosynthetic Surgery in Osteoporosis

Koji Nozaka, Naohisa Miyakoshi, and Yoichi Shimada

Abstract Teriparatide (TPTD), consisting of amino acids 1–34 of human parathyroid hormone (PTH), is a powerful systemic bone anabolic agent that increases osteoblastic activity, decreases osteoblast apoptosis, and improves bone quality. TPTD enhances cancellous bone healing at the site of osteotomy with, at least in part, a local regulating action that increases osteoblastogenesis and decreases adipocytogenesis. In addition, TPTD administered before osteosynthesis stimulates cancellous bone union in rat. TPTD treatment may also have positive effects on bone-hydroxyapatite (HA) block bonding in patients with osteoporosis by increasing cancellous bone formation and enhancing cancellous bone healing around the HA block. Use of TPTD accelerated the fusion rate and shortened the duration of fusion after instrumented lumbar posterolateral fusion in women with postmenopausal osteoporosis. Furthermore, TPTD led to early clinical and radiological improvement of chronic nonunion fractures of the upper and lower extremities, with subsequent complete healing. In bisphosphonate-associated atypical femoral fractures (AFFs), TPTD treatment appears to significantly shorten the postoperative time to fracture healing and reduces rates of delayed healing or nonunion after bisphosphonate-associated AFFs.

Keywords Teriparatide • Osteosynthetic surgery • Bone union

10.1 TPTD as a Bone Anabolic Agent

10.1.1 TPTD Results in a Skeletal Anabolic Response

Teriparatide (TPTD), a portion of human parathyroid hormone (PTH) consisting of amino acid sequences 1 through 34, is a powerful systemic bone anabolic agent that increases osteoblastic activity, decreases osteoblast apoptosis, and improves bone

K. Nozaka, M.D., Ph.D. (✉) • N. Miyakoshi • Y. Shimada
Department of Orthopedic Surgery, Akita University Graduate School of Medicine, 1-1-1 Hondo, Akita 010-8543, Japan
e-mail: nozakak@doc.med.akita-u.ac.jp

Y. Shimada, N. Miyakoshi (eds.), *Osteoporosis in Orthopedics*,
DOI 10.1007/978-4-431-55778-4_10

quality [1, 2]. Parathyroid cells sense extracellular calcium concentration via the calcium-sensing receptors and secrete PTH in response to calcium level decrease [3]. Subsequently, TPTD mobilizes calcium from skeletal stores, stimulates release of calcium (and phosphate) by activation of bone resorption, increases renal tubular calcium reabsorption, and indirectly enhances intestinal calcium absorption via its stimulatory action on renal 1α-cholecalciferol hydroxylase [4]. TPTD is considered to have mixed catabolic and anabolic effects on the skeleton. Long-standing hyperparathyroidism causes osteoporosis of predominantly cortical bone (forearm and hip), while it relatively preserves cancellous bone (spine) [3]. On the other hand, intermittent administration of low-dose TPTD results in a skeletal anabolic response, more obvious in the cancellous than in the cortical bone, due to direct effects on cells of the osteoblastic lineage and indirect effects through the regulation of selected skeletal growth factors [5]. However, little is known about the effects of TPTD on cancellous bone healing after cancellous bone fractures or osteotomies [6–8]. There is increasing evidence from animal research [9] and small clinical series [10–13] that TPTD can enhance fracture healing, which suggests that it may be a useful adjuvant in the treatment of nonunion fractures. In 1999, Andreassen et al. reported that intermittent administration of a high dose of TPTD (200 μg of PTH(1–34)/kg/day) is able to enhance callus volume and the mechanical strength of fractures after both 20 and 40 days of healing [14]. A lower TPTD dose (60 μg of PTH (1–34)/kg/day) in the dose range normally used when investigating the anabolic effects of TPTD on rats does not influence healing of fractures after the first 20 days, but after 40 days of healing, this dose causes a substantial increase in callus volume and the mechanical strength of the fractures.

10.1.2 TPTD Enhances Fracture Strength

In old rats, Andreassen et al. reported the effects of intermittent administration of TPTD on callus formation and mechanical strength of tibial fractures in 27-month-old rats after 3 and 8 weeks of healing [14]. TPTD treatment enhances fracture strength, callus volume, and callus bone mineral content (BMC) after 3 and 8 weeks of healing. Currently, TPTD is the only proven bone anabolic therapy [3], whereas data attributing bone anabolic properties to classic antiresorptive agents, such as bisphosphonates [15, 16] or the strontium ranelate (originally considered as a mixed agent) [17], are not consistently replicated [18]. Alkhiary et al. reported that TPTD enhances fracture healing by increasing BMC and density and strength, and it produces a sustained anabolic effect throughout the remodeling phase of fracture healing [18]. A systemically administered drug that enhances bone repair could have widespread applications to promote the healing of fractures and arthrodesis sites and to promote osteointegration in porous implants. TPTD is the first bone formation agent shown to be effective for the systemic treatment of a bone disease and may represent an attractive new modality for the management of these musculoskeletal conditions.

10.1.3 TPTD Increases Bone Mineral Density and Bone Quality

Intermittent TPTD administration exerts its effects via several molecular actions [5], including but not limited to prevention of osteoblast apoptosis [20], induction of insulin-like growth factor I(IGF-1) synthesis [1, 21], inhibition of sclerostin expression [22],activation of Wnt signaling [23], and induction of transcriptional factors, such as Runx2 [24]. TPTD affects the synthesis of many osteogenic growth factors and cytokines, such as basic fibroblast growth factor and transforming growth factor-β [25]. These anabolic effects of TPTD result in the enhancement of fracture healing by accelerating callus formation and remodeling in rats [14] and monkeys [26]. In humans, TPTD can improve cancellous bone microarchitecture [27], increase vertebral bone mineral density (BMD) [28], and decrease the risk of vertebral and nonvertebral fractures. In addition, several studies have reported that intermittent administration of TPTD also enhances fracture healing of cortical and cancellous bones in osteoporotic conditions induced by estrogen deficiency [19, 29]. Intermittent TPTD has been shown to increase the osteoblast number and their activity, the bone remodeling rate along with the amount of bone deposited in each remodeling cycle, trabecular thickness and trabecular connectivity, and cortical thickness and bone size [4]. Thus, TPTD increases not only bone mass but also bone quality by improving microarchitecture and geometry [2, 30, 31]. TPTD increased the total contents of immature and mature enzymatic cross-links, which contributed significantly to cancellous bone strength [31]. This mode of action is different from that of antiresorptives, which mainly act by maintaining skeletal architecture and decelerating bone turnover. TPTD could also be considered in the treatment of male osteoporosis [32] as well as in glucocorticoid-induced osteoporosis [33]. Another debatable issue is the effect of TPTD treatment on the cortical bone; either no change or a decrease in BMD at cortical bone sites (radius) has been reported with TPTD treatment [28].

10.1.4 Fracture Risk Reduction with TPTD

Intermittent daily administration of 20 or 40 μg of TPTD over a median duration of 19 months was associated with a statistically significant reduction in vertebral and nonvertebral fractures in women with low bone mass [28]. Since the higher dose scheme was associated with a similar effect on bone fragility but a significantly higher risk of adverse events (such as hypercalcemia and hypercalciuria), the 20 μg dose per day, associated with a 65 % reduction in radiographic vertebral fractures, was selected for commercial use. These changes may be attributed to a decrease in secondary mineralization of newly formed osteoid and are probably counteracted by an increase in cortical bone diameter [3].

10.2 TPTD Enhances Bone Union in Animal Study

10.2.1 TPTD Enhances Cancellous Bone Union

In the clinical setting, osteoporotic fractures frequently occur in cancellous bone-rich sites rather than in cortical bone-rich sites [34]. We reported a cancellous bone osteotomy model in normal and ovariectomized (OVX) rats to evaluate the in vivo effects of intermittent administration of TPTD on cancellous bone healing at the osteotomy site under normal and osteoporotic conditions [6]. In addition, the rate of bone union at the surgical site was evaluated after TPTD treatment. Furthermore, to elucidate the mechanisms of cancellous bone healing induced by TPTD, the proliferation kinetics of bone marrow cells and adipose cells surrounding the site of osteotomy were evaluated in combination with conventional cancellous bone histomorphometry. Assessment of cancellous bone union at the osteotomy site (Fig. 10.1), the rate of cellular proliferation as determined by proliferating cell nuclear antigen (PCNA) immunostaining, and adipocytes in the surrounding bone marrow were evaluated. TPTD increased cancellous bone volume by stimulating bone formation in both normal and OVX rats and suppressing adipocyte volume. The percentage of PCNA-positive cells at the osteotomy site after TPTD treatment was two- to threefold higher than that of vehicle treatment controls both in sham-operated and OVX rats (Fig. 10.2). The magnitude of increase in the percentage of

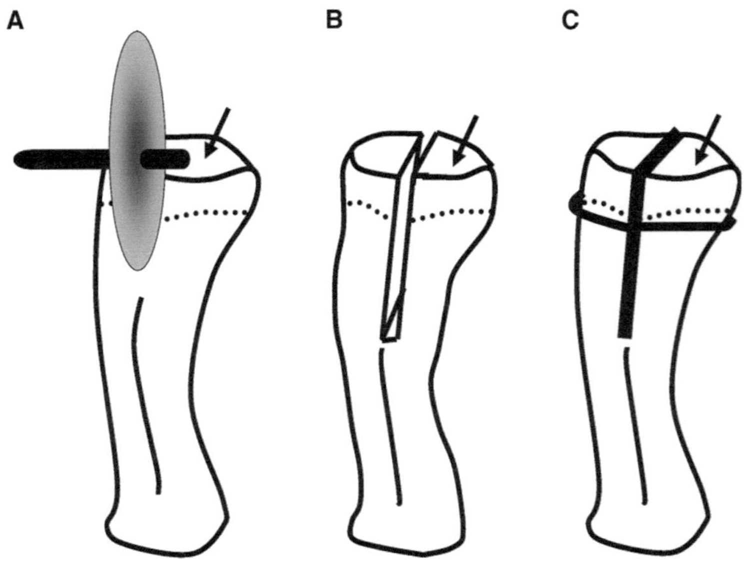

Fig. 10.1 Schema of surgical procedure of cancellous bone osteotomy. Complete midsagittal osteotomy from the knee joint surface (*small arrow*) to the tibial diaphysis was performed using an electrically powered bone saw (**a**, **b**). The osteotomized proximal tibia was then fixed with a cerclage wiring (0.4 mm diameter) circumferentially (**c**). The *dotted line* indicates the growth plate of the proximal tibia (Reprinted with permission)

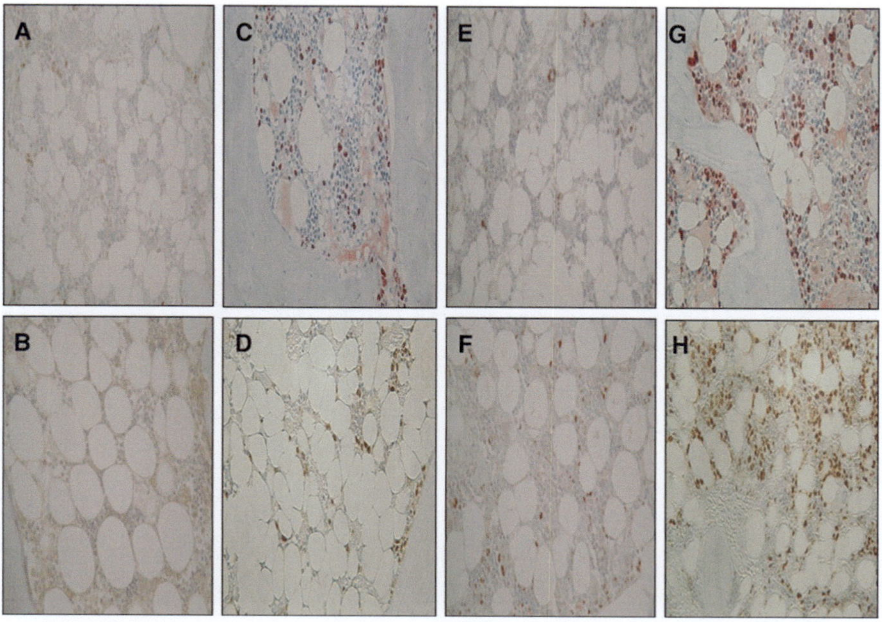

Fig. 10.2 Higher magnification of immunohistochemical analysis of PCNA at the non-osteotomy site and osteotomy site. Five randomized ROIs were analyzed at the bone marrow between the osteotomy line and endosteal surface in the proximal tibia, which corresponded to the measurement area of fat histomorphometry. PCNA-positive cells are identified as the cells stained with *dark reddish-brown dye* in the bone marrow. Sections at the non-osteotomy site from the vehicle-treated sham group (**a**), vehicle-treated OVX group (**b**), TPTD-treated sham group (**e**), and TPTD-treated OVX group (**f**). Sections at the osteotomy site from the vehicle-treated sham group (**c**), vehicle-treated OVX group (**d**), TPTD-treated sham group (**g**), and TPTD-treated OVX group (**h**). A large amount of PCNA-positive cells is observed in the sections from the osteotomy site (**c**, **d**, **g**, and **h**), especially in the sections from the TPTD-treated animals (**g** and **h**) (Reprinted with permission)

PCNA-positive cells after TPTD treatment at the osteotomy site was twice that at the non-osteotomy site. Furthermore, TPTD treatment increased cancellous bone union after osteotomy both in sham-operated and OVX rats. These results suggest that TPTD enhances cancellous bone healing at the site of osteotomy with, at least in part, a local regulating action that increases osteoblastogenesis and decreases adipocytogenesis at and around the osteotomy.

10.2.2 TPTD Before Osteosynthesis Stimulates Cancellous Bone Union

It has been reported that intermittent administration of TPTD promotes bone healing after surgery for osteoporotic fractures [6]. If bone healing is promoted by the administration of TPTD during the preoperative waiting period, prolonged

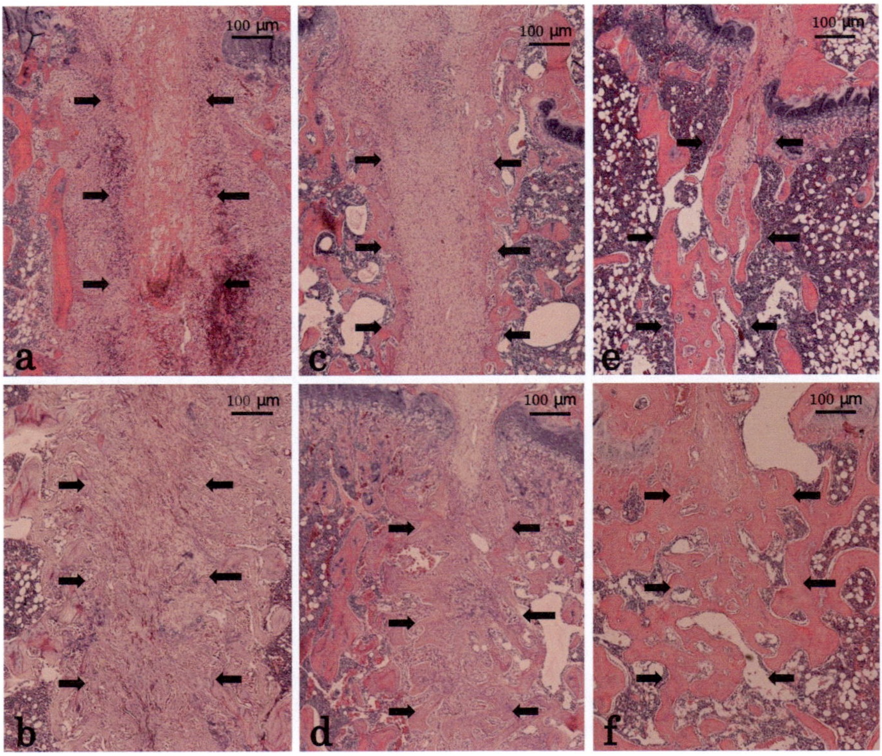

Fig. 10.3 Histological sections stained with hematoxylin and eosin at the osteotomy site. Shown are the histological sections stained with hematoxylin and eosin at the osteotomy site with a magnification of 40 x. Osteotomy sites are showed by *arrows*. One week after the osteotomy, the amount of new cartilage and woven bone produced in the TPTD group (**b**) was greater than that in the vehicle group (**a**). Two weeks after the osteotomy, the amount of remodeled new cancellous bones observed at the osteotomy site in the TPTD-TPTD group (**d**) was greater than that in the vehicle-vehicle group (**c**). Four weeks after the osteotomy, bone union was almost finished in both the TPTD-TPTD (**f**) group and vehicle-vehicle (**e**) group (Reprinted with permission)

bed rest can be prevented. Conversely, it has also been reported that pretreatment with intermittent TPTD administration is not effective for bone union [29]. However, Tsuchie et al. evaluated the effects of TPTD treatment on bone union in the period before osteosynthesis surgery after a fracture occurred [8]. Wire fixation surgery resulted in significant enhancement of bone union after an osteotomy of the proximal tibia over that of sham surgery, with an obvious effect on cancellous bone union after osteosynthesis surgery (Fig. 10.1) [6]. OVX rats underwent an osteotomy of the proximal tibia as a fracture model, and TPTD or vehicle was administered as a preoperative treatment for 1 week. After treatment, the tibiae were fixed with wire for osteosynthesis, and TPTD or vehicle was administered. A number of parameters were investigated: bone histomorphometry, Alcian Blue/hematoxylin staining, and PCNA, Sox9, and Runx2 (Figs. 10.3 and 10.4). Preoperative treatment with TPTD significantly increased bone volume, bone union, and

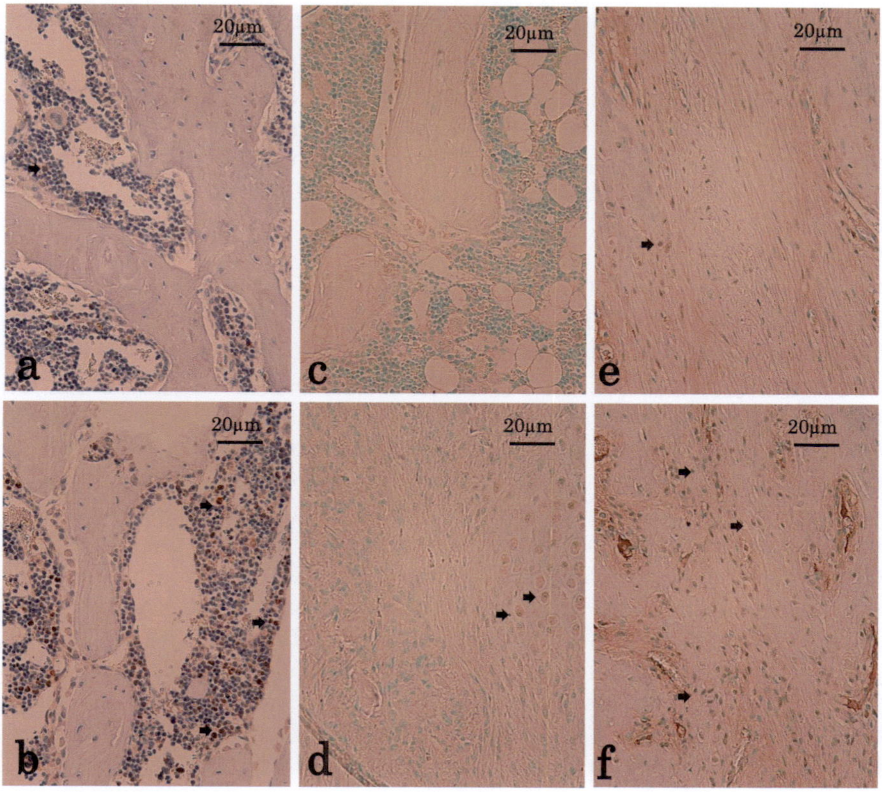

Fig. 10.4 Immunostaining for PCNA, Sox9, and Runx2 at the osteotomy site. Shown are the sections immunostained with antibodies against PCNA (**a** and **b**), Sox9 (**c** and **d**), and Runx2 (**e** and **f**) at the osteotomy site with a magnification of 200 x. Immunostained positive cells stained *dark reddish-brown dye* (some of them are showed by *arrows*). Four weeks after the osteotomy, PCNA-positive cell numbers in the TPTD-TPTD group (**b**) were higher than those in the vehicle-vehicle (**a**) group. Some Sox9-positive cells were observed in the TPTD group at 1 week (**d**), but there were hardly any Sox9-positive cells in the TPTD-TPTD group at 4 weeks (**c**). Two weeks after the osteotomy, Runx2-positive cell numbers in the TPTD-TPTD group (**f**) were higher than those in the vehicle-vehicle (**e**) group (Reprinted with permission)

cartilage volume. Bone union was also promoted by pre- to postoperative treatment with TPTD for 2 weeks. This treatment also significantly increased the percentage of cells positive for Runx2, but not PCNA or Sox9. Preoperative administration of TPTD enhances bone union by promoting cartilage formation and cell differentiation to osteoblasts, but not by promoting cell proliferation. A number of factors are thought to be involved in the stimulation of bone formation by TPTD, such as the promotion of Runx2, IGF-1, and activating protein-I, and the suppression of sclerostin and Smad ubiquitin regulatory factor (Smurf) [21, 35–39]. The Wnt family has also been implicated in the actions of TPTD on the bone [40].

10.2.3 TPTD Improves Bone-Hydroxyapatite Block Bonding

HA blocks have been widely used for the reconstruction of bone defects and as a bone substitute. Bone-implant bonding depends on both implant-related factors and patient variables. Kamo et al. evaluated whether intermittent TPTD administration enhances bone-HA block bonding in normal versus OVX rats. Cancellous bone osteotomy and HA-block implantation were performed in rats (Fig. 10.5) [7]. Newly formed cancellous bone around the HA block and bone-HA block bonding were evaluated. The administration of TPTD significantly increased cancellous bone volume by stimulating bone formation in OVX rats. Although bone-HA block bonding was significantly decreased in OVX rats compared with that of sham-operated rats, TPTD improved the bone-HA block bonding in OVX rats (Fig. 10.6). These results suggest that TPTD treatment may improve bone-HA bonding in osteoporosis by restoring cancellous bone volume and enhancing cancellous bone formation around the HA block. Figure 10.7 illustrates the HA block interface with fluorescent labels under UV light. Most of the fluorescent label at the newly formed trabecular bone on the HA blocks was observed in the sham-vehicle (Fig. 10.7a) and sham-TPTD (Fig. 10.7b) groups. TPTD treatment stimulated fluorescent labeling on the newly formed trabecular bone on the HA blocks even in the OVX groups (Fig. 10.7d). More osteoid was observed in the OVX-TPTD group (Fig. 10.7d), but not in the OVX-vehicle group (Fig. 10.7c), at the newly formed trabecular bone on the HA blocks compared to those in sham-vehicle (Fig. 10.7a) or sham-TPTD groups (Fig. 10.7b). However, there were no fluorescent labels at the interface between HA blocks and trabecular bones in any group.

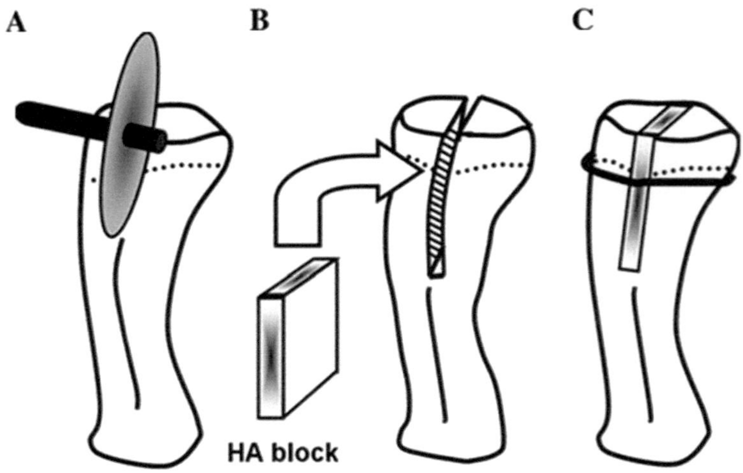

Fig. 10.5 Schema of cancellous bone osteotomy and implantation of HA block. Complete midsagittal osteotomy from the knee joint surface to the tibial diaphysis was performed using an electrically powered bone saw (**a**). The osteotomized proximal tibia was opened bilaterally, and the HA block was placed in the osteotomy site (**b**) and then fixed with a cerclage wiring (0.4 mm diameter) circumferentially (**c**). The *dotted line* indicates the growth plate of the proximal tibia (Reprinted with permission)

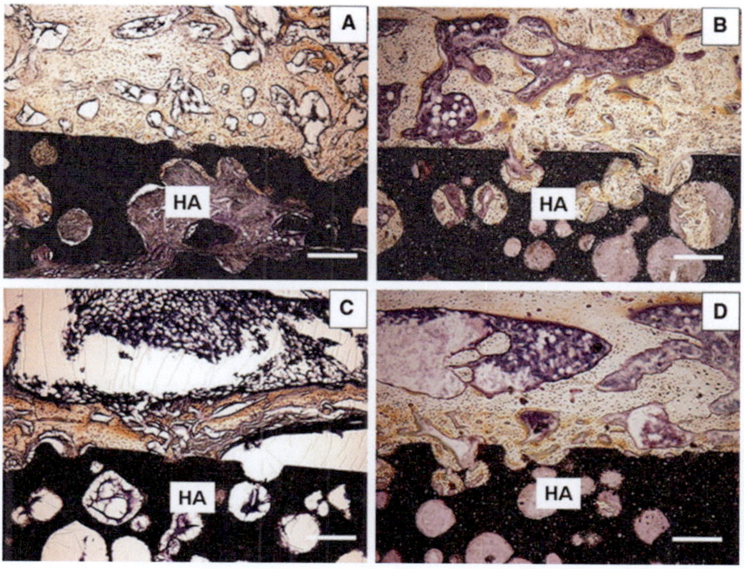

Fig. 10.6 Mid-frontal sections of the HA block interface stained with Villanueva bone stain. (**a**) Sham-vehicle group, (**b**) sham-TPTD group, (**c**) OVX-vehicle group, (**d**) OVX-TPTD group. *Bars* 300 μm. *HA* hydroxyapatite block (×40) (Reprinted with permission)

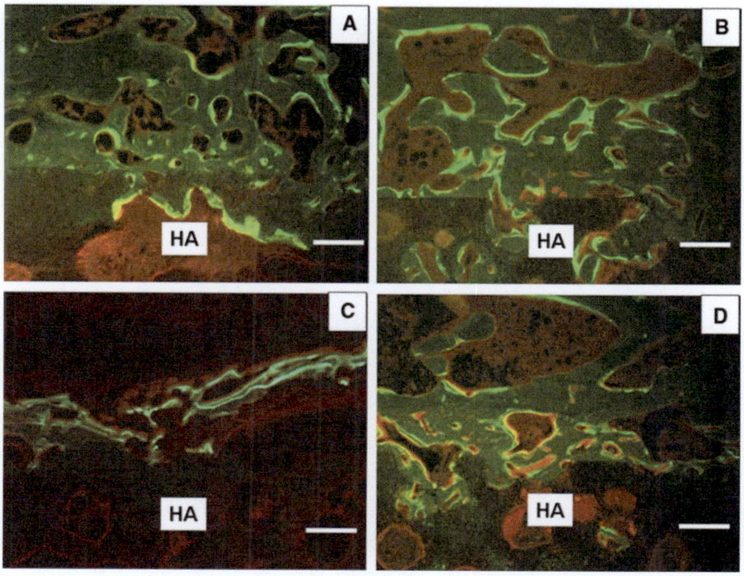

Fig. 10.7 Mid-frontal sections of the HA block interface with fluorescent labels under UV light. (**a**) Sham-vehicle group, (**b**) sham-TPTD group, (**c**) OVX-vehicle group, (**d**) OVX-TPTD group. *Bars* 300 μm. *HA* hydroxyapatite block (×40) (Reprinted with permission)

10.3 TPTD for Spine Surgery

10.3.1 TPTD Accelerates Lumbar Posterolateral Fusion

TPTD has been shown to enhance spinal fusion in women with coexisting postmenopausal osteoporosis when given after surgery for spondylolisthesis and to be more effective than oral bisphosphonates. Use of TPTD accelerated the fusion rate and shortened the duration of fusion after instrumented lumbar posterolateral fusion in women with postmenopausal osteoporosis. Ohtori et al. concluded that if other bone substitutes are not available, TPTD may be an option for improvement of spinal fusion. Preclinical data also support the use of TPTD for lumbar spinal fusion: in a rabbit model of posterolateral intertransverse arthrodesis, TPTD was shown to enhance spinal fusion after an autogenous iliac crest bone graft [41–43]. Lehman et al. reported that TPTD enhances spinal fusion, while calcitonin has a neutral effect [42]. TPTD elicited the best histologic fusion rate, while the calcitonin was similar to saline controls. Although not significant, TPTD treatment showed a strong trend toward superior radiographic fusion over calcitonin treatment in a rabbit spinal fusion model. TPTD administration increased posterolateral fusion success in rabbits [43]. Fusion bone mass and histologic determinants were also improved with TPTD treatment. These results suggest that TPTD shows promise for use as an adjunctive agent to improve spinal fusion in clinical medicine [41, 44]. Additional studies, in rats that underwent posterolateral spinal arthrodesis surgery using autologous bone grafts, showed that intermittent administration of TPTD enhanced bone turnover dominantly on bone formation at the graft site, accelerating spinal fusion [45]. This study suggests that intermittent injection of TPTD might be an efficient adjuvant intervention in spinal arthrodesis surgery and other skeletal reconstruction surgeries requiring bone grafts. Together, these studies suggest that TPTD may be one of the options for enhancing spinal fusion in women with postmenopausal osteoporosis.

10.3.2 TPTD Increases the Insertional Torque of Pedicle Screws During Fusion Surgery

The use of pedicle screws has become common in spinal surgery. However, Inoue et al. reported that, despite their clinical usefulness, they are associated with mechanical problems, such as implant breakage, screw loosening, and other related failures, sometimes requiring revision surgery [44]. The frequency of screw loosening reported in the literature varies from 0.6 to 27 % [46–49]. Considerable problems exist both with the mechanical properties of the implants and with the standardization and accuracy of the operative techniques used. Osteoporosis is a very important risk factor for pedicle screw failure because BMD is reported to be highly correlated with the stability of the pedicle screw [50, 51]. Inoue et al. reported a study where postmenopausal women with osteoporosis underwent instrumented fusion surgery with or without at least 1 month of preoperative TPTD treatment [44]. TPTD significantly increased pedicle screw insertional torque during surgery compared with the values in patients who did not receive preoperative TPTD therapy (controls). The biomechanical pullout strength of pedicle screw fixation was in direct proportion to the torque at the time of screw insertion. A high correlation was found between insertional torque and BMD. Insertional torque is significantly lower in patients with osteoporosis than in those without osteoporosis, with a negative relationship reported between insertional torque and the grade of osteoporosis [44]. TPTD affects insertional torque regardless of screw length, but the effect is greater with longer screws. TPTD, administered daily for 2 months before surgery, reduced the incidence of pedicle screw loosening after instrumented lumbar fusion in postmenopausal women with osteoporosis, suggesting that TPTD increased not only bone mass but also the quality of the pedicle cortex.

10.4 TPTD for Fractures of Extremities

10.4.1 TPTD as a Systemic Treatment for Extremity Fractures

A clinical trial using TPTD for treatment of distal radial fractures was reported in [52]. Postmenopausal women who had sustained a dorsally angulated distal radial fracture in need of dosed reduction, but without surgery, were randomly assigned to 8 weeks of placebo or TPTD. The investigators concluded that the time to healing was shorter in the TPTD-treated group. Average periods of bone union and fusion rate in the TPTD group, as evaluated by radiographic imaging and by CT, were significantly superior to those in the placebo group. Systemic administration of TPTD to accelerate fracture union is an attractive option, which becomes particularly relevant in situations in which a high surgical risk exists.

10.4.2 TPTD for Nonunion/Delayed Fractures

Most adult fractures of the extremity necessitate surgical treatment. High-energy trauma, significant soft tissue injury, inaccurate reduction, unstable fixation, infection, alcohol abuse, advanced age, diabetes, corticosteroid treatment, and osteoporosis have been reported as risk factors of nonunion [53, 54]. Use of TPTD for the treatment of nonunion, particularly atrophic nonunion, is based on its osteogenic effect and has been demonstrated in case series [10–13]. The high prevalence of nonunions in spite of improved surgical techniques has directed research efforts toward development of novel treatments to increase bone formation and accelerate fracture repair [55].

Mancilla EE et al. reported a retrospective series of patients treated for nonunion fractures of the lower extremity to evaluate the efficacy of TPTD on fracture healing and union as well as bone remodeling [56]. TPTD is approved for postmenopausal osteoporosis and glucocorticoid-induced osteoporosis in patients with high risk for fractures; therefore, this was an off-label use in most cases. TPTD led to early clinical and radiological improvement of chronic nonunion fractures of the lower extremities, with complete healing over 3–9 months. Two randomized case control trials examined whether TPTD might accelerate fracture healing when used during the initial treatment of fractures [52, 57]. On the other hand, there are only clinical case reports of one to three patients that describe the use of TPTD for management of fracture nonunion. Improved healing was observed with TPTD treatment in two cases of metatarsal stress fractures, three patients with type III odontoid fractures, an atrophic femoral nonunion, a sternal nonunion, three femoral fractures, one tibial fracture, and a humeral shaft nonunion [10, 12, 13, 58–62]. In relation to the form and dose of TPTD, most reports describe the use of TPTD, and all the trials and case reports in humans have employed doses of TPTD that are approved for treatment of postmenopausal osteoporosis. The standard parenteral dose of TPTD appears to be safe and effective in accelerating healing of lower extremity nonunion/delayed union fractures.

10.4.3 Combined Therapy with Low-Intensity Pulsed Ultrasound and TPTD for Fracture Healing

Few options exist for the conservative treatment of delayed union and nonunion fractures, including low-intensity pulsed ultrasound (LIPUS), electrical stimulation, and extracorporeal shock waves [63]. Recently, LIPUS was used for the treatment for Alagille syndrome, Charcot joint, and leg lengthening [64–68]. The good clinical healing in the present case indicates that these mechanisms are induced by LIPUS and that the effects are enough for the healing of fractures associated with this condition. Warden et al. reported that there were no interactions between TPTD and LIPUS indicating that their effects were additive rather than synergistic [69]. These additive effects were contrasting with LIPUS primarily increasing total callus volume (TV) without influencing BMC and TPTD having the opposite effect of increasing BMC without influencing TV. TPTD may have utility in the treatment of acute bone fractures, whereas LIPUS does not appear to be indicated in the management of closed, diaphyseal fractures in rat studies. Fracture healing is a complex biologic process and is impacted by multiple factors [59]. We reported a case of diaphyseal nonunion with deterioration of bone quality in long bone resolved with LIPUS and TPTD [70]. A combination of LIPUS and TPTD without a second surgical intervention was found to accelerate fracture-healing processes, with no side effects, in a nonunion patient with deteriorated bone quality.

10.4.4 Treatment of Atypical Femoral Fractures (AFFs) with TPTD

Bone remodeling suppressants like the bisphosphonates reduce bone loss and slow progression of structural decay. As remodeling removes damaged bone, when remodeling suppression is protracted, bone quality may be compromised predisposing to microdamage accumulation and atypical femoral fractures. Chiang CY et al. reported TPTD therapy assists in healing of atypical fractures and improves bone quality in patients with bisphosphonate-associated atypical femoral fractures [71]. TPTD treatment increases bone remodeling resulting in the removal of more completely mineralized bone and replacement with newly synthesized and less densely mineralized bone, the opposite sequence of events produced by remodeling suppressants [72, 73]. While remodeling intensity is increased, there is net deposition of the bone within each of the greater numbers of remodeling units as TPTD promotes the differentiation, work, and lifespan of osteoblasts in existing and newly created bone remodeling units [74]. TPTD also increases bone formation on quiescent bone surfaces [75].

Miyakoshi et al. retrospectively reviewed the medical records of 45 consecutive AFFs in 34 Japanese patients who had received oral bisphosphonates for osteoporosis before AFF and had been followed [76]. Bisphosphonates were stopped at diagnosis. Based on TPTD use after fracture, AFFs were divided into non-TPTD and TPTD groups. Time to fracture healing and frequency of delayed healing or nonunion were compared between groups. In subanalyses for all AFFs treated surgically, mean time to fracture healing was significantly better in the TPTD group than in the non-TPTD group, and the frequency of delayed healing or nonunion was significantly lower in the TPTD group than in the non-TPTD group. Subanalyses for surgically treated complete AFFs yielded similar results. TPTD treatment appears to significantly shorten the postoperative time to fracture healing and reduces rates of delayed healing or nonunion after bisphosphonate-associated AFF.

References

1. Miyakoshi N (2004) Effects of parathyroid hormone on cancellous bone mass and structure in osteoporosis. Curr Pharm Des 10:2615–2627
2. Borggrefe J, Graeff C, Nickelsen TN et al (2010) Quantitative computed tomographic assessment of the effects of 24 months of teriparatide treatment on 3D femoral neck bone distribution, geometry, and bone strength: results from the EUROFORS study. J Bone Miner Res 25:472–481
3. Toulis KA, Anastasilakis AD, Polyzos SA et al (2011) Targeting the osteoblast: approved and experimental anabolic agents for the treatment of osteoporosis. Hormones 10:174–195
4. Hodsman AB, Bauer DC, Dempster DW et al (2005) Parathyroid hormone and teriparatide for the treatment of osteoporosis: a review of the evidence and suggested guidelines for its use. Endocr Rev 26:688–703

5. Jilka RL (2007) Molecular and cellular mechanisms of the anabolic effect of intermittent PTH. Bone 40:1434–1446
6. Nozaka K, Miyakoshi N, Kasukawa Y et al (2008) Intermittent administration of human parathyroid hormone enhances bone formation and union at the site of cancellous bone osteotomy in normal and ovariectomized rats. Bone 42:90–97
7. Kamo K, Miyakoshi N, Kasukawa Y et al (2010) Intermittent weekly administration of human parathyroid hormone (1–34) improves bone-hydroxyapatite block bonding in ovariectomized rats. J Bone Miner Metab 28:634–640. doi:10.1007/s00774-010-0178-z
8. Tsuchie H, Miyakoshi N, Kasukawa Y et al (2013) Intermittent administration of human parathyroid hormone before osteosynthesis stimulates cancellous bone union in ovariectomized rats. Tohoku J Exp Med 229:19–28
9. Sato M, Vahle J, Schmidt A et al (2002) Abnormal bone architecture and biomechanical properties with near-lifetime treatment of rats with PTH. Endocrinology 143:3230–3242
10. Oteo-Alvaro A, Moreno E (2010) Atrophic humeral shaft nonunion treated with teriparatide (rh PTH 1–34): a case report. J Shoulder Elb Surg 19:e22–e28. doi:10.1016/j.jse.2010.05.005
11. Rubery PT, Bukata SV (2010) Teriparatide may accelerate healing in delayed unions of type III odontoid fractures: a report of 3 cases. J Spinal Disord Tech 23:151–155. doi:10.1097/BSD.0b013e31819a8b7a
12. Chintamaneni S, Finzel K, Gruber BL (2010) Successful treatment of sternal fracture nonunion with teriparatide. Osteoporos Int 21:1059–1063. doi:10.1007/s00198-009-1061-4
13. Lee YK, Ha YC, Koo KH (2012) Teriparatide, a nonsurgical solution for femoral nonunion? A report of three cases. Osteoporos Int 23:2897–2900. doi:10.1007/s00198-012-2172-x
14. Andreassen TT, Ejersted C, Oxlund H (1999) Intermittent parathyroid hormone (1–34) treatment increases callus formation and mechanical strength of healing rat fractures. J Bone Miner Res 14:960–968
15. Corrado A, Neve A, Maruotti N et al (2011) Dose-dependent metabolic effect of zoledronate on primary human osteoblastic cell cultures. Clin Exp Rheumatol 28:873–879
16. Allen MR, Follet H, Khurana M et al (2006) Antiremodeling agents influence osteoblast activity differently in modeling and remodeling sites of canine rib. Calcif Tissue Int 79:255–261
17. Lyritis GP, Georgoulas T, Zafeiris CP (2010) Bone anabolic versus bone anticatabolic treatment of postmenopausal osteoporosis. Ann N Y Acad Sci 1205:277–283
18. Ma YL, Zeng QQ, Porras LL et al (2011) Teriparatide [rhPTH (1–34)], but not strontium ranelate, demonstrated bone anabolic efficacy in mature, osteopenic, ovariectomized rats. Endocrinology 152:1767–1778
19. Alkhiary YM, Gerstenfeld LC, Krall E et al (2005) Enhancement of experimental fracture-healing by systemic administration of recombinant human parathyroid hormone (PTH 1–34). J Bone Joint Surg Am 87:731–741
20. Jilka RL, Weinstein RS, Bellido T et al (1999) Increased bone formation by prevention of osteoblast apoptosis with parathyroid hormone. J Clin Invest 104:439–446
21. Miyakoshi N, Kasukawa Y, Linkhart TA et al (2001) Evidence that anabolic effects of PTH on bone require IGF-I in growing mice. Endocrinology 142:4349–4356
22. Keller H, Kneissel M (2005) SOST is a target gene for PTH in bone. Bone 37:148–158
23. Canalis E (2010) Update in new anabolic therapies for osteoporosis. J Clin Endocrinol Metab 95:1496–1504
24. Martin TJ, Sims NA, Ng KW et al (2008) Regulatory pathways revealing new approaches to the development of anabolic drugs for osteoporosis. Osteoporos Int 19:1125–1138
25. Sowa H, Kaji H, Iu MF et al (2003) Parathyroid hormone-Smad3 axis exerts anti-apoptotic action and augments anabolic action of transforming growth factor beta in osteoblasts. J Biol Chem 26:52240–52252
26. Manabe T, Mori S, Mashiba T et al (2007) Human parathyroid hormone (1–34) accelerates natural fracture healing process in the femoral osteotomy model of cynomolgus monkeys. Bone 40:1475–1482

27. Dempster DW, Cosman F, Kurland ES et al (2001) Effects of daily treatment with parathyroid hormone on bone microarchitecture and turnover in patients with osteoporosis: a paired biopsy study. J Bone Miner Res 16:1846–1853
28. Neer RM, Arnaud CD, Zanchetta JR et al (2001) Effect of parathyroid hormone (1–34) on fractures and bone mineral density in postmenopausal women with osteoporosis. N Engl J Med 344:1434–1441
29. Komatsubara S, Mori S, Mashiba T et al (2005) Human parathyroid hormone (1–34) accelerates the fracture healing process of woven to lamellar bone replacement and new cortical shell formation in rat femora. Bone 36:678–687
30. Trivedi R, Mithal A, Chattopadhyay N et al (2010) Anabolics in osteoporosis: the emerging therapeutic tool. Curr Mol Med 10:14–28
31. Saito M, Marumo K, Kida Y et al (2011) Changes in the contents of enzymatic immature, mature, and non-enzymatic senescent cross-links of collagen after once-weekly treatment with human parathyroid hormone (1–34) for 18 months contribute to improvement of bone strength in ovariectomized monkeys. Osteoporos Int 22:2373–2383. doi:10.1007/s00198-010-1454-4
32. Orwoll ES, Scheele WH, Paul S et al (2003) The effect of teriparatide [human parathyroid hormone (1–34)] therapy on bone density in men with osteoporosis. J Bone Miner Res 18:9–17
33. Saag KG, Zanchetta JR, Devogelaer JP et al (2009) Effects of teriparatide versus alendronate for treating glucocorticoid-induced osteoporosis: thirty-six-month results of a randomized, double-blind, controlled trial. Arthritis Rheum 60:3346–3355
34. Loveridge N, Power J, Reeve J et al (2004) Bone mineralization density and femoral neck fragility. Bone 35:929–941
35. Tintut Y, Parhami F, Le V et al (1999) Inhibition of osteoblast-specific transcription factor Cbfal by the cAMP pathway in osteoblastic cells. J Biol Chem 274:28875–28879
36. Bellido T, Ali AA, Plotkin LI et al (2003) Proteasomal degradation of Runx2 shortens parathyroid hormone-induced anti-apoptotic signaling in osteoblasts. A putative explanation for why intermittent administration is needed for bone anabolism. J Biol Chem 278:50259–50272
37. Krishnan V, Moore TL, Ma YL et al (2003) Parathyroid hormone bone anabolic action requires Cbfa1/Runx2-dependent signaling. Mol Endocrinol 17:423–435
38. Qin L, Qiu P, Wang L et al (2003) Gene expression profiles and transcription factors involved in parathyroid hormone signaling in osteoblasts revealed by microarray and bioinformatics. J Biol Chem 278:19723–19731
39. Sutherland MK, Geoghegan JC, Yu C et al (2004) Sclerostin promotes the apoptosis of human osteoblastic cells: a novel regulation of bone formation. Bone 35:828–835
40. Kakar S, Einhorn TA, Vora S et al (2007) Enhanced chondrogenesis and Wnt signaling in PTH-treated fractures. J Bone Miner Res 22:1903–1912
41. Ohtori S, Inoue G, Orita S et al (2012) Teriparatide accelerates lumbar posterolateral fusion in women with postmenopausal osteoporosis: prospective study. Spine (Phila Pa 1976) 37:1464–1468. doi:10.1097/BRS.0b013e31826ca2a8
42. Lehman RA Jr, Dmitriev AE, Cardoso MJ et al (2010) Effect of teriparatide [rhPTH(1,34)] and calcitonin on intertransverse process fusion in a rabbit model. Spine (Phila Pa 1976) 35:146–152. doi:10.1097/BRS.0b013e3181b71a96
43. O'Loughlin PF, Cunningham ME, Bukata SV et al (2009) Parathyroid hormone (1–34) augments spinal fusion, fusion mass volume, and fusion mass quality in a rabbit spinal fusion model. Spine (Phila Pa 1976) 34:121–130. doi:10.1097/BRS.0b013e318191e687
44. Inoue G, Ueno M, Nakazawa T et al (2014) Teriparatide increases the insertional torque of pedicle screws during fusion surgery in patients with postmenopausal osteoporosis. J Neurosurg Spine 21:425–431. doi:10.3171/2014.5.SPINE13656
45. Abe Y, Takahata M, Ito M et al (2007) Enhancement of graft bone healing by intermittent administration of human parathyroid hormone (1–34) in a rat spinal arthrodesis model. Bone 41:775–785

46. Esses SI, Sachs BL, Dreyzin V et al (1993) Complications associated with the technique of pedicle screw fixation. A selected survey of ABS members. Spine (Phila Pa 1976) 18:2231–2239
47. Ohlin A, Karlsson M, Düppe H et al (1994) Complications after transpedicular stabilization of the spine. A survivorship analysis of 163 cases. Spine (Phila Pa 1976) 19:2774–2779
48. Pihlajämaki H, Myllynen P, Böstman O (1997) Complications of transpedicular lumbosacral fixation for non-traumatic disorders. J Bone Joint Surg (Br) 79:183–189
49. Soini J, Laine T, Pohjolainen T et al (1993) Spondylodesis augmented by transpedicular fixation in the treatment of olisthetic and degenerative conditions of the lumbar spine. Clin Orthop Relat Res 297:111–116
50. Lee JH, Lee JH, Park JW et al (2012) The insertional torque of a pedicle screw has a positive correlation with bone mineral density in posterior lumbar pedicle screw fixation. J Bone Joint Surg (Br) 94:93–97
51. Okuyama K, Abe E, Suzuki T et al (2000) Can insertional torque predict screw loosening and related failures? An in vivo study of pedicle screw fixation augment- ing posterior lumbar interbody fusion. Spine (Phila Pa 1976) 25:858–864
52. Aspenberg P, Genant HK, Johansson T et al (2010) Teriparatide for acceleration of fracture repair in humans: a prospective, randomized, double-blind study of 102 postmenopausal women with distal radial fractures. J Bone Miner Res 25:404–414. doi:10.1359/jbmr.090731
53. Barnes GL, Kakar S, Vora S et al (2008) Stimulation of fracture-healing with systemic intermittent parathyroid hormone treatment. J Bone Joint Surg Am 90(Suppl 1):120–127. doi:10.2106/JBJS.G.01443
54. Lewallen RP, Peterson HA (1985) Nonunion of long bone fractures in children: a review of 30 cases. J Pediatr Orthop 5:135–142
55. Goldhahn J, Feron JM, Kanis J et al (2012) Implications for fracture healing of current and new osteoporosis treatments: an ESCEO consensus paper. Calcif Tissue Int 90:343–353
56. Mancilla EE, Brodsky JL, Mehta S et al (2014) Teriparatide as a systemic treatment for lower extremity non-union fractures: a case series. Endocr Pract 8:1–22
57. Peichl P, Holzer LA, Maier R et al (2011) Parathyroid hormone 1–84 accelerates fracture-healing in pubic bones of elderly osteoporotic women. J Bone Joint Surg Am 93:1583–1587. doi:10.2106/JBJS.J.01379
58. Raghavan P, Christofides E (2012) Role of teriparatide in accelerating metatarsal stress fracture healing: a case series and review of literature. Clin Med Insights Endocrinol Diabetes 5:39–45
59. Giannotti S, Bottai V, Dell'Osso G et al (2013) Atrophic femoral nonunion successfully treated with teriparatide. Eur J Orthop Surg Traumatol 23(Suppl 2):291–294
60. Corrigan RA, Miller A, McNally MA et al (2013) Treatment of fracture non-union in a young adult with combination anabolic and anti-resorptive bone therapy. Rheumatology (Oxford) 52:1147–1149
61. Tamai K, Takamatsu K, Kazuki K (2013) Successful treatment of nonunion with teriparatide after failed ankle arthrodesis for Charcot arthropathy. Osteoporos Int 24:2729–2732
62. Ochi K, Ikari K, Naomi A et al (2013) Administration of teriparatide treatment for a challenging case of nonunion of periprosthetic fracture after total knee arthroplasty. Arch Osteoporos 8:159
63. Walker NA, Denegar CR, Preische J (2007) Low-intensity pulsed ultrasound and pulsed electromagnetic field in the treatment of tibial fractures: a systematic review. J Athl Train 42:530–535
64. Nozaka K, Shimada Y, Miyakoshi N et al (2014) Pathological fracture of the femur in Alagille syndrome that was treated with low-intensity pulsed ultrasound stimulation and an Ilizarov ring fixator: a case report. BMC Musculoskelet Disord 15:225. doi:10.1186/1471-2474-15-225
65. Gebauer D, Correll J (2005) Pulsed low-intensity ultrasound: a new salvage procedure for delayed unions and nonunions after leg lengthening in children. J Pediatr Orthop 25:750–754

66. Sato W, Matsushita T, Nakamura K (1999) Acceleration of increase in bone mineral content by low-intensity ultrasound energy in leg lengthening. J Ultrasound Med 18:699–702
67. Nozaka K, Shimada Y, Kimura Y et al (2014) Successful treatment of nonunion with an Ilizarov ring fixator after ankle fracture for Charcot arthropathy: a case report. BMC Res Notes 7:503. doi:10.1186/1756-0500-7-503
68. Strauss E, Gonya G (1998) Adjunct low intensity ultrasound in Charcot neuroarthropathy. Clin Orthop 349:132–138
69. Warden SJ, Komatsu DE, Rydberg J et al (2009) Recombinant human parathyroid hormone (PTH 1–34) and low-intensity pulsed ultrasound have contrasting additive effects during fracture healing. Bone 44:485–494. doi:10.1016/j.bone.2008.11.007
70. Nozaka K, Shimada Y, Miyakoshi N et al (2014) Combined effect of teriparatide and low-intensity pulsed ultrasound for nonunion: a case report. BMC Res Notes 7:317. doi:10.1186/1756-0500-7-317
71. Chiang CY, Zebaze RM, Ghasem-Zadeh A et al (2013) Teriparatide improves bone quality and healing of atypical femoral fractures associated with bisphosphonate therapy. Bone 52:360–365
72. Jobke B, Muche B, Burghardt AJ et al (2013) Teriparatide in bisphosphonate-resistant osteoporosis: microarchitectural changes and clinical results after 6 and 18 months. Calcif Tissue Int 89:130–139
73. Koh JS, Goh SK, Png MA et al (2013) Femoral cortical stress lesions in long-term bisphosphonate therapy: a herald of impending fracture? J Orthop Trauma 24:75–81
74. Ma YL, Zeng Q, Donley DW et al (2006) Teriparatide increases bone formation in modeling and remodelling osteons and enhances IGF-II immunoreactivity in postmenopausal women with osteoporosis. J Bone Miner Res 21:855–864
75. Lindsay R, Cosman F, Zhou H et al (2006) A novel tetracycline labeling schedule for longitudinal evaluation of the short-term effects of anabolic therapy with a single iliac crest bone biopsy: early actions of teriparatide. J Bone Miner Res 21:366–373
76. Miyakoshi N, Aizawa T, Sasaki S et al (2014) Healing of bisphosphonate-associated atypical femoral fractures in patients with osteoporosis: a comparison between treatment with and without teriparatide. J Bone Miner Metab. doi:10.1007/s00774-014-0617-3

Part IV
Exercise and Osteoporosis

Chapter 11
Exercise and Fall Prevention

Jun Iwamoto

Abstract The prevention of falls and subsequent osteoporotic fractures can reduce disability, improve quality of life, and reduce the costs of health care for older adults. Exercise plays an important role in preventing falls. A consensus has been reached that exercise programs that include balance and muscle-strengthening exercises, but not brisk walking, reduce the incidence of falls among older adults, especially among those with an increased risk of falls. However, muscle power as assessed by measuring the chair-rising time has been emphasized as a key factor in preventing falls among older adults, since the chair-rising test evaluates the power of the vertical movement and the hip muscles as the most important neuromuscular risk factor for falls and fall-related fractures. Muscle power exercises are superior to balance exercises for improving physical function, and a multidisciplinary exercise program aimed at improving flexibility, body balance, muscle power, and walking ability has been reported to prevent falls among older adults. Vitamin D supplementation has also been shown to reduce the incidence of falls. Older adults with osteoporosis often have sarcopenia (sarco-osteoporosis), and muscle-strengthening and muscle power exercises, together with adequate protein and vitamin D intake, should be recommended to improve sarcopenia. In conclusion, programs that include balance, muscle-strengthening, and muscle power exercises, but not brisk walking, together with adequate protein and vitamin D intake appear to be useful for preventing falls among older adults.

Keywords Muscle strength • Muscle power • Body balance • Whole-body vibration exercise • Osteoporosis

J. Iwamoto (✉)
Institute for Integrated Sports Medicine, Keio University School of Medicine, 35 Shinanomachi, Shinjuku-ku, Tokyo 160-8582, Japan
e-mail: jiwamoto@keio.jp

Y. Shimada, N. Miyakoshi (eds.), *Osteoporosis in Orthopedics*,
DOI 10.1007/978-4-431-55778-4_11

11.1 Introduction

Fall-related injuries such as osteoporotic fractures are serious problems among older adults, since fractures in patients with osteoporosis often lead to disability and increase the risk of mortality [1, 2]. Thus, the prevention of falls and subsequent osteoporotic fractures is a crucial issue for older adults.

The American College of Sports Medicine (ACSM) Position Stand has showed that although no amount of physical activity can stop the biological aging process, there is evidence that regular exercise can minimize the physiological effects of an otherwise sedentary lifestyle and increase active life expectancy by limiting the development and progression of chronic disease and disabling conditions [3]. Consequently, exercises aimed at improving physical function and preventing falls appear to be important for increasing the active life expectancy of older individuals.

A review of randomized controlled trials (RCTs) by Gardner et al. [4] showed that exercise was effective in lowering the fall risk in older adults, and the subsequent reduction in fall-related injuries could reduce health care costs. The risk of clinical, mainly appendicular, fractures is elevated in women with a combination of low bone mineral density (BMD) and incident falls [5]. Thus, effective interventional strategies should be established for target populations to prevent falls and fall-related fractures. The incidence of osteoporotic fractures, i.e., vertebral fractures, increases after menopause, and older women ($\geq$70 years) with osteoporosis have a risk of both vertebral and hip fractures [6, 7]. The objective of the present review was to clarify the role of exercise in the prevention of falls among older adults, focusing mainly on older women with an increased risk of fractures because of the presence of osteoporosis.

11.2 Exercises for Preventing Falls Among Older Adults

11.2.1 Osteoporosis and Exercise in Older Adults: Position Stand of the ACSM and Recommendation by the OSC

According to the ACSM Position Stand on Osteoporosis and Exercise [8], (1) -weight-bearing physical activity is essential for the normal development and maintenance of a healthy skeleton. Activities that focus on increasing muscle strength may also be beneficial, particularly for non-weight-bearing bones. (2) Sedentary women may increase bone mass slightly by becoming more active, but the primary benefit of the increased activity may be in avoiding the further loss of bone that occurs with inactivity. (3) Exercise cannot be recommended as a substitute for hormone replacement therapy at the time of menopause. (4) An optimal program for older women would include activities that improve strength, flexibility, and coordination and that may indirectly but effectively decrease the incidence of osteoporotic fractures by lessening the likelihood of falling.

According to the recommendations developed by the Scientific Advisory Board of the Osteoporosis Society of Canada (OSC) in its Consensus Conference [9], moderate physical activity in patients with osteoporosis can reduce the risk of falls and fractures, decrease pain, and improve fitness and overall quality of life. It may also stimulate bone gain and decrease bone loss. During any exercise program, proper nutrition is necessary to prevent excessive weight loss and impaired immune function resulting from inadequate protein, vitamin, and mineral intake.

11.2.2 Comprehensive Care for Preventing Fall-Related Fractures in Older Adults

The risk of falls increases with age, and thus a large proportion of older adults experience one or more falls per year [10]. In addition to skeletal fragility, falls are a major factor contributing to the occurrence of symptomatic fractures in older adults. Thus, the aim of exercise in older adults with osteoporosis should focus primarily on preventing falls. Since there is no evidence that exercise prevents hip fractures in postmenopausal women with osteoporosis, exercise should be considered in conjunction with pharmacotherapy such as alendronate, risedronate, zoledronic acid, and denosumab, together with calcium and vitamin D supplementation, to reduce the risk of fall-related fractures, including hip fractures [11]. Vitamin D supplementation is useful for reducing the incidence of falls in older adults, as vitamin D supplementation has been reported to reduce the risk of falls by more than 20 % among ambulatory or institutionalized older individuals with stable health [12] Thus, proper exercise programs, together with vitamin D supplementation and pharmacotherapy, play an important role in the prevention of falls and fall-related fractures among older adults with osteoporosis.

11.2.3 Systematic Review and Meta-Analysis of RCTs

The effect of exercise on the incidence of falls has been verified in older adults. Gillespie et al. [13] reported that a multicomponent group exercise program reduced the risk of falls (relative risk [RR] 0.85, 95 % confidence interval [CI] 0.76–0.96), as did a multicomponent home-based exercise (RR 0.78, 95 % CI 0.64–0.94) and Tai Chi (RR 0.71, 95 % CI 0.57–0.87), and that exercise interventions successfully reduced the risk of sustaining a fall-related fracture (RR 0.34, 95 % CI 0.18–0.63). Karlsson et al. [14] reported that physical exercise that included several training modalities, especially balance and muscle-strengthening exercises, was the only intervention program that reduced both the number of fallers and the number of falls among community dwellers (RR [95 % CI] for number of falls: 0.78 [0.71–0.86] for group exercise and 0.66 [0.53–0.82] for home exercise), while Tai Chi reduced the number of falls (RR 0.63, 95 % CI 0.52–0.78). A program consisting of balance and muscle-strengthening exercises appears to be effective for preventing falls among older adults, especially those with an increased risk of falls in terms of a history of falls [15]. Brisk walking appeared to increase the risk of upper limb fractures in women [16], since brisk walking itself may increase the risk of falls. On the other hand, a cohort study by Feskanich et al. [17] showed that among postmenopausal women, walking for at least 4 h per week was associated with a 41 % lower risk of hip fracture, compared with less than 1 h per week. The effect of exercise through walking on the incidence of falls has been controversial. Based on the hierarchy of evidence, however, we have placed greater belief in the results of systematic reviews.

11.3 RCTs Conducted in Japan

11.3.1 Strategy for Preventing Falls in Older Adults

Impairments of muscle strength and muscle power of the lower extremities, balance/postural control, and walking ability have been recognized as important risk factors for falls [18]. These parameters are known to be impaired with aging [19]. In particular, a decline in muscle function in terms of muscle power may be more evident than sarcopenia [20]. In female muscle tissue, the proportion of type I (slow twitch) fibers significantly increases and that of type II (fast twitch) fibers significantly decreases with age [21]. Muscle strength should be distinguished from muscle power; muscle strength [N] is defined as the maximal force that a muscle can produce against a given resistance, while muscle power [W] is defined as the product of force and speed (muscle strength [N] x velocity [m/s]) [18, 22]. The former parameter is related to bone strength, whereas the latter is related to falling [18, 22–24]. Thus, the improvement of muscle power, rather than muscle strength, is likely to be important for preventing falls among older adults. Muscle power can be evaluated simply using the chair-rising time (usually the five-repetition chair-rising time). Theoretically, the improvement of muscle power in the lower extremities as well as balance/postural control and walking ability through exercise is considered to be important for preventing falls among older adults. A recent study showed the effects of a targeted multimodal exercise program incorporating high-speed power training on physical function in older adults [25], suggesting the importance of muscle power exercises for preventing falls.

Neuromuscular parameters that describe locomotion are indispensable variables for the diagnosis and treatment of frailty, fall risk, and osteoporosis. A scientifically based standardized locomotor assessment should be an essential part of medical examinations in research and clinical practice. Runge et al. [22] proposed the following tests for a standardized locomotor assessment: (1) self-selected gait velocity as the single best measure of general locomotor status and a good predictor of age-related adverse events; (2) chair-rising test (five timed chair-rises), which measures the power of the vertical movement and the hip muscles as the most important neuromuscular risk factor for falls and fall-related fractures; (3) tandem standing and tandem walking to measure postural capacity (balance) to the side; (4) timed-up-and-go (TUG) test as a global screening procedure; and (5) clinical gait analysis, with special focus on regularity. Thus, gait velocity, chair-rising time (muscle power), tandem standing time (static body balance), tandem gait time, tandem step number, and TUG (dynamic body balance) are thought to be clinically important parameters in the assessment of physical function in older adults. In Japan, however, the one-leg standing time is usually used to evaluate static body balance [26].

11.3.2 Balance Exercise and Fall Prevention

Sakamoto et al. [26] conducted a 6-month RCT and showed that a balance exercise consisting of a one-leg standing exercise (so-called dynamic flamingo exercise) performed for 1 min, three times a day, increased the one-leg standing time and reduced the incidence of falls (14.2 % for the exercise group and 20.7 % for the control group) among older women ($\geq$75 years, mean age: 80 years) who were unable to stand on one leg for $\leq$15 s (Fig. 11.1).

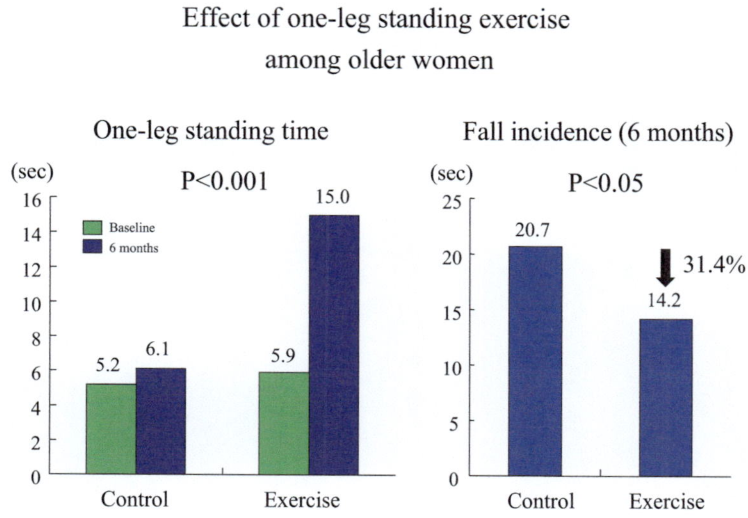

Fig. 11.1 Effect of one-leg standing exercise among older women. A one-leg standing exercise (balance exercise: performed for 1 min, 3 sets per day for 6 months) increased the one-leg standing time and reduced the incidence of falls among older women with poor body balance [26]. A paired-*t* test was used to compare the means between two groups, and the McNemar's test was used to compare the proportions between two groups

11.3.3 Power Exercise and Physical Function Improvement

Because the chair-rising exercise, which is categorized as a muscle power exercise, trains the quadriceps and gluteus medius muscles, this exercise likely improves not only muscle power, but also body balance. An RCT was conducted to compare the effect of a one-leg standing exercise (balance exercise) and the chair-rising exercise (muscle power exercise) on physical function among older patients with locomotive disorders (mean age: 67 years) [27]. The daily exercise program consisted of a one-leg standing exercise (1 min × three sets for each leg per day) in the one-leg standing exercise group and the chair-rising exercise (10 times × three sets per day) in the chair-rising exercise group (Fig. 11.2). The exercises were performed 3 days per week. After the completion of the 5-month exercise program, TUG, the one-leg standing time, and the tandem gait time had improved in the one-leg standing exercise group, while the walking time and the chair-rising time in addition to the above parameters had improved in the chair-rising exercise group. The improvements in the chair-rising time as well as the walking time and the tandem gait time were greater in the chair-rising exercise group than in the one-leg standing exercise group (Fig. 11.3). Thus, the chair-rising exercise was found to be more effective than the one-leg standing exercise for improving muscle power (chair-rising time) as well as walking velocity and dynamic body balance (tandem gait time). However, the effect of chair-rising exercises on the incidence of falls remains to be established.

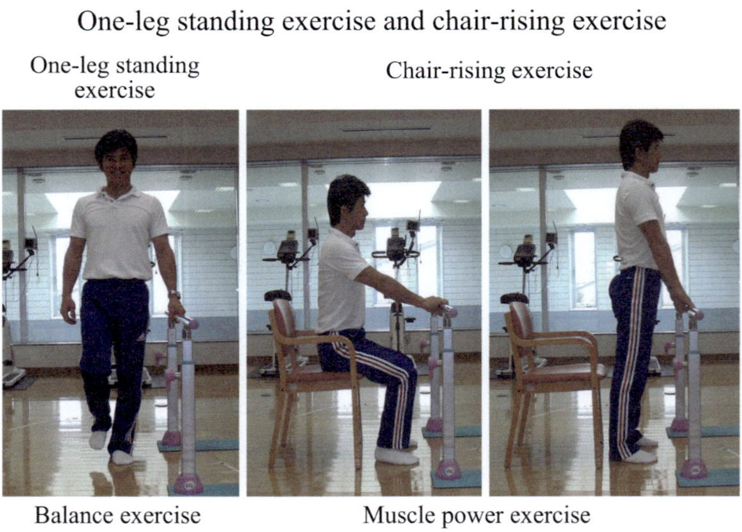

Fig. 11.2 One-leg standing exercise and chair-rising exercise. The one-leg standing exercise is a balance exercise and the chair-rising exercise is muscle power exercise

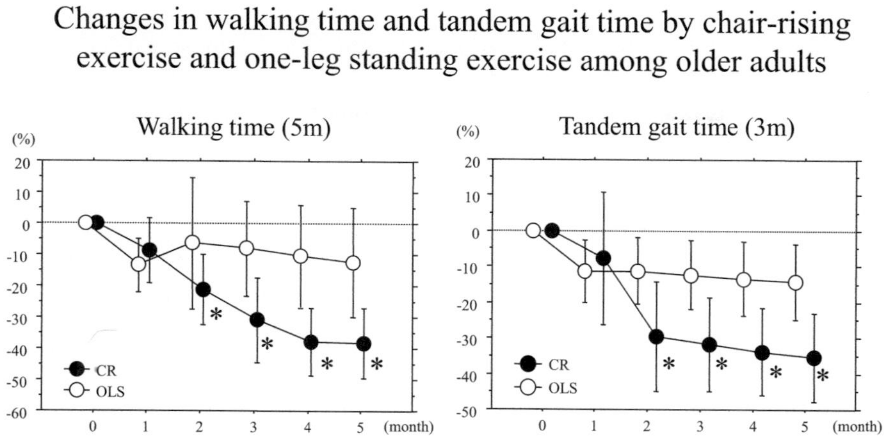

Fig. 11.3 Changes in walking time and tandem gait time by chair-rising exercise and one-leg standing exercise among older adults. The effect of a one-leg standing exercise and the chair-rising exercise on physical function was compared among older patients with locomotive disorders. After the completion of the 5-month exercise program, the chair-rising exercise was more effective than the one-leg standing exercise for improving muscle power (chair-rising time) as well as walking velocity and dynamic body balance (tandem gait time) [27]. $^{*}P < 0.01$ vs. baseline by an analysis of variance with the Fisher PLSD test

Table 11.1 Multidisciplinary exercise program

1. Calisthenics	Anterior, right, left, and posterior flexion of the body: five times in each direction per day
2. Body-balance training	Tandem standing (3 min in each leg forward: two sets per day)
	Tandem gait (ten steps: five sets a day)
	Unipedal standing (3 min in each leg: two sets per day)
3. Muscle power training	Chair-rising training (ten times: three sets per day)
4. Walking-ability training (stepping)	Having one step in the forward, back, right, and left directions: ten times for each stepping per day

All the exercises were supervised and performed in the clinics or hospitals 3 days per week as a multidisciplinary exercise by taking about 30 min

11.3.4 Multidisciplinary Exercise and Fall Prevention

Both one-leg standing exercise (balance exercise) and chair-rising exercise (muscle power exercise) regimens can be utilized in combination for fall-prevention exercise programs. An RCT was conducted to determine the effect of exercise on the prevention of falls in older adults (mean age: 76.4 years), with the aim of improving flexibility, body balance, muscle power, and walking ability (Table 11.1) [28]. All the exercises were supervised and performed in clinics or hospitals 3 days per week in the exercise group and took about 30 min to complete [28]. The exercise program improved flexibility (finger-floor distance with the body flexed in the right and left directions), static body balance (one-leg standing time and tandem standing time), dynamic body balance (TUG and tandem gait step number), muscle power (chair-rising time), and walking ability (10-m walking time and step length), leading to a reduced incidence of falls (exercise group 0.0 % vs. control group 12.1 %), thereby confirming the beneficial effect of the abovementioned exercise program for preventing falls among older adults.

11.3.5 Whole-Body Vibration (WBV) Exercise and Physical Function Improvement

WBV exercise has been developed as a new modality in the field of physiotherapy and has been used to improve physical function in older adults [29–31]. Several available systematic reviews and meta-analyses have discussed the effectiveness of WBV exercise [32–35]. Rogan et al. [32] concluded that a vertical sinusoidal WBV produced small effects on static and dynamic balance, while a side-alternating WBV produced small to moderate improvements in the same balance requirements in older adults. Lau et al. [34] found that WBV exercise was beneficial for enhancing leg muscle strength among older adults.

WBV exercise can be performed using a Galileo machine (G-900; Novotec, Pforzheim, Germany). The Galileo machine is a unique device for applying whole-body vibration/oscillatory muscle stimulation (Fig. 11.4). The subject stands with bent knees and hips on a rocking platform with a sagittal axle, which alternately thrusts the right and left legs upward and downward, thereby promoting the lengthening of the extensor muscles of the lower extremities. This type of training provides reflex muscle stimulation with no serious adverse events. A chain of rapid muscle contractions during the exercise directly activates the neuromuscular system in the lower extremities. The exercise elicits an acute hormonal profile (growth hormone), and neuromuscular performance responses immediately after the exercise [36].

An RCT was conducted to determine the effect of 6 months of WBV exercise (2 days per week) on physical function in older osteoporotic women treated with alendronate (mean age: 74.2 years) [37]. Each WBV exercise session was set at a frequency of 20 Hz and had a duration of 4 min. This frequency was thought to be comfortable and safe for older people. The 6 months of WBV exercise was well tolerated and improved static body balance (one-leg standing time and tandem standing time) and walking velocity, but not dynamic body balance (TUG) or muscle power (chair-rising time), when compared with the results in control subjects. Thus, the benefit and safety of WBV exercise for improving physical function were confirmed in older osteoporotic women treated with alendronate.

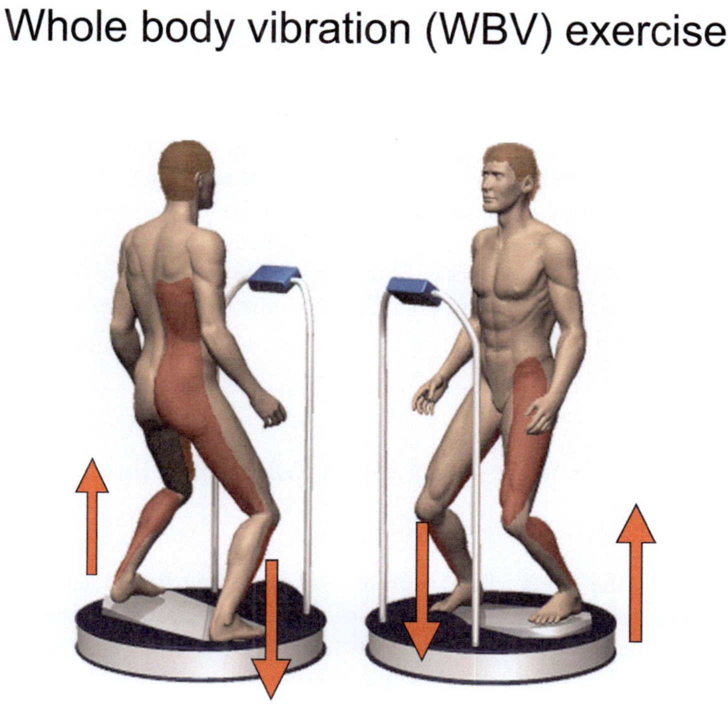

Fig. 11.4 Whole-body vibration (WBV) exercise. The Galileo machine (Novotec, Pforzheim, Germany) is a unique device for applying whole-body vibration/oscillatory muscle stimulation. The subject stands with bent knees and hips on a rocking platform with a sagittal axle, which alternately thrusts the *right* and *left legs* upward and downward, thereby promoting lengthening of the lower extremity muscles. The reaction of the neuromuscular system is a chain of rapid muscle contractions

11.3.6 WBV Plus Power Exercise and Physical Function Improvement

WBV exercise improved static body balance and walking velocity, but not dynamic body balance and muscle power, in older osteoporotic women treated with alendronate [37]. The chair-rising exercise was more effective than a one-leg standing exercise for improving muscle power as well as walking velocity and dynamic body balance in older patients with locomotive disorder [27]. A squatting exercise, which mimics the chair-rising exercise, may train the quadriceps and gluteus medius muscles and improve joint movement in the lower extremities. Thus, it was hypothesized that a combination of WBV exercise and squatting would be more effective than WBV exercise alone for improving physical function, especially in terms of dynamic body balance and muscle power, in older adults.

An RCT was conducted to clarify the beneficial effect of 6 months of WBV exercise plus squatting (4 min per day, 2 days per week) on physical function including body balance, muscle power, and walking ability in older adults (mean age: 72.4 years) [38]. In the squatting group, a dynamic squatting exercise was added on the rocking platform of a Galileo machine during the 4-min WBV exercise session. Both knees and hips were bent from 45° to 60° and extended from 60° to 45° 20 times/min for 4 min. WBV exercise alone improved the indices of body balance and walking velocity from the baseline values. However, WBV exercise plus the squatting exercise was more effective for improving the tandem gait step number (dynamic body balance) and the chair-rising time (muscle power), compared with WBV exercise alone. Thus, the benefit and safety of WBV exercise plus a squatting exercise for improving physical function were confirmed in terms of body balance and muscle power in older adults.

11.4 Feasible Exercises for Elderly Adults in Clinical Practice

For older adults, the safety of an exercise is an important factor. The purpose of exercise in older adults with an increased risk of fractures should be focused on the prevention of falls. Because there is no evidence that exercise prevents hip fractures in postmenopausal women with osteoporosis, exercise should be considered in conjunction with pharmacotherapy in older adults with an increased risk of fractures. Improvement of the vitamin D status is important (intake $\geq$ 800 IU/day and 25-hydroxyvitamin D $\geq$ 30 ng/mL) for reducing the incidence of falls and fractures [39, 40]. Thus, the addition of vitamin D supplementation and pharmacotherapy to exercise programs for preventing falls and subsequent osteoporotic fractures in older adults should be considered.

According to an up-to-date meta-analysis and the best-practice recommendations for exercises to prevent falls among older adults, exercise can prevent falls (RR 0.84, 95 % CI 0.71–0.91), programs that include balance exercises (higher doses: at least 2 h/week; $\geq$ 50 h over the trial period) but do not include walking exercises have the greatest effect on reducing falls, and high-risk individuals should not be prescribed brisk walking programs [41]. Mild-to-moderate-intensity walking exercises are acceptable for older adults with an increased risk of falls, but the aims of walking exercises should be not only the maintenance of general health conditions through aerobic weight-bearing exercise, but also an improvement in the vitamin D status through sunlight exposure [42]. Muscle-strengthening exercises (at least two to three times per week) are also important for preventing falls in older adults [43]. Teixeira et al. [44] reported that an 18-week progressive load training regimen targeting the quadricep muscle (50 % up to 80 % of 1 RM [one maximum repetition]) and proprioception training twice a week decreased the number of falls (RR [95 % CI]: 0.263 [0.10–0.68]) in postmenopausal women with osteoporosis.

Thus, a consensus has been reached that exercise programs that include balance and muscle-strengthening exercises, but not walking exercises, reduce the incidence of falls among older adults, especially among those with an increased risk of falls. However, exercise aimed at improving muscle power is important for preventing falls, because muscle power (muscle strength x velocity) is related to falling [18, 22–24]. A one-leg standing exercise (balance exercise: performed for 1 min, 3 sets per day) was useful for reducing the incidence of falls in older women with poor body balance [26], while the chair-rising exercise (muscle power exercise: 10 times, 3 sets per day) was superior to the one-leg standing exercise (balance exercise) for improving physical function, i.e., muscle power, as well as walking velocity and dynamic body balance in older adults [27]. Both exercise regimens (one-leg standing and chair-rising exercises) can be utilized in combination for fall-prevention exercise programs. A multidisciplinary exercise program aimed at improving flexibility, body balance, muscle power, and walking ability (30 min per day, 3 days per week) reportedly prevents falls among older adults [28].

Exercise can reduce the incidence of falls, fall-related fractures, and several risk factors for falls in older adults [13–15]. Older adults with osteoporosis often have sarcopenia (sarco-osteoporosis). The prevalence of low muscle mass in Japanese women (age: 40–88 years) with a normal BMD, osteopenia, and osteoporosis was 9.0 %, 17.8 %, and 29.7 %, respectively [45], suggesting a significant association between low muscle mass and osteopenia and osteoporosis. Sarcopenia is characterized by an age-related decline in skeletal muscle mass as well as muscle function (defined by muscle strength or physical performance), which may result in a reduced physical capability and a poorer quality of life, impaired cardiopulmonary performance, unfavorable metabolic effects, falls, disability, and mortality in older adults, as well as high health care expenditures [46]. Muscle-strengthening and muscle power exercises, together with adequate protein and vitamin D intake, should be recommended to improve sarcopenia [47, 48]. Programs that include balance, muscle-strengthening, and muscle power exercises, but that do not include brisk walking, together with adequate protein and vitamin D intake appear to be useful for preventing falls in older adults. Exercises should be performed at least two to three times per week [42].

Among older adults who have difficulty performing exercise programs, WBV exercise (2 days per week at a frequency of 20 Hz and for a duration of 4 min) can be utilized [37]. This intensity and frequency of the exercise program were considered to be reasonable for older osteoporotic women, enabling the exercise to be continued without any fatigue or difficulty. WBV exercise was not only effective for improving physical function, i.e., the indices for flexibility, body balance, and walking velocity, but was also considered to be safe and well tolerated. Although WBV exercise improves physical function, it remains uncertain whether it prevents falls in older adults.

11.5 Conclusions

A consensus has been reached that exercise programs that include balance and muscle-strengthening exercises, but not brisk walking exercise, reduce the incidence of falls among older adults, especially those with an increased risk of falls. However, muscle power as assessed by measuring the chair-rising time should be emphasized as a key factor in preventing falls among older adults, since the chair-rising test evaluates the power of the vertical movement and the hip muscles as the most important neuromuscular risk factor for falls and fall-related fractures. Muscle power exercises are superior to balance exercises for improving physical function, and a multidisciplinary exercise program aimed at improving flexibility, body balance, muscle power, and walking ability prevented falls in older adults. Vitamin D supplementation has been shown to reduce the incidence of falls among older adults. In conclusion, programs that include balance, muscle-strengthening, and muscle power exercises, but do not including brisk walking, together with adequate protein and vitamin D intake appear to be useful for preventing falls among older adults.

Conflict of Interest and Disclosure We have no conflict of interest and disclosure.

References

1. Ensrud KE, Thompson DE, Cauley JA, Nevitt MC, Kado DM, Hochberg MC, Santora AC 2nd, Black DM (2000) Prevalent vertebral deformities predict mortality and hospitalization in older women with low bone mass. J Am Geriatr Soc 48:241–249
2. Kanis JA, Oden A, Johnell O, De Laet C, Jonsson B, Oglesby AK (2003) The components of excess mortality after hip fracture. Bone 32:468–473
3. Chodzko-Zajko WJ, Proctor DN, Fiatarone Singh MA, Minson CT, Nigg CR, Salem GJ, Skinner JS (2009) American College of Sports Medicine position stand. Exercise and physical activity for older adults. Med Sci Sports Exerc 41:1510–1530
4. Gardner MM, Robertson MC, Campbell AJ (2000) Exercise in preventing falls and fall related injuries in older people: a review of randomised controlled trials. Br J Sports Med 34:7–17
5. Geusens P, Autier P, Boonen S, Vanhoof J, Declerck K, Raus J (2002) The relationship among history of falls, osteoporosis, and fractures in postmenopausal women. Arch Phys Med Rehabil 83:903–906
6. Fujiwara S (2005) Epidemiology of osteoporosis in Japan. J Bone Miner Metab 23 (Suppl):81–83
7. Orimo H, Yaegashi Y, Onoda T, Fukushima Y, Hosoi T, Sakata K (2009) Hip fracture incidence in Japan: estimates of new patients in 2007 and 20-year trends. Arch Osteoporos 4:71–77
8. American College Sports Medicine (1995) American college sports medicine position stand on osteoporosis and exercise. Med Sci Sports Exerc 27:1–5
9. Prior JC, Barr SI, Chow R, Faulkner RA (1996) Prevention and management of osteoporosis: consensus statements from the Scientific Advisory Board of the Osteoporosis Society of Canada. 5. Physical activity as therapy for osteoporosis. CMAJ 155:940–944

10. Tinetti ME (2003) Clinical practice. Preventing falls in elderly persons. N Engl J Med 348:42–49
11. Murad MH, Drake MT, Mullan RJ, Mauck KF, Stuart LM, Lane MA, Abu Elnour NO, Erwin PJ, Hazem A, Puhan MA, Li T, Montori VM (2012) Clinical review. Comparative effectiveness of drug treatments to prevent fragility fractures: a systematic review and network meta-analysis. J Clin Endocrinol Metab 97:1871–1880
12. Bischoff-Ferrari HA, Dawson-Hughes B, Willett WC, Staehelin HB, Bazemore MG, Zee RY, Wong JB (2004) Effect of Vitamin D on falls: a meta-analysis. JAMA 291:1999–2006
13. Gillespie LD, Robertson MC, Gillespie WJ, Sherrington C, Gates S, Clemson LM, Lamb SE (2012) Interventions for preventing falls in older people living in the community. Cochrane Database Syst Rev 9:CD007146
14. Karlsson MK, Vonschewelov T, Karlsson C, Cöster M, Rosengen BE (2013) Prevention of falls in the elderly: a review. Scand J Public Health 41:442–454
15. Gillespie LD, Robertson MC, Gillespie WJ, Lamb SE, Gates S, Cumming RG, Rowe BH (2009) Interventions for preventing falls in older people living in the community. Cochrane Database Syst Rev 2:CD007146
16. Gillespie LD, Gillespie WJ, Robertson MC, Lamb SE, Cumming RG, Rowe BH (2001) Interventions for preventing falls in elderly people. Cochrane Database Syst Rev 3:CD000340
17. Feskanich D, Willett W, Colditz G (2002) Walking and leisure-time activity and risk of hip fracture in postmenopausal women. JAMA 288:2300–2306
18. Runge M, Rehfeld G, Resnicek E (2001) Balance training and exercise in geriatric patients. J Musculoskelt Neuronal Interact 1:61–65
19. Asmussen E (1980) Aging and exercise. Environ Physiol 3:419–428
20. Runge M, Rittweger J, Russo CR, Schiessl H, Felsenberg D (2004) Is muscle power output a key factor in the age-related decline in physical performance? A comparison of muscle cross section, chair-rising test and jumping power. Clin Physiol Funct Imaging 24:335–340
21. Fayet G, Rouche A, Hogrel JY, Tome FM, Fardeau M (2001) Age-related morphological changes of the deltoid muscle from 50 to 79 years of age. Acta Neuropathol 101:358–366
22. Runge M, Hunter G (2006) Determinants of musculoskeletal frailty and the risk of falls in old age. J Musculoskelt Neuronal Interact 6:167–173
23. Frost HM (1997) Defining osteopenias and osteoporosis: another view (with insights from a new paradigm). Bone 20:385–391
24. Schiessl H, Frost HM, Jee WSS (1998) Estrogen and bone-muscle strength and mass relationship. Bone 22:1–6
25. Gianoudis J, Bailey CA, Ebeling PR, Nowson CA, Sanders KM, Hill K, Daly RM (2014) Effects of a targeted multimodal exercise program incorporating high-speed power training on falls and fracture risk factors in older adults: a community-based randomized controlled trial. J Bone Miner Res 29:183–191
26. Sakamoto K, Endo N, Harada A, Sakada T, Tsushita K, Kita K, Hagino H, Sakai A, Yamamoto N, Okamoto T, Liu M, Kokaze A, Suzuki H (2013) Why not use your own body weight to prevent falls? A randomized, controlled trial of balance therapy to prevent falls and fractures for elderly people who can stand on one leg for $\leq$15 s. J Orthop Sci 18:110–120
27. Yamashita F, Iwamoto J, Osugi T, Yamazaki M, Takakuwa M (2012) Chair rising exercise is more effective than one-leg standing exercise in improving dynamic body balance: a randomized controlled trial. J Musculoskelet Neuronal Interact 12:74–79
28. Iwamoto J, Suzuki H, Tanaka K, Kumakubo T, Hirabayashi H, Miyazaki Y, Sato Y, Takeda T, Matsumoto H (2009) Preventative effect of exercise against falls in the elderly: a randomized controlled trial. Osteoporos Int 20:1233–1240
29. Iwamoto J, Otaka Y, Kudo Y, Takeda T, Uzawa M, Hirabayashi K (2004) Efficacy of training program for ambulatory competence in elderly women. Keio J Med 53:85–89
30. Kawanabe K, Kawashima A, Sashimoto I, Takeda T, Sato Y, Iwamoto J (2007) Effect of whole-body vibration exercise and muscle strengthening, balance, and walking exercises on walking ability in the elderly. Keio J Med 56:28–33

31. Kawanabe K, Kawashima A, Sashimoto I, Abe K, Takeda T, Matsumoto H, Iwamoto J (2008) Influence of vibration exercise on the effect of muscle strengthening and balance training in the frail elderly. Jpn J Orthop Sports Med 28:242–248
32. Rogan S, Hilfiker R, Herren K, Radlinger L, de Bruin ED (2011) Effects of whole-body vibration on postural control in elderly: a systematic review and meta-analysis. BMC Geriatr 11:72
33. Slatkovska L, Alibhai SM, Beyene J, Cheung AM (2010) Effect of whole-body vibration on BMD: a systematic review and meta-analysis. Osteoporos Int 21:1969–1980
34. Lau RW, Liao LR, Yu F, Teo T, Chung RC, Pang MY (2011) The effects of whole body vibration therapy on bone mineral density and leg muscle strength in older adults: a systematic review and meta-analysis. Clin Rehabil 25:975–988
35. Conway GE, Szalma JL, Hancock PA (2007) A quantitative meta-analytic examination of whole-body vibration effects on human performance. Ergonomics 50:228–245
36. Bosco C, Iacovelli M, Tsarpela O, Cardinale M, Bonifazi M, Tihanyi J, Viru M, De Lorenzo A, Viru A (2000) Hormonal responses to whole-body vibration in men. Eur J Appl Physiol 81:449–454
37. Iwamoto J, Sato Y, Takeda T, Matsumoto H (2012) Whole body vibration exercise improves body balance and walking velocity in postmenopausal osteoporotic women treated with alendronate: Galileo and Alendronate Intervention Trail (GAIT). J Musculoskelet Neuronal Interact 12:136–143
38. Osugi T, Iwamoto J, Yamazaki M, Takakuwa M (2014) Effect of a combination of whole body vibration exercise and squat training on body balance, muscle power, and walking ability in the elderly. Ther Clin Risk Manag 10:131–138
39. Bischoff-Ferrari HA, Giovannucci E, Willett WC, Dietrich T, Dawson-Hughes B (2006) Estimation of optimal serum concentrations of 25-hydroxyvitamin D for multiple health outcomes. Am J Clin Nutr 84:18–28
40. Holick MF (2007) Vitamin D, deficiency. N Engl J Med 357:266–281
41. Sherrington C, Tiedemann A, Fairhall N, Close JC, Lord SR (2011) Exercise to prevent falls in older adults: an updated meta-analysis and best practice recommendations. NSW Public Health Bull 22:78–83
42. Miyauchi M, Hirai C, Nakajima H (2013) The solar exposure time required for vitamin D_3 synthesis in the human body estimated by numerical simulation and observation in Japan. J Nutr Sci Vitaminol (Tokyo) 59:257–263
43. de Kam D, Smulders E, Weerdesteyn V, Smits-Engelsman BC (2009) Exercise interventions to reduce fall-related fractures and their risk factors in individuals with low bone density: a systematic review of randomized controlled trials. Osteoporos Int 20:2111–2125
44. Teixeira LE, Sileva KN, Imoto AM, Teixeira TJ, Kayo AH, Montenegro-Rodrigues R, Peccin MS, Trevisani VF (2010) Progressive load training for the quadriceps muscle associated with proprioception exercises for the prevention of falls in postmenopausal women with osteoporosis: a randomized controlled trial. Osteoporos Int 21:589–596
45. Miyakoshi N, Hongo M, Mizutani Y, Shimada Y (2013) Prevalence of sarcopenia in Japanese women with osteopenia and osteoporosis. J Bone Miner Metab 31:556–561
46. Chen LK, Liu LK, Woo J, Assantachai P, Auyeung TW, Bahyah KS, Chou MY, Chen LY, Hsu PS, Krairit O, Lee JS, Lee WJ, Lee Y, Liang CK, Limpawattana P, Lin CS, Peng LN, Satake S, Suzuki T, Won CW, Wu CH, Wu SN, Zhang T, Zeng P, Akishita M, Arai H (2014) Sarcopenia in Asia: consensus report of the Asian Working Group for Sarcopenia. J Am Med Dir Assoc 15:95–101
47. Walston JD (2012) Sarcopenia in older adults. Curr Opin Rheumatol 24:623–627
48. Aagaard P, Suetta C, Caserotti P, Magnusson SP, Kjaer M (2010) Role of the nervous system in sarcopenia and muscle atrophy with aging: strength training as a countermeasure. Scand J Med Sci Sports 20:49–64

Chapter 12
Back Extensor Strengthening Exercise and Osteoporosis

Michio Hongo, Naohisa Miyakoshi, and Yoichi Shimada

Abstract Vertebral deformities associated with osteoporosis are the major cause of kyphosis. Kyphosis progresses with advancing age and has been found to be associated with multiple geriatric health-related problems, including not only those affecting locomotive organs but also internal organs. Back extensor strength has been significantly associated with physical activity, bone density, degree of kyphosis, and multiple factors in the elderly population. Back-strengthening exercise was introduced as a potentially effective method to improve several impaired health conditions induced by kyphosis. Since the exercise prescription for patients with kyphosis is commonly potentially hazardous due to the fragility of the elderly, the optimum intensity and frequency of the exercise need to be determined. Furthermore, several orthoses have been reported for improving kyphosis. This chapter covers the etiology and clinical presentation of kyphosis and the rehabilitation of trunk muscles for the treatment of kyphosis.

Keywords Osteoporosis • Kyphosis • Back extensor strength • Exercise

12.1 Osteoporosis and Kyphosis

Vertebral deformities associated with osteoporosis are the major cause of kyphosis; however, the increase in kyphosis occurs as a result of multiple contributing factors, including deformation of vertebral bodies and intervertebral disks, and other factors such as decreased muscle strength and ligamentous degeneration [1, 2]. Kyphosis has been described as associated with back pain, impaired physical functioning, pulmonary function, gastrointestinal disorders, loss of quality of life, and mortality.

M. Hongo, M.D., Ph.D. (✉) • N. Miyakoshi, M.D., Ph.D. • Y. Shimada, M.D., Ph.D.
Department of Orthopedic Surgery, Akita University Graduate School of Medicine,
1-1-1 Hondo, Akita 010-8543, Japan
e-mail: mhongo@doc.med.akita-u.ac.jp

Y. Shimada, N. Miyakoshi (eds.), *Osteoporosis in Orthopedics*,
DOI 10.1007/978-4-431-55778-4_12

12.1.1 Etiology of Kyphosis

Kyphosis progresses with advancing age. Vertebral fractures and osteoporosis have been considered as notable causes. Spinal osteoporosis and associated vertebral fractures are associated with increased kyphosis and height loss [3]. It is known that women who develop a vertebral fracture are at substantial risk for additional fractures within the next year [4]. However, several studies demonstrated that hyperkyphosis could occur in the absence of underlying osteoporosis and vertebral fractures. One study showed that vertebral fractures explained only about 42–48 % of kyphosis variance [5]. Schneider et al. examined the association of radiographically defined kyphosis with vertebral fractures and found that the majority of men and women with exaggerated kyphosis had no evidence of thoracic vertebral fractures or osteoporosis [6].

The other possible cause of kyphosis is degeneration of intervertebral disks. Dehydration and loss of elasticity in the annulus fibrosus and nucleus pulposus produce loss of height of the intervertebral disk. Other known factors which likely influence the change in kyphosis are trunk muscle strength and the appearance of ligamentous structure.

12.1.2 Kyphosis and Mortality

Kyphosis has been reported to be significantly associated with mortality. Prevalent vertebral deformities in older women with low bone mass are associated with increased risks of mortality and hospitalization [7]. Kado et al. reported that hyperkyphosis predicted an increased risk for death, independent of underlying spinal osteoporosis and the extent and severity of vertebral fractures in older women with vertebral fractures [8]. Their findings suggested that it is not enough to look for vertebral fractures alone.

12.1.3 Kyphosis and Pulmonary Function

Previous studies have demonstrated that increased kyphosis is associated with decreased pulmonary function. Harrison et al. conducted a systematic review to examine the relationships among osteoporotic vertebral fractures, kyphosis, and pulmonary function [9]. However, there were only four studies left after applying their eligibility criteria. Their findings suggested modest but predictable declines in vital capacity related to the degree of kyphosis. These studies reported reductions in vital capacity, with values ranging from 68 to 94 % of predicted values. This was quantified as a 9 % reduction in predicted vital capacity per vertebral fracture [10]. The degree of kyphosis clinically or radiographically correlated with decreases in vital capacity [10–13]; impairments were most notable at kyphotic angles > 55°[11]. On the basis of available studies, declines in vital capacity secondary to kyphosis seem modest and directly related to the number of vertebral fractures or the degree of kyphosis.

12.1.4 Kyphosis and Gastrointestinal Disorders

Hyperkyphosis has been reported to be associated with dysphagia [14, 15], reflux esophagitis or hiatus hernia [16–19], and intrathoracic stomach [20]. Miyakoshi et al. examined whether gastroesophageal reflux disease is affected by spinal kyphosis in the presence of oral pharmacotherapy in 112 patients with osteoporosis [17]. On multivariate analysis, the angle of lumbar kyphosis and the number of lumbar vertebral fractures were identified as indices affecting the presence of gastroesophageal reflux disease.

12.1.5 Kyphosis and Quality of Life

Women with osteoporosis have lower health-related quality of life (QOL) compared with those without osteoporosis, irrespective of a history of previous fracture [21]. A cross-sectional survey by van Schoor et al. assessed the impact of vertebral deformities and osteoarthritis on QOL in a population-based sample and compared this with the impact of six other important chronic diseases on QOL. After adjustment for age, sex, and other chronic diseases, severe osteoporosis of the vertebrae significantly reduced QOL in the general population as much as cardiac disease, peripheral arterial disease, and diabetes mellitus [22]. QOL decreased significantly with an increasing number of prevalent vertebral fractures [23], and QOL scores are dependent on the types of spinal deformity.

Postural deformities were classified into five groups: round back, hollow round back, whole kyphosis, lower acute kyphosis, and normal posture [24, 25] (Fig. 12.1). Miyakoshi et al. described that patients with postural deformities had significantly lower QOL scores than those with normal posture when total QOL scores were evaluated using the Japanese Osteoporosis QOL Questionnaire [26]. QOL scores were the lowest in the group with whole kyphosis. Multiple regression analysis showed that spinal range of motion correlated best with the total QOL score. They concluded that QOL in patients with osteoporosis was impaired by postural deformities, especially by whole kyphosis, and that spinal mobility has a strong effect on QOL in these patients. At the next stage of their study, they evaluated the possible factors affecting spinal mobility, and they found that back extensor strength was the most significant contributor to spinal mobility on multiple regression analysis [27].

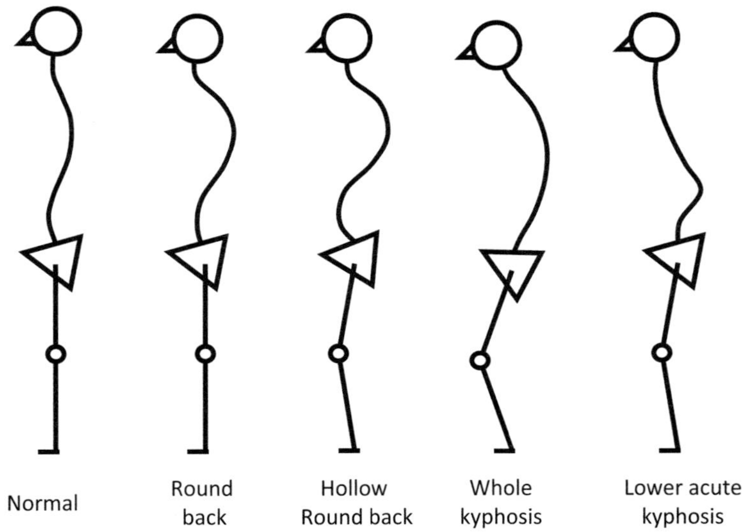

Fig. 12.1 Classification of spinal deformities (Modified from Itoi E.[24] with permission)

12.1.6 Kyphosis and Back Extensor Strength

Spinal column is supported and moved with four major muscle groups including extensors, flexors, lateral flexors, and rotators [28]. Back extensor muscles are the main supportive muscles, which extend the spine and maintain the posture. Back extensor strength has been considered highly important in patients with osteoporosis. Osteoporotic women have been found to have significantly lower back extensor strength than healthy women [29], and back extensor strength demonstrated a negative correlation with kyphosis [30, 31].

Sinaki et al. evaluated back extensor strength, bone mineral density (BMD), and physical activity scores in a cross-sectional study involving 65 women [30]. Back extensor strength had a significant negative correlation with thoracic kyphosis and positive correlations with lumbar lordosis and sacral inclination. However, BMD and physical activity scores did not show any significant correlations with the radiographic factors. These results indicated that the stronger the back extensors, the smaller the thoracic kyphosis and the larger the lumbar lordosis and sacral inclination. In another cross-sectional study by Mika et al., 189 female subjects were grouped by their BMD, and various parameters were compared between the groups [31]. Multivariate analyses of back extensor strength and BMD showed that only back extensor strength affected thoracic kyphosis. There was no correlation between back extensor strength and BMD. A significant difference in back extensor strength was observed only between the osteoporotic and osteopenic groups. They concluded that the severity of thoracic kyphosis might be especially affected by changes in back extensor strength.

Besides these articles that demonstrated significant correlations between back extensor strength and thoracic kyphosis, we have demonstrated associations between lumbar lordosis and back extensor strength [32]. We assessed the association of osteoporotic spinal deformities with back strength in a total of 206 elderly women in Akita, Japan, and in Minnesota, USA. We found that thoracic kyphosis and lumbar lordosis were higher in the Minnesota group than in the Akita group. In the Akita group, multiple regression analysis showed that the angle of lumbar lordosis correlated significantly with back extensor strength, indicating the potential importance of strengthening the back extensors for improving or maintaining lumbar lordosis. The differences identified in the shape of sagittal spinal curvature from two geographic areas of the world might be due to the difference in race and lifestyles.

Based on these findings from several studies, back extensor strength is an important determinant of posture, and preparing strong, natural extrinsic support for the spine seems to be important to decrease the incidence of spinal deformity.

12.1.7 Measurement of Back Extensor Strength

Appropriate measurement of trunk muscle strength is required for the correct evaluation of the performance of the spine. Measurement of muscle strength is roughly classified into isometric and isokinetic procedures. Isokinetic measurement of muscle strength can evaluate physiologic muscle contracture with spinal motion, but the measurements were demonstrated to vary depending on the posture, and the apparatus is relatively expensive. On the other hand, measurement of isometric muscle strength provides reliable and accurate results with the appropriate device, and the device is relatively simple and easy to move. Smith evaluated the repeatability of the methods comparing the isometric and isokinetic strengths of trunk extensors, flexors, and rotators and concluded that the strength data were reliable, and there was no significant difference between the procedures [33].

Measurements of back extensor strength and back-strengthening exercises are better if specific instruments are used to measure trunk strength in sitting positions with various spinal postures [34]. However, the authors' techniques used for measurement of back extensor strength and procedures for back-strengthening exercises in a prone position have been previously established as safe and reliable. During measurement and exercise, a prone position allows back extensors to work without contributions from the musculature of the lower extremities.

The authors use a custom-made strain gauge type back isometric dynamometer. The concept was originally described by Limburg et al. [35]. Subjects lie prone with the hips and knees in the neutral position and the arms fully extended at the elbow. No immobilizing straps are necessary with proper placement of the padded transducer head. Its upper edge is aligned with the superior borders of the scapulae across the midline. During the measurements, subjects raise their hands from the table to prevent the unwanted contribution of upper extremity musculature to the

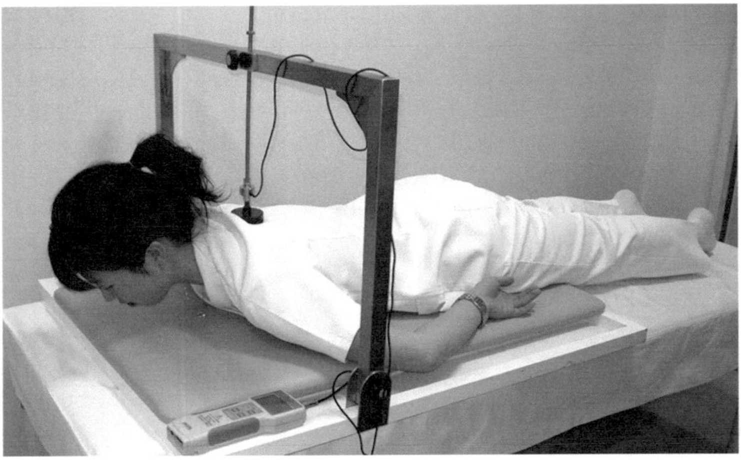

Fig. 12.2 Measurement of isometric back extensor strength with custom-made apparatus with dynamometer

upward force generated by the trunk against the transducer head. Direct contract between the pelvis and the table must be maintained throughout the measurements. The extensor muscles are contracted for 5 s, with no initial upward jerking motions directed at the transducer. The maximum force generated during exertion is processed by the measuring device. The patient is allowed one warm-up trial, which is followed by three successive maximal effort trials separated by 1-min resting periods. The maximal force achieved is then recorded (Fig. 12.2). A more convenient and easy method for evaluating isometric back extensor strength in daily clinical practice has also been reported. A handheld dynamometer fixed with a tripod has been reported to be reliable for the assessment of back extensor strength in women with osteoporosis and vertebral fractures [36].

12.2 Effects of Back-Strengthening Exercise

12.2.1 Bone Mineral Density

Back extensor strength demonstrated a positive correlation with BMD of the spine [37–39]. Iki et al. reported that greater trunk extensor torque reduced bone loss independently of age, body size, and vitamin D receptor genotype [37]. Zhou showed a correlation between muscle strength and BMD using isometric and isokinetic testing modes, demonstrating an age-dependent reduction in BMD and muscle strength throughout early menopause [40]. Sinaki et al. conducted a randomized, controlled trial evaluating the effect of a less demanding exercise program for back extensor muscles using a backpack on muscle strength and bone mineral density [41]. They found that postmenopausal bone loss was unaffected by a modest exercise program despite an increase in muscle strength and concluded that back muscle exercises might be ineffective in retarding vertebral bone loss in ambulatory, healthy, postmenopausal women.

12.2.2 Posture

Several studies have demonstrated the effect of exercise on posture [42–51]. Itoi and Sinaki conducted a study evaluating the effect of a back-strengthening exercise with a weighted backpack for 2 years on spinal curvature [42]. They randomly assigned 60 subjects to either an exercise or a control group and found that back extensor strength increased significantly in both the exercise and the control groups, but no radiographic measurements were significantly different between these groups. The significant increase in back extensor strength in both groups of healthy women suggested that the original grouping did not accurately reflect the amount of exercise. Thus, the 60 subjects were reclassified for comparison on the basis of increase in back extensor strength: 27 with more than or equal to the mean increase of 21.1 kg and 33 with less than 21.1 kg. Furthermore, each of these groups of subjects was subdivided on the basis of degree of thoracic kyphosis. Among the subjects with substantial thoracic kyphosis, those with a significant increase in back extensor strength had a significant decrease in thoracic kyphosis, whereas those with a small increase in strength had a nonsignificant increase in thoracic kyphosis. The authors concluded that increasing the back extensor strength in healthy estrogen-deficient women helps decrease thoracic kyphosis.

Pilates exercise is a "mind-body exercise" that has been used since early in the twentieth century. It focuses on improving strength, core stability, flexibility, muscle control, posture, and breathing [52]. Kuo et al. assessed the changes in sagittal spinal posture in 34 older volunteers after a Pilates-based exercise program for 10 weeks [45]. They found that immediately after the exercise program, participants stood with slightly decreased thoracic flexion and sat with slightly increased lumbar extension. The individually designed Pilates-based exercise program was feasible for healthy older adults, and the high attendance rate supports the suitability of the exercise program over a long period.

Greendale et al. conducted a randomized, controlled trial involving 118 participants with a kyphosis angle of at least 40° and assessed whether a specifically designed yoga intervention could reduce hyperkyphosis [53]. The active treatment group attended hour-long yoga classes 3 days per week for 24 weeks. At the final follow-up, participants randomized to yoga experienced a 4.4 % improvement in kyphosis angle. Based on the results of this study, the decrease in the flexicurve kyphosis angle in the yoga treatment group showed that hyperkyphosis is remediable, a critical first step in the pathway to treating or preventing this condition. However, Sinaki reported three healthy persons with low bone mass who developed new pain and fractures after participation in yoga flexion exercises and cautioned

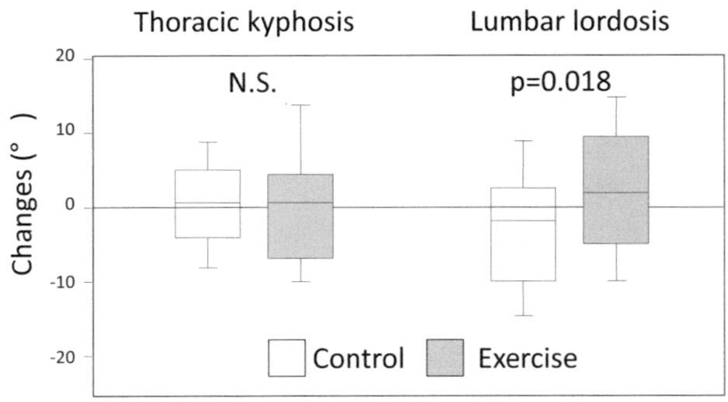

Fig. 12.3 Changes in thoracic kyphosis and lumbar lordosis after back exercise intervention for 4 months (Modified from Hongo et al. [51] with permission)

that flexion yoga positions in patients with osteopenia or osteoporosis could lead to an increased risk of vertebral fractures [54].

Benedetti et al. performed a clinical study to systematically compare the effects of a physical activity program that specifically addressed the flexed posture with a nonspecific exercise program for 3 months and concluded that the program significantly improved postural alignment and musculoskeletal impairment of the elderly [47].

Ball et al. evaluated the progression of kyphosis with age and found that kyphosis increased with age in healthy women, with the greatest difference observed between women 50 and 59 years of age. They then conducted a 1-year prospective, descriptive analysis of the effect of extension exercises on posture in women 50–59 years of age. The progression of kyphosis was greater in women who did not perform extension exercises than in those who performed extension exercises three times per week for 1 year [46].

We have conducted a randomized study assessing the effect of back extensor strength on spinal sagittal curvature [51]. Lumbar lordosis at the neutral position significantly increased in the exercise group. The increase in lumbar lordosis was also significantly larger compared with the control group (Fig. 12.3). However, no significant change was found in thoracic kyphosis. In this study, back-strengthening exercise was shown to be effective in improving spinal deformity by increasing lumbar lordosis.

12.2.3 Vertebral Fractures

A cross-sectional study of patients with osteoporosis showed a negative association between back extensor strength and both kyphosis and the number of vertebral fractures, suggesting that increasing back strength could reduce the risk of vertebral fracture for the osteoporotic spine [55].

As described above, Itoi et al. evaluated the effect of back-strengthening exercise on improvement of kyphosis and found that kyphosis improved with the exercise at the 2-year follow-up [42]. The authors then investigated the long-term protective effect of strengthening the back muscles on vertebral fractures. Subjects

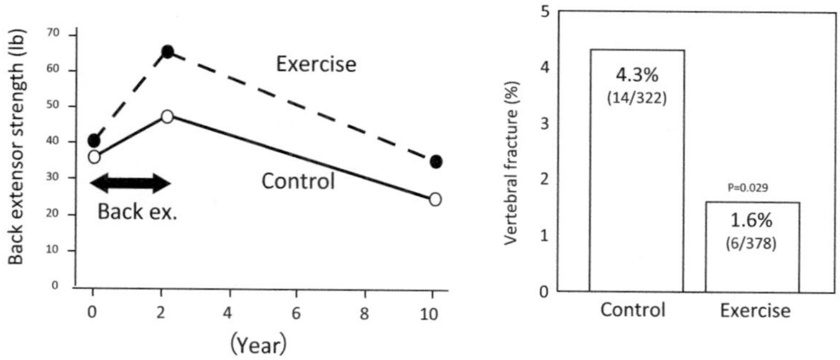

Fig. 12.4 (**a**) Change in back extensor strength at 10-year follow-up after cessation of exercise for 2 years. (**b**) Incident of vertebral fractures at 10-year follow-up (Modified from Sinaki et al. [56] with permission)

performed progressive, resistive back-strengthening exercises for 2 years and were followed up at 2 years and 10 years. The authors found that the back extensor strength in the exercise group was still significantly higher even 8 years after cessation (Fig.12.4a) and the relative risk of compression fracture was 2.7 times higher in the control group than in the exercise group (Fig. 12.4b). They concluded that stronger back extensors achieved through exercises reduced the risk of vertebral compression fractures (Fig. 12.4a, b) [56].

Another study also showed the effect of back-strengthening exercise on the reduction of re-fracture after percutaneous vertebroplasty. In this retrospective analysis, the authors reviewed the data of patients with osteoporosis treated by vertebroplasty. The results showed that an exercise program for osteoporosis including back strengthening after percutaneous vertebroplasty decreased fracture recurrence [57].

Sinaki and Mikkelsen conducted a study comparing treatment programs with extension exercises, flexion exercises, combined exercises, and no therapeutic exercises [58]. The study suggested that a significantly higher number of vertebral compression fractures occurred in patients with postmenopausal osteoporosis who followed a flexion exercise program compared with those using extension exercises. They concluded that extension or isometric exercises seem to be more appropriate for patients with osteoporosis.

12.2.4 Quality of Life

There have been multiple studies describing the effects of interventions on health-related QOL in older women with low bone mass [59–62]. Home-based exercises have been shown to improve QOL scores [61, 62]. Group treatment including trunk extension exercises also improved psychological status, which is considered part of

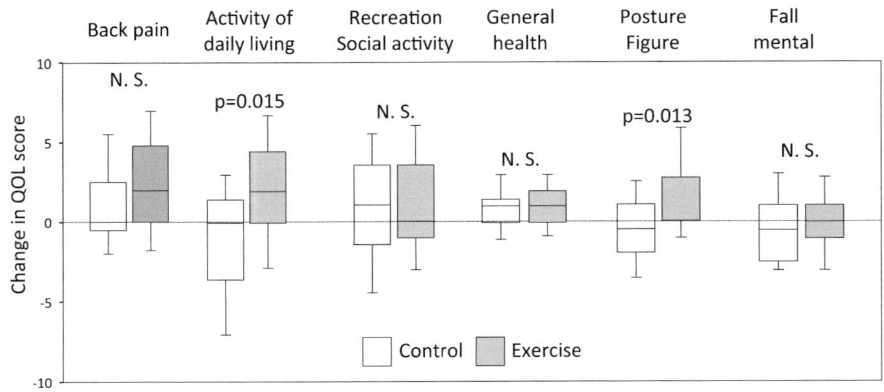

Fig. 12.5 Change in each QOL score (Adapted from Hongo et al. [51] with permission)

QOL [59]. However, the participants were instructed to engage in the home-based or institutional-based exercise for 45–60 min per day.

We conducted a randomized, controlled study in 80 postmenopausal women with osteoporosis to investigate the effect of a home-based, simple, low-intensity exercise. QOL scores increased significantly in the exercise group, while they remained unchanged in the control group. Significant improvements were observed in the scores for activities of daily living and posture in the exercise group compared with control group. Back pain also improved in both groups; however, there was no difference in the improvement of back pain between the groups (Fig. 12.5). Since physical activity was reported to correlate with back extensor strength, enhancing back extensor strength may have a direct effect on improvement of QOL [63]. In this study, the implementation of exercise was relatively favorable, with compliance of 73 % and no major adverse events; the exercise regimen can be safe and sustainable for elderly persons. However, this exercise may not be suitable for kyphotic patients who are unable to lie in a prone position.

Miyakoshi et al. then evaluated the effect of a simple and lower intensity back-strengthening exercise that can be performed by participants who are unable to lie in the prone position [64]. Two types of simple and low-intensity back extension exercises were performed by 31 postmenopausal elderly women. The authors found that 6 months of simple, low-intensity back extension exercises improved QOL and back extensor strength in patients with postmenopausal osteoporosis and vertebral fractures.

12.2.5 Optimum Intensity and Frequency of the Exercise

There have been some concerns related to the exercise prescription. Subjects in the previous studies were all healthy postmenopausal women, and the average weight used in these studies of healthy postmenopausal women was 22 kg, which was equivalent to 30 % of the maximum strength of the back extensors [41]. The same intensity of exercise is not recommended for patients with osteoporosis. As in any weight-lifting exercise program, the exercises need to be modified for osteoporotic patients to avoid pain and/or fracture. As long as it is effective in increasing the back extensor strength, a reduction in the intensity of exercise may be beneficial for patients with osteoporosis.

The effect of less resistance training on achieving significant improvements in trunk muscle strength is not well understood for elderly populations. Swezey et al. reported brief, progressively resisted, trunk isometric exercises with use of an inflatable vinyl ball for postmenopausal women with osteopenia and osteoporosis and found an improvement in trunk extensor strength [65]. Vincent et al. compared muscle strength after low-intensity (50 % of one repetition maximum (1RM)) and high-intensity lumbar exercises (80 % of 1RM) in 60- to 83-year-old adults [66]. It is interesting to note that the magnitude of the increases in lumbar extensor strength was greater with low-intensity lumbar exercise than with high-intensity lumbar exercise. These results suggest that lower intensity exercise provides a similar effect on muscular strength in elderly persons to high-intensity exercise. The authors demonstrated that exercise using a reduced weight was less effective in improving back extensor strength than exercise with an average weight of 14 kg, which was equivalent to 30 % of the maximum back extensor strength in a study with young women volunteers [67].

12.2.6 Author's Recommendation: Low-Intensity Back-Strengthening Exercise

The low-intensity back-strengthening exercise regimen could be performed at home for a duration of approximately 5 min, and it has been demonstrated to be feasible, safe, and effective with high compliance for elderly individuals [63]. In the study, the exercise group with no additional weight had a significant increase in back extensor strength compared with the control group.

The back exercise regimen with low resistance should be considered in terms of feasibility, safety, and effectiveness for the elderly population with osteoporosis. In 1982, it was reported that the combination of a few exercises with avoidance of flexion can safely and effectively strengthen the fragile osteoporotic spine [68]. The author's recommendation for the back exercise is just one exercise for back strength without performing the full program described in the initial study.

The selected single home-based exercise is done according to the procedure described previously [67–69]. Subjects are asked to lie in a prone position on a bed with a pillow under the abdomen such that the spine is slightly flexed. Following a warm-up exercise in which the spine is slowly extended with the aid of both arms ten times, the subjects are then asked to lift the upper trunk off the bed toward the neutral position for 5 s, with a 10-s interval between the contractions (Fig. 12.6). Each

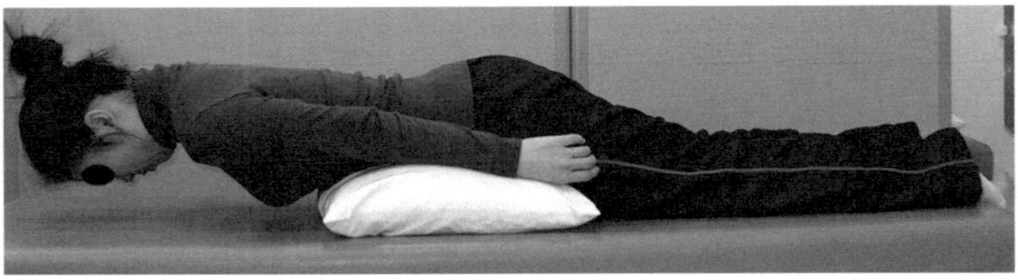

Fig. 12.6 Low-intensity back-strengthening exercise. Subjects are asked to lift the upper trunk off the bed toward the neutral position for 5 s [63]

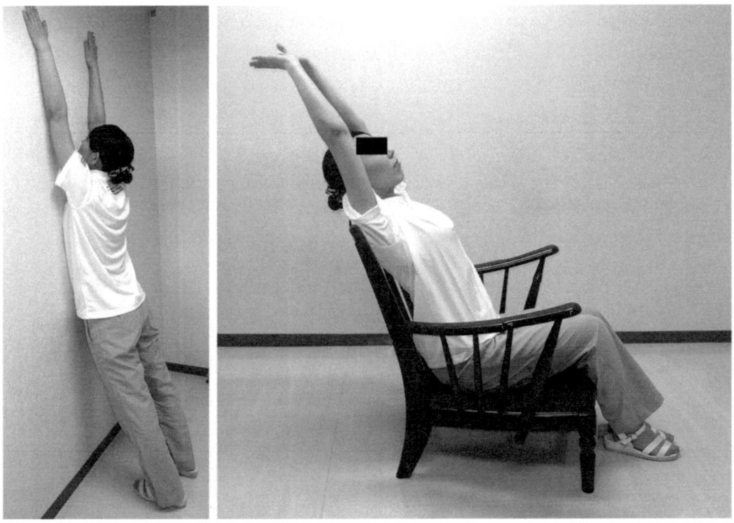

Fig. 12.7 (**a**) Back exercise in standing positions. (**b**) Back exercise in sitting position

contraction is repeated 10 times as a set, with the duration of exercise ranging from 3 to 5 min. It is recommended that this exercise be performed as one set a day, 5 days a week. Back extensor strength and QOL, including physical activity, pain, and posture, can be expected to eventually improve [51, 63]. This effect was considered to be based on the weight of the head, upper extremity, and thoracic trunk.

However, since the posture during these exercises to improve back extensor strength requires lying in a prone position, patients with increased kyphosis have difficulty performing the exercise with the appropriate posture. Therefore, two types of exercise prescriptions in the sitting or standing positions were introduced by Miyakoshi et al. [64]. In one exercise, patients were instructed to stand facing a wall with their feet 30 cm from the wall. Then, with arms elevated and touching the wall, the subject had to lower the chest as close to the wall as possible to extend the back (Fig. 12.7a). In the other exercise, the subject sat in a sturdy chair or sofa with hands behind the neck and then extended the back while leaning on the backrest to extend the back as much as possible (Fig. 12.7b). The authors reported its effectiveness in increasing QOL and back extensor strength.

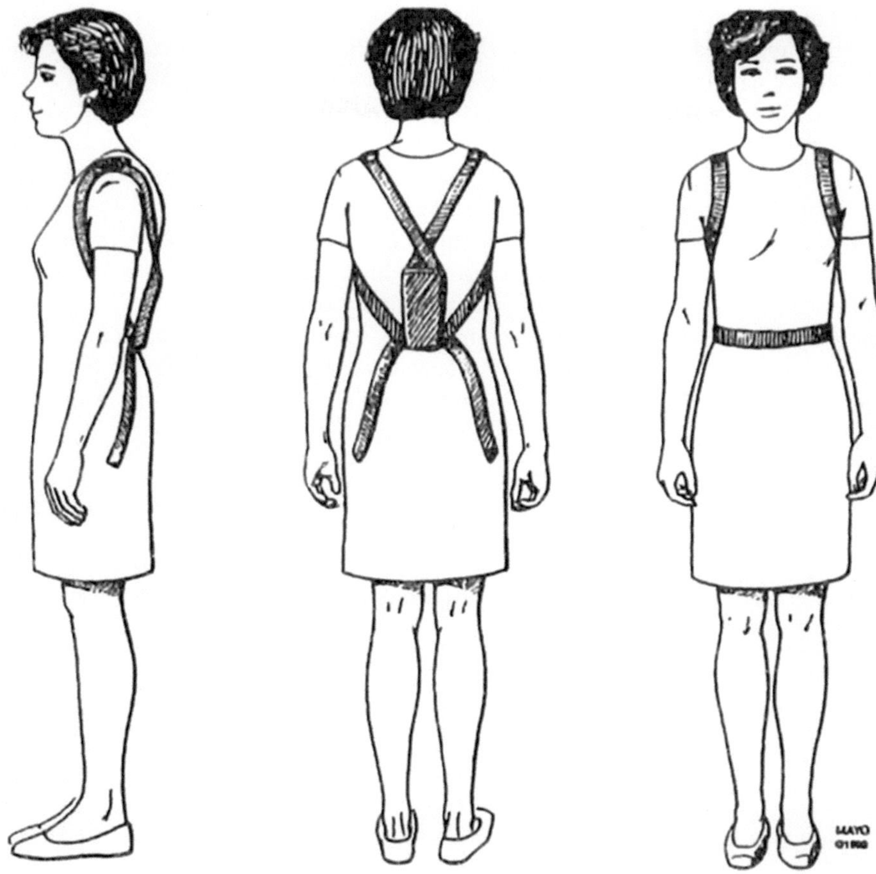

Fig. 12.8 Posture training support (Adapted from Sinaki et al. with permission)

12.2.7 Spinal Orthosis and Back Extensor Strength

There have been few studies evaluating the use of a spinal orthosis and its effect on posture or other outcomes. Kaplan et al. investigated the effect of application of back supports and postural exercise on back strength in comparison with conventional thoracolumbar support in subjects with osteoporosis [70]. They found better compliance with the use of posture training support than with the thoracolumbar support. They also reported an increase in back extensor strength in patients who comply with posture training support and the postural exercise program. Sinaki et al. assessed the effect of a proprioceptive dynamic posture training program on balance in osteoporotic women with kyphotic posture. Subjects undergoing the program were instructed to perform back extensor strengthening exercises, as well as using a 2-pound weighted kypho-orthosis to be worn daily for 2 h only during ambulatory activity, which was called training support. They found that subjects who had abnormal balance and used the proprioceptive dynamic posture training program improved their balance [71] (Fig. 12.8). Pfeifer et al. evaluated the efficacy of a newly developed spinal orthosis in patients with osteoporotic vertebral fractures and found that wearing the orthosis for a 6-month period was associated with a 73 % increase in back extensor strength, a 58 % increase in abdominal flexor strength, an 11 % decrease in angle of kyphosis, a 25 % decrease in body sway, a 7 % increase in vital capacity, a 38 % decrease in average pain, a 15 % increase in well-being, and a 27 % decrease in limitations of daily living [72, 73]. Another randomized, controlled study evaluated the efficacy of a flexible spinal orthosis without any stabilizing components in terms of posture improvement and found that the orthosis with air chamber pads significantly improved posture in women with osteoporosis [74]. Since the device contained no rigid stabilizing elements, the authors considered that the change in posture was a result of muscle activation.

References

1. Kado DM (2009) The rehabilitation of hyperkyphotic posture in the elderly. Eur J Phys Rehabil Med 45:583–593
2. Hinman MR (2004) Comparison of thoracic kyphosis and postural stiffness in younger and older women. Spine J 4:413–417
3. Ensrud KE, Black DM, Harris F, Ettinger B, Cummings SR (1997) Correlates of kyphosis in older women. The Fracture Intervention Trial Research Group. J Am Geriatr Soc 45:682–687
4. Lindsay R, Silverman SL, Cooper C, Hanley DA, Barton I, Broy SB, Licata A, Benhamou L, Geusens P, Flowers K, Stracke H, Seeman E (2001) Risk of new vertebral fracture in the year following a fracture. JAMA 285:320–323
5. Milne JS, Williamson J (1983) A longitudinal study of kyphosis in older people. Age Ageing 12:225–233
6. Schneider DL, von Muhlen D, Barrett-Connor E, Sartoris DJ (2004) Kyphosis does not equal vertebral fractures: the Rancho Bernardo study. J Rheumatol 31:747–752
7. Ensrud KE, Thompson DE, Cauley JA, Nevitt MC, Kado DM, Hochberg MC, Santora AC 2nd, Black DM (2000) Prevalent vertebral deformities predict mortality and hospitalization in older women with low bone mass. Fracture Intervention Trial Research Group. J Am Geriatr Soc 48:241–249
8. Kado DM, Lui LY, Ensrud KE, Fink HA, Karlamangla AS, Cummings SR, Study of Osteoporotic F (2009) Hyperkyphosis predicts mortality independent of vertebral osteoporosis in older women. Ann Intern Med 150:681–687
9. Harrison RA, Siminoski K, Vethanayagam D, Majumdar SR (2007) Osteoporosis-related kyphosis and impairments in pulmonary function: a systematic review. J Bone Miner Res 22:447–457
10. Leech JA, Dulberg C, Kellie S, Pattee L, Gay J (1990) Relationship of lung function to severity of osteoporosis in women. Am Rev Respir Dis 141:68–71
11. Lombardi I Jr, Oliveira LM, Mayer AF, Jardim JR, Natour J (2005) Evaluation of pulmonary function and quality of life in women with osteoporosis. Osteoporos Int 16:1247–1253
12. Culham EG, Jimenez HA, King CE (1994) Thoracic kyphosis, rib mobility, and lung volumes in normal women and women with osteoporosis. Spine (Phila Pa 1976). 19:1250–1255
13. Schlaich C, Minne HW, Bruckner T, Wagner G, Gebest HJ, Grunze M, Ziegler R, Leidig-Bruckner G (1998) Reduced pulmonary function in patients with spinal osteoporotic fractures. Osteoporos Int 8:261–267

14. Goyal N, Narlawar R, Garrett A (2005) Kyphosis, a rare cause of dysphagia. Age Ageing 34:521–522
15. Blechacz B, Gajic O (2008) Images in clinical medicine. Severe kyphosis. N Engl J Med 358, e28
16. Furukawa N, Iwakiri R, Koyama T, Okamoto K, Yoshida T, Kashiwagi Y, Ohyama T, Noda T, Sakata H, Fujimoto K (1999) Proportion of reflux esophagitis in 6010 Japanese adults: prospective evaluation by endoscopy. J Gastroenterol 34:441–444
17. Miyakoshi N, Kasukawa Y, Sasaki H, Kamo K, Shimada Y (2009) Impact of spinal kyphosis on gastroesophageal reflux disease symptoms in patients with osteoporosis. Osteoporos Int 20:1193–1198
18. Kusano M, Hashizume K, Ehara Y, Shimoyama Y, Kawamura O, Mori M (2008) Size of hiatus hernia correlates with severity of kyphosis, not with obesity, in elderly Japanese women. J Clin Gastroenterol 42:345–350
19. Yamaguchi T, Sugimoto T, Yamada H, Kanzawa M, Yano S, Yamauchi M, Chihara K (2002) The presence and severity of vertebral fractures is associated with the presence of esophageal hiatal hernia in postmenopausal women. Osteoporos Int 13:331–336
20. Polomsky M, Siddall KA, Salvador R, Dubecz A, Donahue LA, Raymond D, Jones C, Watson TJ, Peters JH (2009) Association of kyphosis and spinal skeletal abnormalities with intrathoracic stomach: a link toward understanding its pathogenesis. J Am Coll Surg 208:562–569
21. Dhillon V, Hurst N, Hannan J, Nuki G (2005) Association of low general health status, measured prospectively by Euroqol EQ5D, with osteoporosis, independent of a history of prior fracture. Osteoporos Int 16:483–489
22. van Schoor NM, Smit JH, Twisk JW, Lips P (2005) Impact of vertebral deformities, osteoarthritis, and other chronic diseases on quality of life: a population-based study. Osteoporos Int 16:749–756
23. Pluijm SM, Tromp AM, Smit JH, Deeg DJ, Lips P (2000) Consequences of vertebral deformities in older men and women. J Bone Miner Res 15:1564–1572
24. Itoi E (1991) Roentgenographic analysis of posture in spinal osteoporotics. Spine 16:750–756
25. Sato K, Kasama F, Itoi E (1988) Clinical features of spinal osteoporosis: spinal deformity and pertinent back pain. Contemp Orthop 16:23–30
26. Miyakoshi N, Itoi E, Kobayashi M, Kodama H (2003) Impact of postural deformities and spinal mobility on quality of life in postmenopausal osteoporosis. Osteoporos Int 14:1007–1012
27. Miyakoshi N, Hongo M, Maekawa S, Ishikawa Y, Shimada Y, Okada K, Itoi E (2005) Factors related to spinal mobility in patients with postmenopausal osteoporosis. Osteoporos Int 16:1871–1874
28. Beimborn DS, Morrissey MC (1988) A review of the literature related to trunk muscle performance. Spine (Phila Pa 1976). 13:655–660
29. Sinaki M, Khosla S, Limburg PJ, Rogers JW, Murtaugh PA (1993) Muscle strength in osteoporotic versus normal women. Osteoporos Int 3:8–12
30. Sinaki M, Itoi E, Rogers JW, Bergstralh EJ, Wahner HW (1996) Correlation of back extensor strength with thoracic kyphosis and lumbar lordosis in estrogen-deficient women. Am J Phys Med Rehabil 75:370–374
31. Mika A, Unnithan VB, Mika P (2005) Differences in thoracic kyphosis and in back muscle strength in women with bone loss due to osteoporosis. Spine 30:241–246
32. Hongo M, Miyakoshi N, Shimada Y, Sinaki M (2012) Association of spinal curve deformity and back extensor strength in elderly women with osteoporosis in Japan and the United States. Osteoporos Int 23:1029–1034
33. Smith SS, Mayer TG, Gatchel RJ, Becker TJ (1985) Quantification of lumbar function. Part 1: Isometric and multispeed isokinetic trunk strength measures in sagittal and axial planes in normal subjects. Spine (Phila Pa 1976). 10:757–764

34. Graves JE, Pollock ML, Carpenter DM, Leggett SH, Jones A, MacMillan M, Fulton M (1990) Quantitative assessment of full range-of-motion isometric lumbar extension strength. Spine (Phila Pa 1976) 15:289–294
35. Limburg PJ, Sinaki M, Rogers JW, Caskey PE, Pierskalla BK (1991) A useful technique for measurement of back strength in osteoporotic and elderly patients. Mayo Clin Proc 66:39–44
36. Valentin G, Maribo T (2014) Hand-held dynamometry fixated with a tripod is reliable for assessment of back extensor strength in women with osteoporosis. Osteoporos Int 25:2143–2149
37. Iki M, Saito Y, Dohi Y, Kajita E, Nishino H, Yonemasu K, Kusaka Y (2002) Greater trunk muscle torque reduces postmenopausal bone loss at the spine independently of age, body size, and vitamin D receptor genotype in Japanese women. Calcif Tissue Int 71:300–307
38. Sinaki M, Offord KP (1988) Physical activity in postmenopausal women: effect on back muscle strength and bone mineral density of the spine. Arch Phys Med Rehabil 69:277–280
39. Sinaki M, McPhee MC, Hodgson SF, Merritt JM, Offord KP (1986) Relationship between bone mineral density of spine and strength of back extensors in healthy postmenopausal women. Mayo Clin Proc 61:116–122
40. Zhou Z, Zheng L, Wei D, Ye M, Li X (2013) Muscular strength measurements indicate bone mineral density loss in postmenopausal women. Clin Interv Aging 8:1451–1459
41. Sinaki M, Wahner HW, Offord KP, Hodgson SF (1989) Efficacy of nonloading exercises in prevention of vertebral bone loss in postmenopausal women: a controlled trial. Mayo Clin Proc 64:762–769
42. Itoi E, Sinaki M (1994) Effect of back-strengthening exercise on posture in healthy women 49 to 65 years of age. Mayo Clin Proc 69:1054–1059
43. Greendale GA, McDivit A, Carpenter A, Seeger L, Huang MH (2002) Yoga for women with hyperkyphosis: results of a pilot study. Am J Public Health 92:1611–1614
44. Morey MC, Schenkman M, Studenski SA, Chandler JM, Crowley GM, Sullivan RJ Jr, Pieper CF, Doyle ME, Higginbotham MB, Horner RD, MacAller H, Puglisi CM, Morris KG, Weinberger M (1999) Spinal-flexibility-plus-aerobic versus aerobic-only training: effect of a randomized clinical trial on function in at-risk older adults. J Gerontol A Biol Sci Med Sci 54: M335–M342
45. Kuo YL, Tully EA, Galea MP (2009) Sagittal spinal posture after Pilates-based exercise in healthy older adults. Spine (Phila Pa 1976) 34:1046–1051
46. Ball JM, Cagle P, Johnson BE, Lucasey C, Lukert BP (2009) Spinal extension exercises prevent natural progression of kyphosis. Osteoporos Int 20:481–489
47. Benedetti MG, Berti L, Presti C, Frizziero A, Giannini S (2008) Effects of an adapted physical activity program in a group of elderly subjects with flexed posture: clinical and instrumental assessment. J Neuroeng Rehabil 5:32
48. Pawlowsky SB, Hamel KA, Katzman WB (2009) Stability of kyphosis, strength, and physical performance gains 1 year after a group exercise program in community-dwelling hyperkyphotic older women. Arch Phys Med Rehabil 90:358–361
49. Renno AC, Granito RN, Driusso P, Costa D, Oishi J (2005) Effects of an exercise program on respiratory function, posture and on quality of life in osteoporotic women: a pilot study. Physiotherapy 91:113–118
50. Katzman WB, Sellmeyer DE, Stewart AL, Wanek L, Hamel KA (2007) Changes in flexed posture, musculoskeletal impairments, and physical performance after group exercise in community-dwelling older women. Arch Phys Med Rehabil 88:192–199
51. Hongo M, Miyakoshi N, Kasukawa Y, Ishikawa Y, Shimada Y (2014) Effect of back strengthening exercise on back pain and spinal alignment. J Spine Res 5:901–904. (in Japanese)
52. Barker AL, Bird ML, Talevski J (2015) Effect of Pilates exercise for improving balance in older adults: a systematic review with meta-analysis. Arch Phys Med Rehabil 96:715–723

53. Greendale GA, Huang MH, Karlamangla AS, Seeger L, Crawford S (2009) Yoga decreases kyphosis in senior women and men with adult-onset hyperkyphosis: results of a randomized controlled trial. J Am Geriatr Soc 57:1569–1579
54. Sinaki M (2013) Yoga spinal flexion positions and vertebral compression fracture in osteopenia or osteoporosis of spine: case series. Pain Pract 13:68–75
55. Sinaki M, Wollan PC, Scott RW, Gelczer RK (1996) Can strong back extensors prevent vertebral fractures in women with osteoporosis? Mayo Clin Proc 71:951–956
56. Sinaki M, Itoi E, Wahner HW, Wollan P, Gelzcer R, Mullan BP, Collins DA, Hodgson SF (2002) Stronger back muscles reduce the incidence of vertebral fractures: a prospective 10 year follow-up of postmenopausal women. Bone 30:836–841
57. Huntoon EA, Schmidt CK, Sinaki M (2008) Significantly fewer refractures after vertebroplasty in patients who engage in back-extensor-strengthening exercises. Mayo Clin Proc 83:54–57
58. Sinaki M, Mikkelsen BA (1984) Postmenopausal spinal osteoporosis: flexion versus extension exercises. Arch Phys Med Rehabil 65:593–596
59. Gold DT, Shipp KM, Pieper CF, Duncan PW, Martinez S, Lyles KW (2004) Group treatment improves trunk strength and psychological status in older women with vertebral fractures: results of a randomized, clinical trial. J Am Geriatr Soc 52:1471–1478
60. Liu-Ambrose TY, Khan KM, Eng JJ, Lord SR, Lentle B, McKay HA (2005) Both resistance and agility training reduce back pain and improve health-related quality of life in older women with low bone mass. Osteoporos Int 16:1321–1329
61. Chien MY, Yang RS, Tsauo JY (2005) Home-based trunk-strengthening exercise for osteoporotic and osteopenic postmenopausal women without fracture – a pilot study. Clin Rehabil 19:28–36
62. Papaioannou A, Adachi JD, Winegard K, Ferko N, Parkinson W, Cook RJ, Webber C, McCartney N (2003) Efficacy of home-based exercise for improving quality of life among elderly women with symptomatic osteoporosis-related vertebral fractures. Osteoporos Int 14:677–682
63. Hongo M, Itoi E, Sinaki M, Miyakoshi N, Shimada Y, Maekawa S, Okada K, Mizutani Y (2007) Effect of low-intensity back exercise on quality of life and back extensor strength in patients with osteoporosis: a randomized controlled trial. Osteoporos Int 18:1389–1395
64. Miyakoshi N, Horikawa A, Hongo M, Shimada Y (2010) Effects of a simple, low-intensity back extension exercise on quality of life and back extensor strength in patients with osteoporosis and vertebral fractures: a 6-month randomized controlled trial. J Bone Miner Res 25: S342
65. Swezey RL, Swezey A, Adams J (2000) Isometric progressive resistive exercise for osteoporosis. J Rheumatol 27:1260–1264
66. Vincent KR, Braith RW, Feldman RA, Magyari PM, Cutler RB, Persin SA, Lennon SL, Gabr AH, Lowenthal DT (2002) Resistance exercise and physical performance in adults aged 60 to 83. J Am Geriatr Soc 50:1100–1107
67. Hongo M, Itoi E, Sinaki M, Shimada Y, Miyakoshi N, Okada K (2005) Effects of reducing resistance, repetitions, and frequency of back-strengthening exercise in healthy young women: a pilot study. Arch Phys Med Rehabil 86:1299–1303
68. Sinaki M (1982) Postmenopausal spinal osteoporosis: physical therapy and rehabilitation principles. Mayo Clin Proc 57:699–703
69. Sinaki M (1989) Exercise and osteoporosis. Arch Phys Med Rehabil 70:220–229
70. Kaplan RS, Sinaki M, Hameister MD (1996) Effect of back supports on back strength in patients with osteoporosis: a pilot study. Mayo Clin Proc 71:235–241
71. Sinaki M, Lynn SG (2002) Reducing the risk of falls through proprioceptive dynamic posture training in osteoporotic women with kyphotic posturing: a randomized pilot study. Am J Phys Med Rehabil 81:241–246

72. Pfeifer M, Begerow B, Minne HW (2004) Effects of a new spinal orthosis on posture, trunk strength, and quality of life in women with postmenopausal osteoporosis: a randomized trial. Am J Phys Med Rehabil 83:177–186
73. Pfeifer M, Kohlwey L, Begerow B, Minne HW (2011) Effects of two newly developed spinal orthoses on trunk muscle strength, posture, and quality-of-life in women with postmenopausal osteoporosis: a randomized trial. Am J Phys Med Rehabil 90:805–815
74. Vogt L, Hubscher M, Brettmann K, Banzer W, Fink M (2008) Postural correction by osteoporosis orthosis (Osteo-med): a randomized, placebo-controlled trial. Prosthetics Orthot Int 32:103–110

Index

Y. Shimada, N. Miyakoshi (eds.), *Osteoporosis in Orthopedics*,
DOI 10.1007/978-4-431-55778-4

V

W

Y

MIX
Papier aus verantwortungsvollen Quellen
Paper from responsible sources
FSC® C105338
FSC
www.fsc.org

If you have any concerns about our products,
you can contact us on
ProductSafety@springernature.com

In case Publisher is established outside the EU,
the EU authorized representative is:
Springer Nature Customer Service Center GmbH
Europaplatz 3, 69115 Heidelberg, Germany

Printed by Libri Plureos GmbH
in Hamburg, Germany